THE BRAIN
WELLNESS
PLAN

THE BRAIN WELLNESS PLAN

BREAKTHROUGH MEDICAL, NUTRITIONAL, AND IMMUNE-BOOSTING THERAPIES

Dr. Jay Lombard,
Board Certified Neurologist

and Carl Germano, RD, CNS, LDN

Kensington Books
http://www.kensingtonbooks.com

This book is designed to provide accurate and authoritative information in regard to the subject matter covered. It is sold with the understanding that the publisher is not engaged in rendering medical or related professional services and that without personal consultation the authors cannot and do not render judgment or advice about a particular patient or medical condition. If medical advice is required, the services of a competent professional should be sought. While every attempt has been made to provide accurate information, the authors and publisher cannot be held responsible for any errors or omissions.

KENSINGTON BOOKS are published by

Kensington Publishing Corp.
850 Third Avenue
New York, NY 10022

Kensington and the K logo Reg. U.S. Pat. & TM Off.
ISBN 1-57566-293-0

First Revised Printing: June, 2000
10 9 8 7 6 5 4 3 2

Printed in the United States of America

This book is dedicated to my wife, Rita, for her endless devotion and love, and to my parents for teaching me that intellectual curiosity must always be coupled with compassion.

—Jay Lombard

To my wife, Alise, for her inexhaustible love and patience. To my son, Grant, and daughter, Samantha, who give special meaning and cohesion to my life. Lastly, to my mother, Frances, for the wealth of love and support she has provided me. All of you mean the world to me.

—Carl Germano

ACKNOWLEDGMENTS

Thanks to Tracy Bernstein for her patience, insight and remarkable intelligence. Thanks to Neenyah Ostrom for putting the pedal to the metal with me in the process of writing this book. Thanks to Carl Germano who has convinced me that a "cocktail" approach, rather than a "magic bullet" is the only way to treat neurological disease. Also, thank you to my friends and family for their endless love and support. Finally, thank you to countless researchers who have devoted their lives to solving the mystery of disease in the hope of alleviating suffering.

—Jay Lombard

Special thanks to Rand Skolnick for providing me the opportunity to "shine" and work for the supplement company that continues to set the standards for the industry; to Jerry Hickey for bringing Dr. Lombard and me together to complete this important work; to Holly Robinson (and her fax machine), whose touch is felt on every page; to photographer Jill LeVine, for making me look good; to Lee Heiman, for his continued support and valued suggestions; to Tracy Bernstein, for her editing of the manuscript; to Paul Dinas, for working to accommodate my anxiety of getting this book published as quickly as possible; and to Kensington Publishing, for believing in this important work. Most importantly, thanks to all the researchers, nutritional scientists, and physicians who sought to better understand the true meaning of clinical nutrition and functional medicine above and beyond what the establishment led them to believe. Lastly, to the pioneers of progressive nutritional supplementation for the prevention and treatment of disease, I thank you all for your commitment and significant contributions to the field of nutritional medicine.

—Carl Germano

CONTENTS

PREFACE TO THE NEW EDITION

It is with great excitement and some apprehension that I write the preface for the updated version of *The Brain Wellness Plan*. This book was originally written in 1996 and published in 1997. The need for a rewrite is obvious. Since 1996, there has been an explosion of information regarding the brain and neurological illnesses. Researchers are now acknowledging that the brain has the inner potential to heal itself and regenerate, a notion that was regarded as absurd less than one decade ago. Furthermore, the basic molecular underpinnings of neurological diseases have now been isolated and identified, giving scientists an extraordinarily focused target to guide future therapies.

Against this background, *The Brain Wellness Plan* has been revised and expanded. This book will bring readers up to date on the cutting-edge of therapeutic advances in Alzheimer's, Parkinson's, ALS, multiple sclerosis, autism, attention deficit disorder, depression, and chronic fatigue syndrome. With a mild self-congratulatory pat on the back, we take note of our previous cutting-edge recommendations that are now in popular use; these include the use of S-adenosyl methionine in depression, creatine in ALS, and estrogens in Alzheimer's disease. We now look forward to the future with wonder at the new nutraceutical compounds we have identified and mentioned in our book, such as Huperzine A for Alzheimer's and mild cognitive impairment, the use of fetal stem cells in ALS and Parkinson's, vitamin D in multiple sclerosis, and transfer factor in chronic fatigue syndrome, to name only a few.

My apprehension is two-fold: one is that the rapidly advancing field of neuroscience will make some of the discoveries we mention in this book obsolete by the time they are published. We accept that modifications and adjustments to the "cocktail" approach should and will be made over time. The second factor is that people with neurological disease will look at this book as a prescription rather than as an overview of treatment options. This already has been the experience of Dr. Lombard in his capacity as a practicing neurologist and author of *The Brain Wellness Plan*. We recognize that a tightrope of sorts must be walked upon. On this tightrope, a balance needs to be established between basic science research, which is accelerating at a blinding fast pace, and the patient's need. Unfortunately, a good deal of research is still at the level of animal or basic human studies. Researchers cannot leap any further than the currently established guidelines that help propel their work to the greater population of patients. On the other hand, there is the consideration of patients who are suffering and dying with neurodegenerative diseases. ALS is a case in point. The average life expectancy of a patient with ALS after diagnosis is between two and three years. Most ALS drugs in the pipeline are a long way off, perhaps longer than the two to three years that ALS patients currently have to live.

This conflict pits the practical demands of research against the practical demands of human life. It is our opinion that the need to save lives takes precedence over the needs of science. I recognize this is an unorthodox position in the medical world and would like to qualify and preface this assumption with a critical caveat, the Hippocratic oath: "First Do No Harm." In the case of nutritional substances, in most cases the danger of self-administering vitamins and herbal therapies is financial rather physical. In cases where people do not have the luxury of taking a "wait and see" approach to the establishment of a definite relationship between nutritional substances on the course of a neurological disease, we hope this book provides a guideline for the most carefully studied compounds, the rationale for their use, the clinical data to support their efficacy, and future goals of therapy.

Concurrently, we cannot overemphasize our desire and need for nutritional substances to be studied in a scientific and methodical fashion. Nutritional compounds, like their pharmaceutical predecessors, are active compounds that effect specific changes within a cell. The potency of these compounds to influence physiological function and brain function in particular is being increasingly observed by researchers. Unfortunately, however, a large gap still exists between basic science research on nutritional compounds and clinical data. One of the reasons for this gap is financial. Pharmaceutical companies simply will not fund a study investigating, for instance, the effects of creatine in ALS. An additional hope of writing this book is that it will hopefully propel researchers to carefully study the compounds mentioned based upon their physiological effects on vital cell function, as well as to study them in clinical settings in an appropriate manner so we can gain accepted knowledge about the role that these compounds play in neurological diseases.

INTRODUCTION

For too many of us, the prospect of aging is shadowed by gloomy stereotypes. Perhaps we imagine an elderly man who can scarcely maintain his balance as he shuffles outside to retrieve the morning paper, or an older woman so forgetful that she can no longer name her own children, much less drive to the grocery store.

As we age, all of us lose brain cells as a result of genetic weaknesses, infections, injuries, and environmental toxins—the combination of which often leads to brain disease and dysfunction.

And the brain—our body's most complex organ, despite its compact three-pound size—commands everything from memory to sex drive. So it is little wonder that many of us have accepted the notion that we are fated to suffer neurological illnesses and lose brain power as we age.

Thankfully, those days are over. New investigations conducted by top researchers worldwide have led today's most informed health care practitioners to this promising conclusion: The brain has the capacity to heal and regenerate at every stage of our lives.

In *The Brain Wellness Plan,* you will find valuable insights and the most current medical information available about brain health. In addition to offering a practical, two-step "Brain Wellness Plan" for preventing brain disease and boosting brain power through optimum nutrition, this book provides complete treatment protocols for the most common neurological illnesses affecting Americans today.

These protocols—aimed at effectively treating Alzheimer's, Parkinson's, multiple sclerosis, ALS, ADHD, chronic fatigue syndrome, and depression—represent the first of their kind in complementary medicine, integrating breakthrough advances in nutrition with medical and immune-boosting therapies. As such, they highlight how well we can now harness nature in our efforts to prevent and heal brain disease.

Our combined clinical, teaching, and research experience—as a chief neurologist at a New York medical center and private practitioner in neurology and neuropsychiatry, and as a certified nutritionist with nearly two decades of clinical practice and ten years invested in research—has taught us that employing innovative, complementary medicine techniques in preventing and treating neurological illnesses is the best road to brain health.

Our overarching goal in writing *The Brain Wellness Plan* is to give you the tools—and the inspiration—to make informed choices when caring for yourself or someone you love. Join us, and become your own—and your family's—best advocate in maintaining and restoring brain health.

The First Secret to Keeping Our Brains Well: A Healthy Brain-Immune Connection

Thanks to well-documented scientific studies conducted at prestigious medical centers around the world, today we can describe in detail the intricate dance between the brain and the immune system, the brain's most important partner in health.

In the first section of this book, we invite you to fully explore the partnership between the brain and the immune system, and to learn how these two seemingly disparate body systems work as one in health and disease.

The dawning appreciation among health care practitioners of the brain's role as a dynamic organ working in concert with other body systems means that you can now harvest information from the front lines of medicine to maintain optimum health.

In *The Brain Wellness Plan,* you will read that a continuous dialogue exists between our brain and other organ systems, including the immune system, gastrointestinal tract and endocrine systems. This dialogue is made possible by compounds known as messenger molecules and include hormones such as estrogen, DHEA and melatonin, as well as neurotransmitters including serotonin, dopamine and glutamate. Messenger molecules are also derived from the immune system and include cytokines or immunotransmitters. These immunotransmitters not only affect immune system function but also exert a profound influence on our brains in health and disease. In fact, the recent identification of specific immunochemical compounds may hold the key to the very fate of life or death for our brain cells.

Nutritional Therapies with the Power to Heal

Nutritional science is barely more than a century old. Yet, we have already reaped astounding answers to the most essential questions about how the foods we eat have the power to help us live longer, healthier lives.

From the B vitamins to *ginkgo biloba,* some nutritional compounds can profoundly influence all aspects of brain and immune function. In *The Brain Wellness Plan,* we present the results of significant basic research and detail clinical trials documenting specific ways in which these nutritional agents maintain brain health and reverse neurological diseases.

In our two-step plan to brain health, we offer a guide to nutrients with proven potential in promoting the health of your gastrointestinal tract, allowing for better absorption of essential brain-strengthening nutrients, and a comprehensive list of foods and supplements you can start incorporating into your diet immediately to support your overall health.

What About Brain Nutrients?

Besides taking steps to ensure your overall well-being, you can also begin now—no matter what your age—to add the nutrients so essential to supporting brain health and a vital brain-immune connection.

The Brain Wellness Plan provides a comprehensive discussion of "neuroimmunomodulation," the exciting concept of using specific nutrients tailored to smooth the essential two-way chemical dialogue between the brain and the immune system.

After introducing basic neuroimmunomodulators that serve as the foundation for brain health, such as the powerful new generation of brain-protecting antioxidants, we move into Part II of the book. From Alzheimer's to multiple sclerosis, from Lou Gehrig's disease to depression, we devote the entire second section to a detailed discussion of eight common neurological illnesses.

Besides offering you an overview of each disease and its impact on the brain, we present practical ways to ascertain that you or your loved one has received the most accurate, sophisticated diagnosis possible, followed by a complete, disease-specific combined medical and nutritional approach for care, which lists:

1. Recommended dosages of safe, effective nutritional agents you can take immediately to treat that particular neurological disorder, and
2. How to work with your health care provider to incorporate cutting-edge medications and hormonal therapies into a complete disease treatment plan.

Here, you will discover evidence for just how neuroimmunomodulating therapies have proven beneficial in both successfully preventing the root causes of disease and in treating clinical symptoms.

The guidelines developed in *The Brain Wellness Plan* are meant as recommendations, not as prescriptions for treatments. They contain the latest breakthroughs in medical and nutritional science and address the pathophysiological cascade of a particular disorder. These guidelines have a common outline. The first step in treatment is to reduce the underlying disease process, which in most cases involves excessive immune system activity. This excessive immune system activity may be in the form of free radical damage or other pro-inflammatory mechanisms. The second broad-based approach for each disorder is to enhance the energy production of our brain cells. This is accomplished by supporting the mitochondria, the molecular energy factory of our cells. Several nutritional compounds can increase mitochrondrial function and have been suggested as treatment for Parkinson's, Alzheimer's, ALS and other neurological diseases.

Finally, the third category in our guideline for care includes a seemingly futuristic strategy: regenerating the brain and neurotransmitters. Once considered the domain of science fiction, researchers now believe that brain regeneration is possible and probable in our lifetime. By utilizing growth factors, we have come several steps closer to a promise for a cure.

Become a Partner in Building a Better Brain-Immune Connection

Millions of people are affected by the ravages of brain injuries each year. Until recently, neurological diseases were considered irreversible and permanent, and to this day some physicians feel they have nothing to offer in terms of healing them.

Now, armed with new understanding of the biochemical processes involved in the brain-immune connection and ways to modulate those processes, you no longer have to accept the idea that brain disease or dysfunction is inevitable with age. Instead, you can work with your health care practitioners to aggressively prevent neurological disorders and to restore brain health should they occur.

Our ability to maintain brain wellness and to heal ourselves rests on our ability to educate ourselves about the underlying causes of disease, and on our determination to fight back with knowledge. We hope you will use this book as your first step toward preventing and reversing brain disease—and take advantage of this marvelous medical revolution to make the most of your life.

PART I

The Brain-Immune Connection

CHAPTER 1

BRAIN-IMMUNE CONNECTION BASICS

From the earliest moment of development to the last stages of your life, your brain and immune system are involved in a constant, ever-changing dialogue. Each influences the other in specific and profound ways.

The growth of the human brain and its health are dependent on proper immune function from infancy. Conversely, the premature demise of brain cells in diseases such as Alzheimer's, Parkinson's, and ALS is linked to inadvertent or inappropriate immune system activity.

Biological communication between your body's many systems relies on messenger molecules which travel between cells and act in concert with one another. In this chapter, you will learn about the ongoing chemical dialogue between the brain and the immune system, a connection that depends on two languages: the neurotransmitters of the brain, and the immunotransmitters of the immune system.

First, though, let's take a look at the regional control center for monitoring this vital biological dialogue, a brain structure known as the hypothalamus.

The Hypothalamus: Where Brain and Immune System Meet

The hypothalamus is an area of the brain no larger than a pea, yet its complex communication pathways connect your brain with your endocrine, cardiovascular, and immune systems. Like a master conductor in a biological symphony, the hypothalamus orchestrates the production and release of thyroid, stress, growth, and sex hormones. It also controls the amount of insulin released by the pancreas.

Furthermore, this tiny brain structure links our emotions to our bodily responses. For instance, anger, depression, and anxiety are all mediated by chemical communication signals that originate in the hypothalamus. These signals include neurotransmitters and substances known as "hormone-releasing factors," or neuropeptides—protein-like substances which regulate body temperature, level of alertness, blood pressure, respiratory rate, appetite, and reproductive functions.

Now, in addition to commanding this vast spectrum of responses, recent scientific discoveries have linked the hypothalamus to immune function as well. Research has demonstrated that this part of the brain exchanges a significant amount of information with the body's immune system via their respective neurotransmitters and immunotransmitters.

Hypothalamic messengers allow the brain to directly influence the immune system and either increase or decrease its activity. The immune system even has receptor sites for these neurotransmitters. The receptor sites are found on white blood cells, lymph nodes, and various other immune organs.

Conversely, the brain's hypothalamus is directly and continuously influenced by the immune system. Certain brain regions are specifically designed to receive immunotransmitters, and in this way the immune system can profoundly influence brain metabolism, the electrical activity of neurons, and the synthesis and release of neurotransmitters.

This elaborate biological communication network, which we refer to as the brain-immune connection, is the basis of your well-being or your vulnerability to a particular disease. As you will see throughout *The Brain Wellness Plan,* your health depends on the ongoing ability of the brain and the immune system to communicate effectively in both directions.

Neurons: Speaking the Brain's Language

When mystery novelist Agatha Christie's favorite detective, Hercule Poirot, is up against a tough case to solve, he often looks for answers in "the little grey cells." Those little grey cells are the neurons in our brains.

Neuron, the word for the brain's most basic cellular unit, is Greek for "string." Indeed, people during the Greek and Roman eras drew a parallel between man, who is manipulated by the gods, and puppets on strings. However, even early on, physicians such as Hippocrates (*ca.* 460–377 B.C.) managed to persuade at least some in the scientific community that diseases were not punishments from the gods, but the result of natural causes.

Today, we are able to use tools such as digitized computer microscope systems to actually see what is happening in the brain, leading us to understand a great deal about brain function and to closely map specific disease pathways.

Essentially, the brain relies on efficient connections between neighboring neurons to process information it receives from sense organs such as your eyes, ears, and skin, as well as from within your body. That way, your brain can keep track of what's going on in your body's external and internal environments and instruct other bodily systems to respond accordingly.

Your emotional and physical health depends on how well your brain cells communicate with one another—and with the rest of your body—via neurotransmitters.

The Brain's Messengers

Neurotransmitters are the brain's Pony Express messengers, chemicals that leap across the tiny gaps, or synapses, between brain cells. If there is a match between the neurotransmitter's password and the chemical gates of the receptors of the receiving cell, the event causes the receiving neuron to either fire or shut down, depending on the message received.

In other words, each of your neurons has certain receptors on their cell surfaces, which we call membranes, and these receptors act as receiving platforms for messages from various neurotransmitters. This exacting process requires a specific match between the receptor and the neurotransmitter, much as every lock requires a specific key.

Once a specific neurotransmitter binds to a neuron receptor, it sets a chain reaction into motion within the cell. These chemical reactions in turn then regulate and control every cellular process, producing specific biological effects.

Receptors found in neuron membranes are highly specialized in terms of their structure, and that structure is dependent upon the condition of the cell membrane. The cell membrane, which is composed mostly of proteins and lipids, is in a constant state of flux. Changes in cell membranes actually occur from moment to moment, and are uniquely affected by factors such as the emotions, diet, and the immune system. Even slight alterations in this specialized cell membrane design can have negative consequences on the ability of neurotransmitters to produce the desired effects, and can ultimately cause disease.

For example, patients with Alzheimer's suffer massive destruction of the brain cells that release a memory-enhancing neurotransmitter called acetylcholine. That discovery has prompted recent efforts to try to make up for that loss by administering drugs and nutritional agents that boost the brain's acetylcholine content.

In Parkinson's disease, brain damage mainly targets a particular set of dopamine-producing neurons, shortchanging the body of the dopamine neurotransmitter so essential for controlling muscle movements and balance. One of the most effective drug therapies for patients with Parkinson's is L-Dopa, which helps restore a normal level of that crucial neurotransmitter.

In Part II of *The Brain Wellness Plan*, we describe each neurological disease in relationship to the chemical messengers involved in the brain-immune communication relay systems. Right now, though, we'll simply profile a few of the most important neurotransmitters to emerge among the more than fifty to have been discovered and studied in recent years.

A Profile of the Brain's Key Players

• *GABA and Glutamate*

Two of the most abundant neurotransmitters in the central nervous system, glutamate and GABA (gamma-aminobutyric acid) are amino acids that play opposing roles. Because glutamate plays an energizing role while GABA is the calming neurotransmitter, the two are important in maintaining brain health.

In addition to playing an energizing role, glutamate acts to stimulate brain cells. However, if your brain should produce excessive amounts of this excitatory neurotransmitter, healthy neurons may be destroyed. GABA, on the other hand, reduces brain cell activity. Depressed levels of this calming neurotransmitter are associated with anxiety and epileptic seizures.

• *Serotonin*

A neurotransmitter synthesized from the amino acid tryptophan, serotonin is intimately involved in regulating sleep, appetite, sexual behavior, mood, and cardiovascular and immune activity. An imbalance of serotonin may be responsible for depression, autism, obsessive-compulsive disorder, eating disorders, sleep disturbances, and chronic pain syndromes.

• *Acetylcholine*

Acetylcholine is perhaps the most vital neurotransmitter in regulating memory and cognitive abilities. A depressed level of acetylcholine is the key culprit for the symptoms associated with Alzheimer's disease.

• *Dopamine*

Dopamine greatly influences your thought processes and motor activity. Low dopamine levels in the brain cause the tremor, impaired motor control, and poor balance that are hallmark symptoms of Parkinson's.

• Norepinephrine

When you are excited or anxious and feel your heart pounding, it is due to the effects of the brain's norepinephrine messages on your heart. An imbalance of this neurotransmitter may cause impaired physiological responses to stress and other emotional events.

• Prostaglandins

Originally, these hormone-like molecules were not considered in relation to their impact on the brain. Now research has demonstrated that prostaglandins, which are derived from biological fats (phospholipids), influence the activity of receptors and neurotransmitters.

A key prostaglandin in the brain-immune connection is a substance known as arachidonic acid. Derived from specific types of dietary fats known as omega-6 fatty acids, arachidonic acid is involved in promoting the destructive effects of the neurotransmitter glutamate we described earlier.

• Nitric Oxide

The newest neurotransmitter to fall under scientific scrutiny, nitric oxide holds exciting promise for maintaining and mending the brain-immune connection. This tiny molecule has an edge over its larger molecular-weight neurotransmitter cousins for two reasons: its small size allows it to diffuse more rapidly through tissues, and it does not require specific cell membrane binding sites for its activity. Instead, nitric oxide rapidly enters cells and works from within cell membranes, which is why we call it a "rapid response neurotransmitter." As you will see throughout *The Brain Wellness Plan*, nitric oxide is deeply involved in learning and memory, and helps coordinate activity between the brain and immune system.

Before proceeding to a more detailed discussion of these and other neurotransmitters, the role they play in causing and treating specific diseases, and complete protocols for aggressively restoring the body's chemical balances, we want to introduce you to your brain's partner in health: your immune system.

Your Brain's Most Important Partner: The Immune System

The biological complexity of the brain's communication system is matched in intricacy and efficiency by the immune system's complicated communication network. Like the brain, the immune system's different components "speak" to one another—and with the rest of the body—through its chemical messengers, the immunotransmitters.

At its most basic level, the function of the immune system is to protect us from the harmful effects of bacteria, viruses, parasites, and environmental toxins. This enormous task is carried out by various components of the immune system, which must work in close harmony with one another for best results.

The most important of these immune system components are the lymphocytes, or white blood cells, which fight bacteria, fungi, and other foreign bodies. Lymphocytes include both T cells and B cells.

In addition, throughout this book you will read about another important type of white blood cell, the macrophage. Macrophages are the immune system's foot soldiers, capable of engaging in hand-to-hand battle and literally gobbling up invaders to destroy them.

The number of white blood cells called into battle depends, of course, on the severity of the invasion. Your immunotransmitters play a vital role in goading the immune system components into action and in regulating the scope of the battle.

Cytokines: The Immune System's Messengers

Because the immune system plays such a complex role in defending our bodies, it has developed a highly specialized form of communication to allow its various cellular components to coordinate their ferocious activity. This communication relies on immunotransmitters called cytokines.

Cytokines are to the immune system what neurotransmitters are to the brain. Just as the brain relies on neurotransmitters to exchange information among its own neurons and with the rest of the body, so your immune system's ability to relay messages between its components and throughout the body depends on cytokines.

The three types of cytokines you will read about most in this book will be the interleukins, tumor necrosis factor (TNF), and interferons. All these natural proteins are capable of mounting and amplifying immune responses to a variety of biological challenges.

When your body is threatened by invasion, cytokines signal your immune system to mobilize reserve troops of white blood cells. When the invasion is over, it is up to your cytokines to put out the word to stop mobilizing the troops.

In other words, these immunotransmitters coordinate your white blood cells, boosting their activity at times of infection, injury, or other demands and reining them back in after battle. In this regard, we can think of cytokines as the body's Paul Revere molecules, calling the immune system's troops out as needed.

The Brain-Immune Connection: A Two-Way Dialogue

In the past, scientists catalogued neurotransmitters as chemical messengers limited only to transmitting information between neurons in the brain. As we explained earlier, however, recent investigations at top research institutions worldwide have dispelled that notion—we now understand that there is a two-way chemical dialogue between the brain and the immune system. Each can influence the other directly.

For example, the neurotransmitters norepinephrine and serotonin have receptors on various components of the immune system and are therefore able to influence immune response in specific ways.

Conversely, in certain areas of the brain, neurons have receptors for cytokines. As you will see in the next chapter, when cytokines are unleashed by the immune system, they can profoundly alter the way important neurotransmitters are released or inhibited.

Another good example of the brain's influence on the immune system is through the cortisol hormone. Cortisol is produced via the hypothalamus. When you suffer stress, your hypothalamus produces a substance called "corticotropin-releasing factor" (CRF), which then stimulates the release of cortisol from your adrenal glands. Cortisol plays such a pivotal role in the brain-immune connection that it has fallen under close scrutiny for its relationship to such diverse disease states as depression, chronic fatigue syndrome, and Alzheimer's.

Why is cortisol so important? The increased level of cortisol triggered by stress—an adaptive response that no doubt evolved to help us survive attacks by predators or enemy tribes—allows your body to muster a coordinated defense to the event. That defense may include heightened awareness, increased heart rate, and increased blood flow to muscles.

Cortisol has several detrimental effects on brain function, including blocking a brain cell's ability to utilize glucose properly. A persistent state of glucose underutilization by brain cells appears to be a key factor in initiating a detrimental process called "apoptosis."

Apoptosis describes a specific way in which brain cells die. It also occurs in normal cells during aging, to rid the body of senescent cells and make room for new, healthy ones. Apoptosis has also been implicated in the development of several neurological disorders, including Alzheimer's, Parkinson's, and Lou Gehrig's diseases. In each of these disorders, a trigger—which may be a particular environmental agent or genetic factor—initiates a destructive cascade that results in the production of enzymes known as caspases. Caspases degrade essential cell structures by initiating the breakdown of proteins that support the cell. The activation of caspases represents a final common pathway of cell death in Alzheimer's and Parkinson's diseases, and perhaps Lou Gehrig's disease. If scientists unravel the secret to the initiating and propagating factors of apoptosis, they will undoubtedly provide clues to developing sophisticated interventions that may delay—or even cure—neurodegenerative diseases.

The Brain's Own Immune System

You rarely see the immune system's components in the brain, because an overzealous immune response activated to fight off invading toxins or viruses is all too capable of killing off healthy (and irreplaceable) brain cells in the process.

However, as Drs. Wolfgang J. Streit and Carol A. Kincaid-Colton explain in their November 1995 article in *Scientific American*, scientists are in the throes of discovering mounting evidence for an extensive defense network that functions like the brain's own private immune system.

Studies examining the way certain "microglia" cells respond to antibodies in the brain demonstrate that these normally mild-mannered cells can perform amazing, Superman-like feats. Within minutes of disturbances in their environment, microglia cells rush to surround damaged neurons and produce some of the same deadly chemicals that immune system cells manufacture to eat up invaders.

As in the immune system, some of those protective chemicals used by the brain's microglia also end up destroying healthy bystander cells in the course of battle. This has aroused new suspicions that overzealous microglia may contribute to certain neurologic disorders.

The possible good news? Finding ways to specifically inhibit microglia activity or block their products might yield new therapies for treating patients with neurological illnesses.

In general, three broad-based treatment strategies are employed to treat patients with neurological diseases. These include (1) to reduce excessive inflammatory activity, (2) to increase brain mitochondrial activity, and (3) to rebalance neurotransmitter levels.

A very important aspect of treating neurological disease is to turn down the thermostat on an overactive immune system. As we mentioned earlier, an overactive or overzealous immune system has been implicated in the etiologies of Alzheimer's, Parkinson's and Lou Gehrig's diseases, and possibly autism. There are several ways to damp the immune system, through either pharmacological or nutritional methods. Pharmacological strategies to calm an overexcited immune system that may be targeting vital neurological components of the brain can include both medical and nutritional anti-inflammatory compounds.

In the nonsteroidal class of drugs, new compounds known as Cox-II inhibitors have gained wide popularity among physicians because of their safety and how easily they're tolerated. Prescription Cox-II inhibitors include Celebrex and Vioxx. These agents have been approved by the FDA to treat inflammatory conditions like rheumatoid arthritis. Their ability to reduce brain inflammation makes them an excellent candidate for further study in degenerative brain conditions like Alzheimer's disease and perhaps Lou Gehrig's disease. Natural Cox-II inhibitors have also been identified, and are used by nutritionally oriented physicians. These include flavonoids, plant compounds that have been used as anti-inflammatory agents in traditional folk medicine for hundreds of years. The active extracts of these herbs have now been identified and include numerous anti-inflammatory compounds like resveratrol, triterpenoids (including ursolic acid), caffeic acid, and bupleurum.

Resveratrol is found in grapes. It is currently being studied for possible beneficial effects in heart disease and cancer. Most of the triterpenoids are derived from a common plant named *Plantago major*, the extracts of which have demonstrated anti-inflammatory properties. In particular, the *Plantago major* extract ursolic acid significantly inhibits the Cox-II enzyme and is an excellent candidate as a natural anti-inflammatory substance.

Other anti-inflammatory compounds found in nature include vitamin D, estrogen, and the omega-3 fatty acids. Their utility in selectively treating such disorders as Alzheimer's disease, multiple sclerosis, and certain forms of depression is increasingly appreciated.

Efforts to increase mitochondrial function are vital to neurological rescue, especially in neurodegenerative diseases like Alzheimer's and Parkinson's. An overwhelming body of evidence has now implicated mitochondrial impairment in these disorders as well as other conditions, including autism and chronic fatigue syndrome. The mitochondria are necessary for cell function, because they produce the highly energetic compound ATP, which drives all the enzymatic processes of the cell. ATP can be thought of as the essential fuel of cells. Five nutritional compounds have been shown to increase mitochondrial function and have also been suggested as useful in treating neurological diseases. These include creatine and cyclocreatine (a synthetic derivative of creatine) for Lou Gehrig's disease and autism; the compound NADH for Parkinson's disease, Alzheimer's disease, and chronic fatigue syndrome; and Idebenone (a coenzyme Q10 analog) for Alzheimer's disease. Furthermore, ribose (a form of sugar) has also been demonstrated to raise cellular ATP content, especially in muscle and heart cells. It is likely to be beneficial to patients who complain of muscle fatigue, as well as to chronic fatigue syndrome patients. Whether ribose can increase brain ATP levels has not yet been determined. If ribose does demonstrate this effect, it may also become an essential component of mitochrondrial enhancement in treatment strategies for those neurological diseases associated with mitochondrial failure.

Finally, specific neurotransmitter imbalances are associated with given disorders. For example, it is well established that there is a decline of the neurotransmitter acetylcholine in Alzheimer's disease. Thus, pharmacological or nutritional strategies include ways of raising brain acetylcholine levels, which, in turn, improve memory deficits. These strategies include prescription medications, such as the drug Aricept, and new nutritional substances like Huperzine A and CDP choline. In autism, certain neurotransmitters may be increased, while others are deficient. Thus a treatment strategy may be based on adding a medication that blocks dopamine, like Risperidone, and concurrently administering a nutritional substance that raises the neurotransmitter glutamate, such as DMG. In depression, and in some cases of autism, the goal of therapy would include raising brain serotonin levels. This can be accomplished pharmacologically with medications like the selective serotonin reuptake inhibitors (SSRIs) or, nutritionally, through use of supplements like St. John's wort, SAMe, and N-acetyltryptophan. Each of these supplements raises serotonin levels using a different mechanism.

CHAPTER 2

COMMUNICATION BREAKDOWN

Because every disease we discuss in this book is directly influenced by a brain-immune system communication breakdown, in this chapter we focus on just how disturbances in the brain-immune connection are associated with these diseases.

Like any partnership, the brain-immune relationship can become strained and damaging to both parties if communication breaks down. Several important factors appear to be responsible for causing communication to falter between these systems—factors based on the unique characteristics of the two systems involved.

The brain, for instance, is a very fatty substance. Approximately 25 percent of the dry weight of the brain is composed of lipids (fats). These lipids serve many important roles, which include insulating nerve fibers and acting as the building blocks of cell membranes surrounding neurons.

As essential as these brain cell lipids may be to your brain's health, however, the brain's fatty content has a downside as well: it makes the brain an easy target for immune-initiated injury through free radical attack.

Other natural agents called upon by the immune system in defending the body against diseases, infections, toxins, and other stresses may also serve as catalysts for devastating neurological illnesses. These include nitric oxide, one of the newest neurotransmitters to demand the scientific spotlight; cytokines, the

immune system's most important immunotransmitters; and cortisol, the hormone which plays such a principal role in mediating
the body's response to stress.

Contemporary scientific studies in neurology and immunology have demonstrated that the body's own immune system has
the ability to damage healthy brain cells. As you will discover in
The Brain Wellness Plan, the failure of your own body's natural
ability to protect itself against an inappropriate immune response
may lead to neurological illnesses such as Parkinson's, Alzheimer's, and Lou Gehrig's disease.

The Body's Terrorists: Rampaging Free Radicals

When the body fights off an infection, the immune system's
cytokines go to work, sending messages to the brain that cause
more white blood cells to mobilize. The more white blood cells
your body activates, the more free radicals they produce.

These free radicals are among your immune system's most
powerful weapons. Naturally produced by the body as a response
to aging and during times of disease, injury, and emotional stress,
free radicals are chemicals with a single electron molecule, whose
mission it is to find another electron free for pairing. That process
of electron looting is known as "oxidation," and it's the same
process that rusts metal and spoils butter.

Various components of the immune system rely on free radicals to neutralize threatening invaders. Free radicals are like
pellets of poison pinging about in the body, damaging whatever
they hit. These free radicals go to work to destroy invaders by
interfering with their cellular machinery, literally dissolving or
breaking down the genetic material of bacteria, toxins, and
viruses.

When all is going well, the immune system is capable of identifying foreign invaders such as viruses and bacteria by accurately
"reading" molecular codes found on cell surfaces. These molecular codes are like the flags of different armies, and the immune
system will not attack a cell if it sees a flag belonging to the body's
own host army.

Once the immune system has produced antibodies to a certain antigen, or invader, it even develops a "memory" of sorts, so that it can readily respond with the same fighter cells the next time that invader appears.

If functioning properly, then, our immune components do not turn against our own body's cells. Unfortunately, free radicals can interfere with the biological components of our own healthy cells just as they destroy invaders, literally dismantling the body's essential cellular proteins, fatty cell membranes, and DNA. And too often, the cells destroyed by free radicals are in the brain, because the high fat content of the brain's neurons make them particularly vulnerable to free radical attack.

Why is fat so attractive to free radicals? Because fat, by its very chemical makeup—it contains carbon, oxygen, and hydrogen molecules—can readily give up an electron to a free radical in search of a partner. And then that fat molecule, in turn, becomes a free radical, perpetuating the cycle of free radical destruction.

This process is called "lipid peroxidation," which means that the fat literally becomes oxidized and goes from being a stable molecule to an unstable molecule. We see it as a biological uprising, where just one free radical has the ability to attract others to its revolutionary cause and produce instability in the biological government.

The most important natural defenses we have against free radical damage are our body's natural "antioxidants," a broad range of chemical substances that all have one thing in common: they ward off free radical damage to cells because they can safely donate electrons. Pairing those antioxidant electrons with free radicals effectively stops free radicals in their tracks—often in time to prevent damage to healthy cells.

The brain has a highly developed antioxidant security system designed to protect itself against free radical attack. This antioxidant system involves two critical enzymes, superoxide dismutase and glutathione, which you will hear more about later. These two substances are the front line body guards capable of protecting the delicate machinery of neurons from the harmful effects of free radicals.

Unfortunately, in many neurological diseases—including Parkinson's, Alzheimer's, ALS, and multiple sclerosis—the brain's specialized antioxidant mechanisms fail. As you will see in Part II, the cause of this failure might be genetic, environmental, or even dietary, but the consequences are the same: unchecked free radical activity on the brain's cellular machinery.

This free radical attack homes in on the fat-heavy membranes of the brain's neurons. When a neuron membrane undergoes lipid peroxidation, the fats acquire more oxygen and become rancid (peroxidized). This causes a chain reaction, causing those neurons to break down and destroy surrounding healthy brain cells in turn.

Lipid peroxidation appears to be the final common pathway for many neurological illnesses. Specific disease symptoms depend on which area of the brain is under attack.

In Alzheimer's, for instance, the cell membranes of the hippocampus, the brain's memory region, are the ones to fall prey to free radical attack. In Parkinson's disease, on the other hand, the area of the brain to suffer the most damage is the "substantia nigra," which produces dopamine, the neurotransmitter responsible for muscle movement and coordination.

In addition, certain investigators have shown that free radical attack on one of the fatty substances found in brain cells—arachidonic acid—can literally accelerate the free radical injury to brain cells.

Arachidonic acid is normally kept under a tight lock and key by neurons. However, during excessive immune system activity and free radical production, arachidonic acid is released and stimulates a series of injurious steps to brain cells. The most potentially damaging effect of arachidonic acid is its ability to create an extensive amount of glutamate, the excitatory neurotransmitter that researchers have linked to ALS and Parkinson's disease.

The Role of Nitric Oxide in Producing the Most Toxic Free Radical Offender of All

In the last chapter, you read about the value of nitric oxide as a neurotransmitter. Unfortunately, the excessive production of nitric oxide can also be blamed for throwing the brain-immune connection off kilter and causing some of the brain's worst free radical damage.

When the immune system's cytokines activate the macrophages—those important white blood cells capable of gobbling up invading viruses and bacteria—the macrophages produce large amounts of nitric oxide in the course of battle.

Over the past decade, scientists have shown that the production of nitric oxide through the combination of immune and nervous system activity—activity often sparked by an infection, exposure to a toxin, or as part of the aging process—plays a key role in the development of neurological diseases.

The real trouble starts when nitric oxide, through various chemical reactions, produces peroxynitrite, a biologically essential oxidant with the dubious distinction of being the most toxic free radical to the body—and especially to the brain.

For instance, recent studies of human plasma exposed to peroxynitrite show that this free radical terrorist is capable of damaging plasma proteins and depleting such crucial antioxidants as vitamin C, uric acid, coenzyme Q10, and glutathione. Peroxynitrite also has the potential to step up the production of toxic lipid peroxides which further damage cell membranes.

You will read more about peroxynitrite in the next chapter and in our chapter on Parkinson's disease. There, we discuss new scientific evidence supporting the idea that inhibiting nitric oxide synthesis may prevent the loss of dopamine-producing neurons because it slows down peroxynitrite production.

How Cytokines Play a Role in Disease

Cytokines—the immune system's own chemical messengers crafted to deliver warnings to speed up or slow down the immune system's responses—may also play a complex role in causing or promoting neurological illness.

How do they do this? Researchers have discovered that certain cytokines are specifically "offensive" because they ratchet up immune system activity.

In recent years, investigators have identified a large number of cytokines as the cause of quite a few—and sometimes detrimental—effects on brain function. For example, certain cytokines are capable of producing fatigue, slowed thinking, and other depressive symptoms. The gamma interferon cytokine directly inhibits the brain's ability to synthesize serotonin, and low levels of serotonin can cause depression. This may explain why patients with viral illnesses or diseases such as multiple sclerosis experience much higher rates of depression, as low serotonin levels are directly linked to depressive states.

In addition, we now have evidence that the cytokine interleukin-1 promotes sleep and reduces appetite. In patients with Alzheimer's disease, scientists have demonstrated that interleukin-6 is partially responsible for the manufacture of beta amyloid, one of the substances that kills off brain cells and destroys memory.

Cortisol: Too Much of a Good Thing Causes Problems

As you learned in the last chapter, cortisol is the hormone that allows your body to coordinate a response to stress. Typically, when that stress abates, your sensory organs send a message to your brain that it's okay to shut down cortisol production for the time being. However, under some circumstances, the cortisol response ends up perpetuating itself, resulting in a variety of pathological changes in the brain and immune system.

What happens when your body's cells are continually exposed to cortisol? Studies reveal that continued exposure to excessive cortisol may damage specific brain regions involved in mood and memory. In addition, your body's immune mechanisms may automatically shut down when too much cortisol is present.

Preprogrammed Cell Death

In order for the body to stay healthy, millions of our cells sacrifice themselves every minute as part of the brain's natural, ongoing housekeeping process to keep things in order.

Scientists have now discovered that certain groups of brain cells are destined for a preprogrammed cell death. This mysterious form of cell suicide is called "apoptosis," from the Greek for "a flower losing its petals."

A number of brain disorders, including Alzheimer's, Parkinson's, and amyotrophic lateral sclerosis, may result when apoptosis spins out of control and leads to abnormal cell suicide. Investigators believe apoptosis is mediated by specific immune system cytokines known as interleukins. If so, learning to inhibit inappropriate apoptosis with neuroimmunomodulating nutritional substances, hormones, and drugs will no doubt contribute to new therapies for neurological illnesses in the future.

What's Next: Basic Nutritional Guidelines

Now that you know just how important it is to maintain a healthy brain-immune connection, you're probably wondering how to get started on just the right foods and supplements for optimum health.

In the next chapter, we discuss your body's gastrointestinal tract in relation to its brain-supporting role, and present a basic nutritional guideline for brain wellness that every healthy individual should incorporate into a daily nutritional plan.

CHAPTER 3

FOOD FOR THOUGHT

In this chapter, we focus on the first part of our two-step Brain Wellness Plan, the nutritional guidelines any healthy individual must follow to support optimum overall health. First, however, we will take a quick look at the body's digestive tract.

Wait: if this is a book about the brain, why are we bothering to include information on your digestive tract?

Simple. The gastrointestinal (GI) tract carries out three important roles in maintaining an optimum brain-immune connection. First of all, the brain absolutely depends on the GI tract's ability to assimilate and deliver nutrients which act as essential building blocks for neurotransmitters. Secondly, the brain requires the GI tract to remove toxins which have the potential to adversely affect brain-immune function. And, finally, optimum brain health rests on the GI tract's ability to properly regulate immune system activity.

Why Is a Healthy Gastrointestinal Tract so Important for the Brain?

• The Brain Is a Hungry Organ

The idea that your brain's metabolism is highly dependent on your body's overall nutritional status becomes evident if you think about your brain's neurons—like all cells in your body—as tiny factories. Each neuron shoulders the responsibility for producing its own energy and requires certain nutrients to fuel its manufacturing processes.

Every cell is made up of carbohydrate, protein, and fat molecules, and most of a cell's metabolism is carried out within its mitochondria. These tiny organelles are often referred to by biologists as "the powerhouses of the cell" because mitochondria are so important to oxidative phosphorylation—the chemical production of energy and a fundamental process to all living creatures that need oxygen.

Because of their complex communication duties, neurons consume an average of five times more glucose than other cells in the body. For that kind of fuel, the brain must depend on the digestive tract's efficient intestinal digestion and absorption of food.

In recent years, many in the scientific community have devoted their research to documenting the relationship between nutrients and brain cell function. The brain is dependent on adequate gastrointestinal function for delivering the essential nutrients it cannot make on its own. Otherwise, the brain will not be able to keep its biological machinery running.

In addition to providing the essential compounds for cellular energy production, the GI tract must also deliver the ingredients for other critical brain constituents. These include essential fatty acids, or phospholipids, which act as building blocks for cell membranes, hormones, and certain neurotransmitters.

The GI tract also carries B vitamins to the brain. B vitamins are indispensable in synthesizing neurotransmitters and in forming myelin, the insulating substance that sheaths connections between neurons and makes it possible for them to transmit messages effectively.

• The Brain Relies on the GI Tract to Help Clean House

Your gastrointestinal tract always has different types of resident bacteria—some useful to our digestive processes, some harmful. A second, and equally essential, role the GI tract plays in brain function therefore involves maintaining a healthy ecological balance between beneficial and harmful bacteria. The GI tract's natural detoxification processes allow most harmful toxins to exit the body via the liver.

If the GI tract should fail to keep up with its housekeeping chores, a variety of toxins produced by certain strains of bacteria may have detrimental consequences on brain metabolism. These toxins can eventually produce a variety of neurological and psychiatric symptoms, ranging from seizures to behavioral disturbances.

Of all the toxins to reach the brain as a result of impaired GI function, ammonia is the best documented. Normally produced in the GI tract by bacteria as a result of protein digestion, ammonia is cleaned out of healthy bodies through the liver, which serves as the body's major detoxification center.

In patients with liver disease, high levels of ammonia have been linked to deleterious effects on brain function. In fact, patients with elevated ammonia levels due to an impaired GI tract may suffer from personality changes, agitation, hyperactivity, and seizures.

Recently, scientists have also uncovered links between bacterially derived toxins in the GI tract and neurological diseases such as schizophrenia and autism. In schizophrenia, some researchers have speculated that specific substances manufactured by anaerobic bacteria in the GI tract interfere with synaptophysin, an important brain protein required for the release of certain neurotransmitters.

And in patients with autism, specific organic acids released by different strains of bacteria appear to interfere with the brain's ability to properly metabolize glucose.

The Gut–Immune System Connection

Rather than think of the immune system as outside and separate from the gut, think of your GI tract as part of your immune system in the way it protects the body from disease.

Groups of nerve fibers line the intestinal wall from the esopha-

gus to the rectum. More than half of your immune system occu-
pies the space surrounding the gastrointestinal tract, making the
GI tract the largest organ in the body capable of producing
important immune system components such as white blood cells
and cytokines.

Since most microorganisms that threaten the body enter
through the mouth and nose, the GI tract also acts as a main
line of immune defense, preventing microscopic invaders and
other materials contained in the intestinal tract from passing
into the body's internal environment.

Its exposure to many antigens causes the GI tract's immune
response to be activated regularly. If the immune response that
takes place in the GI tract were separate from the rest of the
immune system, this would pose no problem. The gut could
simply respond to an invader without the dramatic domino effect
of gearing up an entire systemic immune response with all of
those potential consequences, like inflammation.

In essence, then, your GI tract acts as a neuroimmunomodulating organ by supporting a healthy immune system response to
infections, toxins, and other stresses. However, if the GI tract is
not healthy, the consequences may be devastating, in that your
entire immune system kicks into gear and affects the rest of
your body systems. Many brain-immune disorders are directly or
indirectly related to dysfunctions in the GI tract—largely because
your gut's failure to do its job of utilizing nutrients and cleansing
the body of harmful substances can result in inappropriate
immune system activation.

How Does the GI Tract Communicate?

Just as the brain and immune system communicate through
chemical messengers, your GI tract relies on specific substances
called peptides to relay information. These are long sequences
of amino acids that we find widely distributed in the brain and
gastrointestinal tract. Peptides can be readily absorbed from the
gastrointestinal tract, entering the bloodstream and eventually
reaching the brain.

Once they have successfully completed their winding journey into the brain, peptides regulate the synthesis of new neurotransmitters, influencing the metabolism of brain cells.

We now believe that peptides are able to modulate our pain, memory, learning, and behavior—which is why peptide function is currently the subject of top-funded clinical and basic science research investigations into neurological disorders.

Food for Thought: From Theory to Practice

The Brain Wellness Plan is a two-step process that focuses on general dietary guidelines. We developed these guidelines to help ensure that you can adequately incorporate and assimilate (1) the nutrients any healthy individual should include in a diet designed to support optimum health and (2) specific brain-supporting substances we recommend for individuals eager to prevent neurological illnesses by boosting the brain-immune connection. We call these therapeutic substances "neuroimmunomodulators."

We will discuss specific neuroimmunomodulators, or Step 2 of *The Brain Wellness Plan,* in the next chapter. They will appear again in relation to specific diseases in Part II of this book.

For now, however, we will focus only on practical, general nutritional guidelines every person should follow as the first step toward maintaining lifelong optimum brain function.

A Nutrition Primer for Brain-Immune Health: Basic Guidelines for the Healthy Individual

Ask your physician, best friends, and family members to describe the perfect diet, and you're likely to get as many different descriptions of an "ideal" regimen as the number of people you ask. This shouldn't be surprising, since even many physicians and clinical nutritionists hotly disagree about the "perfect" foods and nutritional supplements.

What most professionals in nutritional science *will* unite to tell you, however, is that the Recommended Daily Allowances (RDAs) touted for so long by the government as the gold standard of nutrition are really nothing more than a shadowy list of minimum requirements.

The RDA is a guideline for preventing vitamin deficiencies, but shortchanges you when it comes to listing optimum doses of all the nutrients necessary for healthy brain and immune system function. And when it comes to preventing and treating diseases of any kind, the RDAs fail utterly.

At the end of this chapter, you will find a summary chart that serves as a quick source and dosage guide for optimal brain-immune nutrients. You should address specific recommendations with your health care practitioner.

Getting Started on the Road to Health

- Avoid current fad diets and focus on your individual health profile—seek the guidance of a clinical nutritionist.
- Eat a variety of foods, with emphasis on dark-colored fruits and vegetables such as blueberries, cantaloupe, broccoli, kale, tomatoes, and sweet potatoes.
- Eat whole, unrefined, nutrient-dense carbohydrates such as whole grain bread, cereals, pasta, brown rice, oats, barley, etc.
- Eat organic vegetables, meats, or poultry to avoid exposure to excessive hormones and pesticides.
- Limit your fat intake to a maximum of 25 percent of your total daily calories.
  - Limit saturated fats, such as butter and fats found in milk and meat, to no more than 5 percent of your fat intake.
  - Emphasize monounsaturated fats (such as olive oil) and fats high in omega-3 fatty acids (flaxseed oil, fish oils) to constitute the remaining 20 percent of your fat intake.
- Limit red meats to no more than 4 ounces two times per week.
- Emphasize fish, fowl, and low-fat yogurt as protein sources.
- Explore vegetarian sources of protein, including tofu, tempeh, wheat gluten, and grain and bean dishes.

- Limit cholesterol to less than 300 mg daily.
- Avoid sugar and sweets.
- Do not be fooled by the new "low-fat" desserts, as they are usually loaded with sugar.
- Avoid packaged, processed foods that may contain undesirable nutritional constituents such as hydrogenated fats, preservatives, or high amounts of saturated fat or sugar.

How Can You Help Your GI Tract Absorb Brain Nutrients?

As we learned earlier in this chapter, your GI tract plays an indispensable part in absorbing and delivering essential nutrients to the brain. Unfortunately, all it takes is a brief look at the shelves of your local pharmacy to know that most people are not digesting nutrients very well: those stomach remedies, antacids, laxatives, and digestive aids add up to a billion-dollar industry.

In other words, you aren't "what you eat," as perhaps your mother once cautioned you. More accurately, you are "what you use," or what you can digest and absorb.

As you now know, the health of your GI tract affects the digestion, absorption, and function of many nutritional substances. Additionally, your GI tract is the first line of defense against disease-causing bacteria and viruses. Therefore, your GI tract is an integral aspect of your immune defense in maintaining wellness. That's why good digestion is as crucial to your health as optimum nutrition.

Enhancing your GI tract's ability to perform its brain-supporting duties requires a combination of substances, including glutamine, dietary fiber, friendly bacteria, chlorophyll, and nucleotides. While these nutrients may not directly affect brain health, they do support the GI tract functions so essential to brain wellness.

• Glutamine

An important amino acid, glutamine is the major source of energy for cells in the GI tract and important to protein synthesis.

Glutamine helps preserve the integrity of the GI tract by maintaining its mucosal barrier lining and thus keeping toxins out of the bloodstream and away from the brain.

Glutamine is also the primary respiratory fuel for stimulated macrophages and lymphocytes. Finally, it has been identified as a critical nutrient for maintaining the immune system and for preventing bacteria from leaving the gut following injury or other trauma.

While you can find glutamine in protein-containing foods, we recommend supplements of this vital gut-supporting nutrient.

RECOMMENDED DOSE FOR HEALTHY INDIVIDUALS: 1000 mg daily. Take on an empty stomach to maximize absorption.

•Indigestible Fiber

Indigestible fiber helps you eliminate wastes and harmful bacterial toxins from the GI tract. Also, increased intake of these dietary fibers helps stimulate the growth of beneficial bacteria and repair colon cells. The dietary guidelines we recommend here will be useful in providing valuable fibers to the diet.

Using special indigestible fibers such as fructosoligosaccharides (FOS) can provide an important medium in the large intestine for feeding beneficial bacteria. You can purchase FOS by itself or combined with friendly bacteria.

RECOMMENDED DOSE FOR HEALTHY INDIVIDUALS: 4 g of FOS daily in addition to dietary fiber from meals. May be taken in divided doses between meals.

•Friendly Bacteria

The gut's integrity is also maintained by a healthy balance of "friendly" microorganisms such as those found in the lactobacillus and bifido bacteria families. Maintaining high levels of these friendly bacteria in the intestinal tract is critical for detoxification and health. By producing acids and natural antibiotics, warding off pathogens such as viruses and molds, and assisting your GI tract in proper bowel function, these friendly bacteria play important roles in keeping your entire system healthy.

> **RECOMMENDED DOSE FOR HEALTHY INDIVIDUALS:** Look for supplements containing billions of both lactobacillus and bifido strains of the beneficial bacteria. We recommend following the dosages typically found in the product's "suggested use" section. It is best to take these products between meals.

• Chlorophyll

Products such as wheat, barley, and oat grass powders are rich in chlorophyll—a substance known for its power to remove toxins from your intestinal tract.

> **RECOMMENDED DOSE FOR HEALTHY INDIVIDUALS:** We suggest supplementing your diet with a high-chlorophyll drink such as wheat grass juice or barley grass juice once or twice daily, between meals. These are also available in tablets.

• Nucleotides

Nucleotides are the structural units of nucleic acids, and play a major role in almost every one of your body's biochemical processes.

You are probably most familiar with nucleotides as the building blocks of our genetic material: DNA (deoxyribonucleic acid) and RNA (ribonucleic acid). Chemically, nucleotides are known as cytidine, adenosine, guanine, inosine, and uridine.

Essentially, a healthy brain–gut–immune system feedback loop depends on the efficient function of your body's nucleotides, as these acids modify the type and growth of intestinal bacteria. Specifically, nucleotides enhance the growth of "friendly" bacteria, such as lactobacilli and bifido, in the gastrointestinal tract, and suppress the proliferation of the "bad" bacteria that can provoke an immune system response.

Investigators have demonstrated that nucleotides are important for maintaining cellular immune response, and their deficiency may impair that. Today's clinical studies with human subjects confirm the benefits of dietary nucleotides, which are now used to supplement hospital feedings and infant formulas.

All foods with protein contain nucleotides, and infants receive them naturally through breast milk.

RECOMMENDED DOSE FOR HEALTHY INDIVIDUALS: To benefit most from nucleotides—especially when your immune system is challenged during infections—we recommend supplementing your diet with nucleotides in the 1–2 g range. Nucleotides should be taken between meals for the most efficient absorption.

Basic Brain Nutrients

• Multivitamins

The "multi" is the basis for any supplement program and represents an overall "insurance" supplement to the diet by providing a wide array of essential nutrients. You'll find a variety of multis on the market. Basically, multivitamins come in one-, two-, or three-a-day formulas and in tablet or capsule form. Essentially, all cover the same spectrum of nutrients.

RECOMMENDED DOSE FOR HEALTHY INDIVIDUALS: Our preference is for the two- or three-a-day formula multivitamins. Taken in smaller amounts throughout the day, the nutrients are better absorbed and utilized than if taken all at once.

• Antioxidants

A full spectrum of antioxidants—including carotenoids, vitamin E, vitamin C, polyphenols, lipoic acid, n-acetyl-cysteine, tocotrienols, and coenzyme Q10—is your best support against free radical damage to the body. We will discuss specific neuroimmunomodulating antioxidants in greater detail in the next chapter.

RECOMMENDED DOSE FOR HEALTHY INDIVIDUALS: We recommend adding any one of the general antioxidant supplements on the market to the general multiple vitamin, since the antioxidant supplement contains higher quantities and a more complete array of this important class of nutrients.

• Calcium-Magnesium Supplement

While these minerals have been emphasized for healthy bones and marketed to women, calcium and magnesium also play important roles in maintaining brain wellness. Magnesium plays a pivotal role in brain cell energy production by activating crucial enzymes involved in the manufacture of ATP, the energy currency of cells. Magnesium is also an important ingredient for the enzymes essential in producing important neurotransmitters such as serotonin.

In addition, magnesium stabilizes cell membranes and protects them against the harmful effects of excitatory neurotransmitters such as glutamate, and has been documented for its beneficial effects in preventing migraine headaches. Calcium, meanwhile, is a critical mineral for boosting the potential of nerve and muscle cells to communicate through electrical impulses.

RECOMMENDED DOSE FOR HEALTHY INDIVIDUALS: Because calcium and magnesium are too large to be contained in sufficient quantities in the general multivitamin supplements on the market, we recommend taking 1000 mg of calcium and 500 mg of magnesium daily. Each of these minerals is available individually or may be purchased together in a single formulation. For your convenience, you may wish to purchase the combination calcium-magnesium products.

• The B Vitamins: More than Just Deficiency Fighters

The entire group of B vitamins is involved in maintaining a healthy brain-immune connection. The major B vitamins include thiamine (B_1), riboflavin (B_2), niacin (B_3), pyridoxine (B_6), cobalamin (B_{12}), folic acid, pantothenic acid, biotin, choline, and inositol.

The B vitamins work in chorus to promote brain and immune system health by protecting nerve tissue against oxidation, enhancing memory, and insulating nerve cells. Your body also requires B vitamins for producing many neurotransmitters. Choline and phosphatidylcholine, for example, are necessary for the brain's manufacture of acetylcholine, the memory neurotransmitter that runs short in Alzheimer's disease and other disorders.

Scientists have long recognized the symptoms of B vitamin deficiency. Some of those include many of the same symptoms associated with Alzheimer's and other dementias, such as memory loss, emotional instability, and reduced attention span.

For instance, recent studies have shown that the important neurotransmitters GABA and serotonin require adequate levels of vitamin B_6 to be properly synthesized by the brain's neurons.

The brain requires adequate thiamine from the diet to effectively use carbohydrates for energy production. In addition, dietary B_{12} and folic acid are both necessary to form myelin, the insulating substance that sheathes neurons and makes it possible for neurons to transmit messages.

Links between nutritional disorders and neurological clinical symptoms have also been well documented. A severe thiamine deficiency can result in hallucinations and memory disturbances, while a shortage of vitamin B_6 leads to irritability, depression, and seizures. A vitamin B_{12} deficiency can result in memory disturbances and impaired sensations.

We cannot overemphasize the importance of adequate B vitamin intake for a healthy nervous system and proper brain function. The best dietary sources include whole grain breads, cereals, pastas, and meat. We also suggest adding a complete B vitamin supplement to the diet instead of incorporating large doses of individual B vitamins.

RECOMMENDED DOSE FOR HEALTHY INDIVIDUALS: A daily supplement that provides 50 mg each of the entire family of B vitamins.

• Copper, Zinc, Manganese, and Selenium: Essential Micronutrients to Incorporate Into Your Diet

Four of the most important micronutrients that healthy individuals should consider adding as daily supplements are copper, zinc, manganese, and selenium.

The distribution of copper in the brain corresponds directly to the distribution of the neurons that synthesize dopamine and norepinephrine, for example. This makes sense, since the enzyme that serves as an essential ingredient for synthesizing those neurotransmitters is copper-dependent.

Zinc, an essential trace mineral found in protein-rich foods such as meat and whole grains, has a number of important effects on the brain. Among them are zinc's influence on neurotransmitter production and enzyme functioning. It is interesting to note that the brain's highest concentration of zinc is located in the hippocampus, the brain's memory center.

If children suffer a zinc deficiency, they may experience appetite disturbances and growth retardation. Zinc also plays a leading role in preventing brain damage in children exposed to lead at an early age.

A combination of zinc, copper, and manganese is essential in inducing the important cellular antioxidant, superoxidase dismutase (SOD). Like glutathione, SOD is responsible for protecting cells from free radical damage. It is important to note, however, that individuals with Parkinson's disease should avoid taking manganese supplements at all; we discuss this further in our chapter on that illness.

Finally, selenium has the ability to increase the production of glutathione, a key intracellular antioxidant enzyme system responsible for protecting all of the body's cells from free radical damage and detoxifying noxious agents from the body.

RECOMMENDED DOSES FOR HEALTHY INDIVIDUALS: Because these micronutrients are so essential to your health, we recommend adding supplements of each to your daily diet. Look for fully reacted mineral chelates for each of the minerals recommended below.

Copper   2 mg
Zinc   30 mg (adults); 15 mg (children 6–12)

Selenium   200 mcg (Do not exceed this amount.)
Manganese   2 mg (except for those with Parkinson's
            disease)

Each of these nutrients should be taken daily with a meal.

This is just a partial list of the many nutrients we now know are essential to maintaining an optimum brain-immune connection. We have outlined recommended food sources and dosages of all these nutrients in Table 1.

What's Next: Using Neuroimmunomodulators to Mend the Brain-Immune Connection

As you have seen, research conducted at major medical centers and universities around the world has shown that disturbances in the balance of our body's fatty acids and destruction of healthy brain cells by free radicals lie at the heart of disease.

Combining expert knowledge of these culprits with our new-found understanding of the power of nutrients to maintain and restore the brain-immune connection, we now turn our attention to the second step of our Brain Wellness Plan. This step relies on neuroimmunomodulators.

Informed clinicians from around the world are now recommending these nutrients as a means of preventing neurological illness, and are incorporating them into disease therapies designed to treat neurological illnesses.

When combined with advanced medical interventions, these nutritional and hormonal substances have the potential to restore the brain-immune connection. What's more, many are readily available in your local health food store or nutritional oriented pharmacy.

TABLE 1

GENERAL SUPPLEMENT HEALTH PROTOCOL:
A SUMMARY

Nutrient*	Recommended Daily Dose
Multiple vitamin-mineral	Follow label directions.
Chelated calcium	1000 mg, with a meal
Chelated magnesium	500 mg, with a meal
Advanced antioxidant formula	Look for an advanced formula and follow label instructions.

SOD Inducers
(May be obtained individually or found in a single product. Those with Parkinson's should avoid manganese.)

Copper	1 mg, with a meal
Zinc	10 mg, with a meal
Manganese	4 mg, with a meal
Selenium	200 mcg, with a meal (Do not exceed this amount.)

*With regard to all the minerals listed above, look for fully reacted mineral chelates for maximum absorption and utilization.

GENERAL GUT HEALTH PROTOCOL:
A SUMMARY

Nutrient	Recommended Daily Dose
Glutamine	1000 mg, away from food
Multiple strain friendly bacteria	Follow label directions
FOS	4 grams as directed on label
Nucleotides	1–2 grams, away from food
Barley grass/wheat grass	1–2 servings as directed

CHAPTER 4

THE BRAIN
WELLNESS PLAN

The revolution in neuroimmunomodulation combines studies from nutrition, neurology, and immunology to bring us incredible insights into just how food and supplements can positively influence brain and immune system health.

In this book, we have collected the latest research in designing a basic "Brain Wellness Plan" that serves as a preventive measure for healthy individuals.

Medical science has also demonstrated that certain neuroimmunomodulating agents are also therapeutic in treating neurological diseases. In Part II of the book, we will begin describing those agents disease-by-disease, devoting a chapter to each of the most common neurological ilnesses affecting Americans today.

For now, we will begin by describing the three foundations for brain health. These include: (1) anti-inflammatory compounds including key antioxidants, essential fatty acids, DHEA, and phosphatidylserine; (2) mitochondrial supporting agents, including acetyl-L-carnitine (ALC), coenzyme Q10, and creatine; and (3) compounds that restore proper neurotransmitter balance such as the natural substances Huperzine A, CDP choline, SAMe, and St. John's wort.

The First Foundation for Brain Health: Natural Anti-Inflammatories

The first foundation for brain health is to reduce excessive immune activity in the brain. It is now widely appreciated that aging, Alzheimer's disease, Parkinson's disease, multiple sclerosis, Lou Gehrig's disease, chronic fatigue syndrome, depression, and autism are intimately related to brain immune dysregulation. These detrimental effects are initiated and mediated by cortisol and free radicals, proinflammatory agents that wreak havoc on neurons and their mitochondria, in particular.

Antioxidants and Brain Health

As you will recall, with extra electrons available for donating, antioxidants can neutralize free radical attacks by satisfying the free radicals' quest for electrons. Antioxidants are especially important as we age, because they provide the best support against free radical damage to the body's time-weakened cellular structures and machinery.

During any challenge to your immune system—from disease, infections, toxic exposure, stress, or aging—you need extra antioxidants to help scavenge the free radicals naturally produced by the immune system's cells while combating those challenges.

As we discussed earlier, the brain's high fat content renders it especially vulnerable to free radicals, so the body has defined specific ways to protect brain cell fatty acids through special antioxidants. The special power of these antioxidants rests on their ability to cross the blood-brain barrier, the protective physical and chemical structure that surrounds the nervous system.

• Polyphenols and Brain Health

Antioxidants that fall into the polyphenol class (which includes bioflavonoids, the plant chemicals) demonstrate a wide variety of biochemical effects that can directly influence certain disease conditions. One of the primary effects polyphenols have on the body is their readiness for lipid peroxidation warfare:

They're always ready to pair up with a free radical and calm it down. In addition, polyphenols spring into action when it becomes necessary to detoxify the body's blood of certain metals, like iron, that may otherwise promote additional, risky, free radical activity if these metals' levels reach the danger mark.

Finally, polyphenols have a keen knack for slowing down the production of lipo-oxygenase, an enzyme that can turn up the heat under the body's inflammatory and allergic responses.

One interesting polyphenol, epigallocatechingallate, is readily available through drinking green tea. This compound has been studied by the American Health Foundation, which found it to be significantly better at inhibiting deadly peroxynitrite reactions than either vitamin C or glutathione.

Our own food supply is filled with polyphenols. Excellent dietary sources include red wine, green tea, berries and other fruits, soybeans, and brightly colored vegetables. The best supplements include fruit polyphenols; grape seed extract; pine bark extract; Pycnogenol® (a special form of pine bark extract that contains a mixture of important polyphenolic components); and herbs like bilberry, *Ginkgo biloba*, and milk thistle.

RECOMMENDED DOSE FOR HEALTHY INDIVIDUALS: 120 mg daily of either Pycnogenol®, fruit polyphenols or grape seed extract, or the same amount of a supplement that combines at least two into a single formula. Take these supplements with a meal.

•Vitamin E and Brain Health

One of the best-known antioxidants, vitamin E (tocopherol) is widely considered one of the most important fat-soluble antioxidants to date. The rest of the vitamin E story—which measures the chemical relatives of tocopherols called tocotrienols—is only now beginning to unfold.

The tocotrienols, which are found predominantly in rice, bran, and rice or barley oil, possess a unique chemical makeup that allows them to act as efficient free radical hunters by penetrating fatty acids effectively. Tocotrienols prevent oxidative damage of the fatty tissues that make up the brain.

RECOMMENDED DOSE FOR HEALTHY INDIVIDUALS: Since tocotrienols may prove to be better antioxidants than tocopherols, we suggest adding 50 mg of tocotrienols to your daily nutritional program. Additionally, we recommend taking 400 IUs of tocopherols. Take these fat-soluble supplements with a meal.

• Ginkgo biloba *and Brain Health*

The leaves of the ginkgo tree contain a number of important constituents. Researchers examining just how *Ginkgo biloba* extract enhances our physiological functions have discovered that this natural compound has a number of wonderful properties. For example, it can:

- Open the blood flow of arteries, veins, and capillaries.
- Inhibit monoamine oxidase, the enzyme that breaks down certain neurotransmitters in the brain.
- Decrease the clumping of blood in vessels.
- Increase cellular glucose uptake by hungry cells.
- Act as a powerful antioxidant, protecting against lipid peroxidation and enhancing SOD activity.

In clinical trials of *Ginkgo biloba,* patients with a variety of disorders have experienced better health, including improved blood flow, reduced dizziness, improved memory, and fewer headaches and depressive episodes. Thus, as you will see in the chapters that follow, *Ginkgo biloba* extract is an essential ingredient in nutritional protocols for treating a variety of brain disorders.

RECOMMENDED DOSE FOR HEALTHY INDIVIDUALS: 60 mg daily of standardized *Ginkgo biloba* extract, taken with a meal. **Note:** In order to provide a reliable and consistent dose of the active constituents found in this natural substance, purchase only a standardized *Ginkgo biloba* extract.

• *Essential Fatty Acids as Anti-inflammatories in Brain Health*

Omega-3 fatty acids are essential fatty acids derived from either cold-water fish or plant sources. Cold-water fish (like fatty tuna, mackerel, and salmon) contain the essential fatty acids EPA (eico-sapentaenoic acid) and DHA (docosahexanoic acid). Flaxseed oil, derived from the flax plant, contains another omega-3 fatty acid called linoleic acid.

Omega-3 fatty acids are important ingredients for your body's production of prostaglandins, some of which serve to tone down immune response and, therefore, combat inflammation. Additionally, the important omega-3 fatty acid DHA contributes to building up central nervous system lipids, discouraging the formation of certain prostaglandins capable of triggering inflammatory processes, and is essential to good communication between nerve cells.

Therefore, omega-3 fatty acids are natural anti-inflammatories because of their ability to reduce the potentially harmful effects of arachidonic acid and to decrease our pro-inflammatory prostaglandins.

Omega-3 fatty acids have been best studied in bipolar or "manic" depression. In this disorder, patients experience extreme mood swings characterized by either intensely depressed moods or mania (overexcitement). Omega-3 fatty acids may benefit these patients by preventing excessive stimulation or excitement of these cells, as well as stabilizing brain cell membranes. Omega-3 fatty acids also appear to protect the myelin sheaths in multiple sclerosis patients.

RECOMMENDED DOSES FOR HEALTHY INDIVIDUALS:
- DHA: 300 mg with a meal.
- Flaxseed oil: 1 tbsp with a meal.
- Primrose or borage oil: 2 g with a meal.

•DHEA as an Anti-inflammatory in Brain Health

A steroid naturally produced by both your brain and adrenal glands, DHEA (dehydroepiandrosterone) serves several important functions in the brain. For one thing, DHEA is essential for nurturing the growth and function of neuron dendrites, the tiny branching fibers that help brain cells stay in touch with one another and keep your brain's communication network in healthy working order.

Your DHEA level peaks at adolescence and steadily declines as you age. However, you need DHEA just as much, or more, as time passes: DHEA protects you from the damaging effect of hormones produced by your body during times of stress—most notably, from the cortisol hormone. DHEA actually buffers cells against the effects of overzealous cortisol activity, and partially regulates cortisol production.

As you may recall from an earlier chapter, cortisol is a hormone produced during stress that is currently under close scrutiny for its relationship to such diverse neurological diseases as depression and Alzheimer's. Investigators have determined that, when excess cortisol is produced as a result of stress, those high levels of cortisol can cause higher levels of free radicals and thus damage to healthy brain cells, particularly in regions of the brain responsible for memory and learning.

Additionally, human studies testing the effects of DHEA on the immune system have revealed that DHEA can normalize potentially dangerous cytokine levels. DHEA may prove especially beneficial in controlling the cytokine interleukin-6, which is linked to Alzheimer's.

RECOMMENDED DOSE FOR HEALTHY INDIVIDUALS: People interested in adding a DHEA supplement should check with their health care practitioners about the appropriate use and dosage of DHEA for their individual needs.

• Phosphatidylserine (PS) in Brain Health

Another naturally occurring fatty acid in the brain and in all cell membranes, phosphatidylserine (PS) has proved to be a safe, potentially effective therapeutic agent in treating memory deficit disorders such as Alzheimer's disease.

PS enhances enzymes involved in monitoring neurotransmitter production and release. It also increases the brain's energy efficiency because it enhances the brain's ability to metabolize glucose.

Furthermore, PS and DHA can modulate the fluidity of cell membranes—an essential feature if cells are going to "speak" to one another by sending chemical messengers back and forth. PS also increases communication between cells by increasing the number of membrane receptor sites for receiving messages.

As you will see in later chapters, scientific studies have demonstrated that PS supplements can increase the output of acetylcholine, the neurotransmitter so important to memory, and so may enhance the quality of life among Alzheimer's patients. This remarkable substance also has the potential to stimulate the brain to produce dopamine.

Clinical trials with elderly patients suffering memory deficit disorders have shown that adding PS to the daily diet improved the ability of these patients to think and decreased behavioral disturbances. In other studies, PS also improved the performance of patients with age-associated memory impairment, a disorder affecting millions of Americans each year.

Because PS is such an important neuroimmunomodulator, you will find its therapeutic use—and studies supporting that use—related to a number of disorders described throughout this book.

> **RECOMMENDED DOSE FOR HEALTHY INDIVIDUALS:** 100 mg of PS daily with a meal. Look for the trademarked Leci-PS™ from Lucas Meyer on the label of your favorite PS supplement manufacturer.
>
> In addition, take 100 mg daily of DHA, with a meal. Look for the trademarked Neuromins™ from Martek Biosciences Corporation on the label of your favorite DHA supplement manufacturer.

The Second Foundation for Brain Health: Supporting Mitochondria

Mitochondria are vital for all cells. By manufacturing ATP, they provide the biological energy required to drive all enzymatic processes. Conversely, decreased mitochondrial function results in decreased ATP and, ultimately, cell death. Mitochondrial supportive agents include acetyl-L-carnitine (ALC), coenzyme Q10, and creatine. Additionally, D-ribose is emerging as an important player in increasing cellular ATP. Further studies are needed to determine its role in the brain.

• Acetyl-L-Carnitine (ALC) and Brain Health

Of all the amino acids, acetyl-L-carnitine (ALC) has been the one to receive most of the rave reviews for its essential role in transport and delivery of fatty acids into the cell. Once inside the cell membrane, fatty acids can then be used for energy metabolism and structural repair.

ALC is naturally found in meat and milk, and has demonstrated impressive success in protecting the brain from the ravages of aging. Currently, ALC is one of the most important natural substances under scientific scrutiny for its potential clinical applications in memory deficit disorders and maintaining memory in healthy individuals.

In human studies, ALC has been used over the last decade to treat Alzheimer's, with favorable results, and many studies document ALC's role in building up memory and the ability to perform problem-solving tasks.

While you must have an adequate intake of all the essential amino acids—and this is easily accomplished by consuming sufficient quantities of protein—later on in the book, we will talk about manipulating the intake of individual amino acids in relation to treating specific brain diseases.

RECOMMENDED DOSE FOR HEALTHY INDIVIDUALS: 500 mg daily, on an empty stomach.

• Coenzyme Q10 and Brain Health

Found in cell mitochondria, the antioxidant coenzyme Q10 plays a major role in cellular energy production. As you will learn in later chapters on Parkinson's disease and chronic fatigue syndrome, the mitochondria are organisms within all cells responsible for energy production, and they are particularly vulnerable to free radical damage. Coenzyme Q10 is essential in defending them, because it is one of the few antioxidants that can actually penetrate mitochondria and provide a defense against the mito-chondrial membrane.

RECOMMENDED DOSE FOR HEALTHY INDIVIDUALS: 120 mg daily, taken with a meal.

• Creatine and Brain Health

Creatine is an amino acid that is vital for the health of the mitochondria. Creatine increases the production of mitochondrial ATP. It also prevents free radical damage to mitochondria, and has proven beneficial in animal models of neurodegenerative disease in which mitochondrial dysfunction is a key aspect.

RECOMMENDED DOSE FOR HEALTHY INDIVIDUALS: 1g daily.

The Third Foundation of Brain Health: Helping to Restore Neurotransmitter Imbalances

Neurotransmitter imbalances are associated with Alzheimer's disease, Parkinson's disease, depression, and autism. In Alzheimer's disease, we know that too little of the neurotransmitter acetylcholine results in cognitive decline. In Parkinson's disease, too little dopamine is produced, leading to balance defects. In depression and autism, serotonin is clearly implicated.

• Increase Acetylcholine Levels

Low levels of acetylcholine, the memory neurotransmitter, are recognized as contributing to Alzheimer's disease and other forms of dementia. Studies show, however, that when acetylcholine levels increase, memory and other cognitive functions improve. Two natural substances that boost acetylcholine levels are Huperzine A, which blocks the breakdown of acetylcholine, and CDP choline, which stimulates the production of acetylcholine.

Huperzine A and Brain Health Huperzine A, a powerful extract from a rare type of Chinese moss, has been used in traditional Chinese medicine for patients with memory impairment for hundreds of years. Recently, the molecular structure and action of Huperzine A has been discovered, and we've learned that it blocks an enzyme, acetylcholinesterase, that degrades acetylcholine. By inhibiting the acetylcholine enzyme, Huperzine A allows acetylcholine levels in the brain to increase and it thereby enhances memory and cognitive function. Huperzine A has also been shown to protect brain cells from premature cell death.

RECOMMENDED DOSE FOR HEALTHY INDIVIDUALS: 50–200 mcg daily.

CDP Choline and Brain Health CDP choline stimulates the production of the neurotransmitter acetylcholine. Additionally, CDP choline is crucial to the synthesis of phosphatidylcholine, a compound that protects the integrity of brain cell membranes, assisting in cell membrane function and repair. Our brain cell membranes become increasingly fragile as we age (and in neurodegenerative diseases like Alzheimer's disease), and phosphatidylcholine is a phospholipid essential for the integrity of our brain cell membranes.

RECOMMENDED DOSE FOR HEALTHY INDIVIDUALS: 1–2 g daily.

• Increase Dopamine

To increase dopamine, it's important to employ certain amino acids like tyrosine and phenylalanine as well as SAMe (discussed below); additionally, certain dopamine agonist drugs may be more beneficial here than are the natural substances currently available.

• Raise Serotonin Levels

Decreased levels of the neurotransmitter serotonin are implicated in both depression and autism. Furthermore, it's been shown that raising serotonin levels in these two conditions is correlated with a diminution of symptoms. Maintaining healthy levels of serotonin, then, can certainly contribute significantly to brain health (although greatly increased levels of this neurotransmitter can cause potentially serious side effects, which is why prescription drugs that increase serotonin levels should never be taken simultaneously with herbs that do the same). Two natural substances that appear to increase serotonin levels (among their other actions, including increasing levels of other neurotransmitters like acetylcholine and norepinephrine) are St. John's wort and SAMe (s-adenosyl methionine).

SAMe and Brain Health S-adenosyl methionine, or SAMe, occurs naturally in every one of your body's cells. Basically, SAMe is a member of the body's cleanup crew, serving to detoxify cell membranes and synthesize neurotransmitters. SAMe also has beneficial effects on serotonin and norepinephrine, the major neurotransmitters that control mood. By increasing the ability of enzymes to synthesize serotonin and norepinephrine, SAMe acts as a natural antidepressant without the side effects of prescription antidepressants currently on the market.

In addition, SAMe is one of the principal mediators in the formation of glutathione, the major cellular antioxidant. Depletion of glutathione is associated with aging and several neurological diseases. Because of its ability to raise intracellular glutathione levels, SAMe is effective in treating liver disease and other conditions associated with chronic inflammation.

Investigators have discovered that adding SAMe to the diet of aging rats increases the number of acetylcholine receptor sites in the memory centers of those rat brains. Treating aging rats with SAMe also increases the strength and fluidity of cell membranes—that is, how easily crucial nutrients can move into cells and waste can exit.

RECOMMENDED DOSE FOR HEALTHY INDIVIDUALS: 200 mg daily, taken with a meal.

St. John's Wort and Brain Health St. John's wort has been used in European folk medicine for centuries. Extracts of St. John's wort are now widely used for the treatment of depression in Germany, where it is one of the most widely prescribed antidepressants. The mechanism of St. John's wort in depression is not entirely clear, but may be similar to different classes of antidepressants.

Some researchers have suggested that St. John's wort acts like antidepressants called "monoamine oxidase inhibitors." Other researchers speculate that St. John's wort may act similarly to the antidepressants known as selective serotonin reuptake inhibitors (SSRIs). SSRIs such as Prozac and Zoloft block the inactivation of serotonin, so that increased amounts of this neurotransmitter remain in the brain and exert a prolonged effect.

RECOMMENDED DOSE FOR MILD CASES OF DEPRESSION: 240 mg of the standardized extract daily.

Conclusion

While ongoing animal and human studies continue to bring us new insights into the mechanisms by which nutrients and foods influence the brain–immune system connection, research in the emerging field of nutrition science has finally reached the patient bedside.

Today, we have the hard science to back up many theories in "alternative" medicine that were once considered nothing more than old wives' tales or folklore by mainstream physicians and many patients. Just as there are nutrients that promote optimal health, we know with certainty that it is possible to use these neuroimmunomodulators as aggressive nutritional interventions in combination with mainstream medical and hormonal therapies to address specific illnesses.

As prevention becomes the focus of our evolving health care system, we can expect to continue refining nutritional protocols to maintain normal brain and immune system function in both healthy and compromised patients.

TABLE **2**

SUPPLEMENTS FOR OPTIMAL BRAIN HEALTH

Strategy/Nutrient	*Recommended Daily Dose*
Decrease Inflammation	
Antioxidants	
Polyphenols (Pycnogenol®)	120 mg
Vitamin E	400 IU
Ginkgo biloba	60 mg
DHA (essential fatty acid)	100 mg
DHEA	Consult your physician.
Phosphatidylserine	100 mg
Support Mitochondrial Action	
ALC	500 mg
Coenzyme Q10	120 mg
Creatine	1 g
Balance Neurotransmitter Levels	
Huperzine A	50–200 mcg
CDP choline	1–2 g
SAMe	200 mg
St. John's wort	Up to 240 mg daily as recommended by your health care practitioner.

Treating Neurological Illnesses with Breakthrough Medical, Nutritional, and Immune-Boosting Therapies

CHAPTER 5

ALZHEIMER'S DISEASE

After her official retirement, Joan stayed on as a part time consultant in the hospital public relations office where she had worked for over three decades. She enjoyed her job, and the extra money always came in handy. Besides, at sixty-nine she was still in good health and couldn't see the point of wasting all her time in the garden.

Gradually, though, she began to have trouble at work. At first it was the little things: She'd misfile a project, or forget the name of someone she knew in the next office. And one day she forgot her way to the cafeteria, where she'd been having lunch nearly every day since joining the staff.

Her coworkers began to tease her about being so forgetful. Joan made jokes right along with them, but she really wanted to cry. Wait until they got old and forgot things. They'd see how much fun it was.

Finally, one day Joan's supervisor suggested that perhaps it was time she took that retirement after all, and things seemed to go gradually downhill from there.

Joan's daughter brought her to the family doctor, but he dismissed her complaints as symptoms of the normal aging process.

A year went by, and things didn't get any better. Joan had difficulty sleeping, fumbled over routine daily tasks, and was hesitant about driving. She had to look at the daily newspaper to remember the date and kept forgetting the way to the supermarket. Worse still, she accused everyone in her family of hiding things in her house so she couldn't find them, and was so argumentative these days that her grandchildren grumbled about having to go there for Sunday dinners.

However, it wasn't until Joan took a walk one winter afternoon, wearing her best summer dress on a snowy day, that her family finally believed something was seriously wrong.

Alzheimer's Disease: An Overview

Like more than 4 million Americans, Joan suffers from the beginning stages of Alzheimer's disease, the key cause of dementia among people over sixty-five.

The word "dementia" literally means "deprived of mind," and the primary effects of any dementia are cognitive. Over time, those with Alzheimer's experience a progressive loss of mental faculties, beginning with memory, learning, attention, and judgment—in short, all the activities that make us human.

While the symptoms of Alzheimer's in its early stages can mimic depression, psychosis, and various mental illnesses—sometimes causing physicians to make an erroneous early diagnosis—Alzheimer's is in fact a physical disorder whose symptoms are caused by the death and destruction of neurons in very specific areas of the brain.

People who have had Alzheimer's include many whose names you easily recognize, such as the illustrator Norman Rockwell, actress Rita Hayworth, essayist E. B. White, President Ronald Reagan, and film director Otto Preminger. For each of them, as for the people you know with Alzheimer's, the disease came at a devastating cost.

Without effective treatment, most people with Alzheimer's eventually become incapacitated. Experts estimate that about half of the nation's more than 1.3 million nursing home residents today may have Alzheimer's. More than 10 percent of people over sixty-five, and fully half of us who reach eighty-five, will suffer from the disease.

In fact, since being recognized early in the twentieth century as a distinct illness, Alzheimer's is being touted by some health care professionals as "the disease of the century," because we can expect to find a growing number of Alzheimer's patients in our population.

The reason is simple: Alzheimer's patients are predominantly over sixty-five years old, and Americans are living longer than ever before. People over eighty-five now make up the fastest-growing age group in the United States, and the Census Bureau predicted that 5.1 million Americans would be over eighty-five by the year 2000, compared to just 2.5 million in that category in 1982. By the year 2034, we can expect to see three times as many people with Alzheimer's disease as we find in our population today.

About seven out of every ten Alzheimer's patients live with their families, and the emotional, physical, and financial burdens those families suffer are enormous.

The caretakers of Alzheimer's patients are often the hidden victims of the disease. Besides watching the people they love become increasingly forgetful, confused, and unable to function on their own, family members of Alzheimer's patients face the painful task of deciding how to care for their loved ones over the long term. Whether an Alzheimer's patient lives at home or in a nursing home, the cost can reach upward of $47,000 annually—an enormous economic burden to both family and society.

Though we have no cure as yet for Alzheimer's, we have come a long way in understanding some of its possible causes, the abnormalities in the brain underlying the symptoms of Alzheimer's, and ways to slow its progression.

From onset of symptoms to diagnosis, from treatment to hope on the horizon, in this chapter we will discuss Alzheimer's disease in the context of some of the most exciting—and effective—hormonal and nutritional therapies available today. These therapies truly do offer hope to Alzheimer's patients and their families, alleviating disease symptoms by treating chemical imbalances in the brain-immune connection.

The focus of the nutritional therapy we describe here is directed at:

1. Improving memory, language, reasoning, and judgment by providing supplementary compounds that assist with the synthesis and release of neurotransmitters.
2. Reducing the production of cellular toxins in the brain brought on by inadvertent or excessive activation of the immune system.
3. Slowing or stopping oxidative damage to cells.

In addition to discussing medical interventions, we will offer you a guideline for a rigorous, progressive treatment plan which includes medical therapies, hormonal interventions, standardized herb extracts, and vitamins.

As with any therapeutic approach, this multifaceted treatment strategy is most successful when instituted in the early stages of the disease. Additionally, we urge anyone with a family history of Alzheimer's to participate in this diet and supplement program as a preventive measure.

What Goes Wrong in Alzheimer's, and Why

Almost everything we know about Alzheimer's has come from examining the brains of patients who died of the disease and generously donated their organs to science. Looking at one of these brains provides a visual clue to the biology of the disease: the sulci, or valleys between the brain tissue that give the brain its wrinkled appearance, are distinctly wider in the brain of a person with Alzheimer's than they are in healthy brains.

Alzheimer's was first discovered in 1906 by Alois Alzheimer, who observed unusual changes in the brain of a woman who died at age fifty-five, five years after developing dementia. Using special silver stains to more clearly reveal the structure of this woman's brain cells, Alzheimer discovered that the cerebral cortex—the seat of our intellectual functions—contained abnormal nerve cells with tangled fibers and clusters of degenerating nerve endings.

In Alzheimer's disease, the intricate process of communication between nerve cells is derailed owing to loss of connections between nerve cells brought on by neuron dysfunction and the death of neurons. The disease primarily strikes the hippocampus, a structure deep in the brain that is involved with cognition and memory.

1. *A New Gene Provides Clues*

Genes are biologic units located on chromosomes, structures in the nucleus of each cell. Genes transmit hereditary information using the molecule DNA (deoxyribonucleic acid). We now know that even the slightest alterations in the DNA code can produce a faulty protein—and those faulty proteins can lead to cellular weakening or breakdown.

Today's Alzheimer's researchers have linked one gene alteration in particular to the neuron dysfunction leading to Alzheimer's. It involves the apolipoprotein-E, or ApoE, gene, which helps transport cholesterol through the human body and form healthy cellular membranes for the brain's neurons. We all have ApoE, but whether we are susceptible to Alzheimer's or not largely depends on which version of this gene we inherited from our parents: ApoE2, ApoE3, or ApoE4.

Genetic research reveals that people who inherit the gene which encodes for ApoE4 have the highest chance of getting Alzheimer's.

Recently, for example, researchers at the Duke University General Clinical Research Center and the Joseph and Kathleen Bryan Alzheimer's Disease Research Center in Durham, North Carolina, collaborated on studies linking the ApoE4 gene and Alzheimer's. They discovered that the risk for Alzheimer's for people with copies of the ApoE4 gene from both parents is *three times greater* than that for other people.

Meanwhile, scientists at the Mayo Clinic in Rochester, Minnesota, chose to follow a group of older patients who suffered mild memory impairment. They found that over two-thirds of the patients who developed clinical dementia had a copy of the gene for ApoE4, and concluded that the presence of ApoE4 was the best predictor for Alzheimer's.

2. *Faulty ApoE Genes Impair Healthy Cell Membranes*

Just why is a defective ApoE gene linked to Alzheimer's?

Recent studies at the McGill Center for Studies in Aging in Quebec, Canada, suggest that the ApoE gene plays a central role in how effectively the brain's hippocampus responds to injury, particularly when it comes to regulating the transport of the cholesterol and phospholipids so crucial to building strong neuron membranes.

Although we have not yet pinpointed every step of the Alzheimer's pathology, we do know that people who inherit a certain mutation of the ApoE gene are, in effect, getting a faulty version of this otherwise helpful protein. They are therefore missing out on the building blocks of fat so essential to building up healthy cell membranes.

3. *Protein Plaques Form on the Brain*

In Alzheimer's patients, researchers have discovered plaques, or patches of dead cells and other castoff material, lying outside the brain's neurons. Most of these plaques are located in the areas of the brain associated with memory.

At the core of each of these plaques is a potentially deadly substance called beta amyloid, an abnormal protein not usually found in the brain.

Beta amyloid is a protein chopped off from a larger parent molecule known as amyloid precursor protein, or APP, during regular cellular metabolism.

Recently, scientists have reported finding a specific enzyme, known as beta secretase, which is responsible for generating beta amyloid from its parent molecule, amyloid precursor protein, or APP. This is an exciting finding because specific drugs or nutrients can now be identified that inhibit the effects of beta secretase, and thereby can also prevent the deposition of amyloid in Alzheimer's brains.

In a recent paper published in *The New England Journal of*

Medicine, Harvard Medical School researchers explain that APP is normally inserted partially into the membrane, and then the protruding part is cleaved, releasing a soluble form of the precursor protein. That way, an intact beta amyloid peptide is not normally generated. Production of the beta amyloid peptide in the aging brain, or in the brain affected by Alzheimer's, requires a change in the normal processing of APP which, in turn, results in abnormally high levels of beta amyloid.

How do increased levels of the beta amyloid protein contribute to the cascade of steps ultimately resulting in neuron death?

Investigators believe that neurons in the hippocampus die when beta amyloid is added, leading to the hypothesis that this protein is toxic to neurons when freed from its parent substance. In other words, beta amyloid breaks into pieces and sends out free radicals, the unstable molecules that can do the body so much damage.

In summary, then, people who inherit the defective ApoE4 gene have neurons that are inherently less structurally sound and may die more easily. This cell death sets off an immune response characterized by an increased production of fighter white blood cells and their chemical clearing tools to remove castoff fragments of dead or dying nerve cells at the site of injury.

In patients with Alzheimer's, beta amyloid may be viewed by the body as a toxic invader initially responsible for killing off mature neurons and causing further damage to neuron cell membranes. The immune system responds to the accumulation of damage accordingly.

As the plaques form, the immune system's messengers, the cytokines, amplify the body's response. In particular, the immune system calls upon a cytokine known as interleukin-6, which has the power to cleave APP, the amyloid precursor protein, thus releasing beta amyloid and damaging vulnerable neurons.

If, indeed, it is true that the neurons of Alzheimer's patients are being killed off as a direct consequence of beta amyloid, new research efforts will focus on developing certain drugs which may act as amyloid protease inhibitors. We hope someday to develop therapies that successfully block the production of this toxic protein and thus alleviate the symptoms of Alzheimer's.

TABLE 3

WHAT CAUSES ALZHEIMER'S?

- A defective apolipoprotein-E gene (ApoE4) is inherited.

- This defective gene causes ineffective synthesis of cell membranes responsible for protecting the brain's neurons from injury.

- An inadvertent, overzealous immune system response occurs owing to faulty cell membranes.

- The immune system messenger cytokine, interleukin-6, is overproduced.

- Increased levels of interleukin-6 stimulate beta amyloid to break off from its parent molecule, amyloid precursor protein (APP).

- Beta secretase, a protein, stimulates beta amyloid to break off from its parent molecule, amyloid precursor protein.

- Beta amyloid causes free radical injury to cells, promoting neuron death in the area of the brain responsible for producing acetylcholine, a neurotransmitter essential for memory and cognition.

4. *The Brain's Ability to Produce Acetylcholine Is Impaired*

Ultimately, then, the brain's neurons die off in Alzheimer's disease owing to the effects of beta amyloid and free radicals. The brain region of greatest injury appears to be in the hippocampus's nucleus basalis of Mynert, the brain's central processing plant for the neurotransmitter acetylcholine.

Acetylcholine is the chemical essential for communication between neurons responsible for memory and cognitive thinking. When acetylcholine levels fall dramatically, we see the memory loss and faulty reasoning that are hallmark symptoms of Alzheimer's.

What About Environmental Suspects in Alzheimer's?

Although researchers have studied a number of environmental suspects as causal factors in Alzheimer's disease—particularly zinc and aluminum—the scientific community is still debating the effects of these elements. While zinc is an essential mineral that plays numerous roles in health and disease, it may be negatively associated with Alzheimer's disease.

The theory that using aluminum cookware or drinking water treated with aluminum may be a risk factor dates back to the 1970s, when scientists first discovered traces of aluminum and iron in the brain plaques of people with Alzheimer's. Subsequent studies since then have produced conflicting results, however.

While researchers at the Mount Sinai School of Medicine's Department of Pathology were able to use atomic absorption spectrometry to show that the diseased brain tissue of certain Alzheimer's patients had a two- to three-fold increase in aluminum, others have demonstrated that groups of people exposed to unnaturally high levels of aluminum show no increased risk of Alzheimer's.

Nevertheless, aluminum is a neurotoxin that can impair cognition, and has been found to interfere with more than fifty neurochemical reactions. Because of this, and because brain aluminum levels are increased in patients with Alzheimer's, it would be sensible to avoid as much aluminum as possible. From aluminum cookware to aluminum-based deodorants and antacids, we encourage you to read labels and make educated choices.

Zinc has also been linked to Alzheimer's in controversial ways. Some scientists suggest that too little zinc is at fault, while others hypothesize that too much zinc can contribute to neuron death by causing soluble beta amyloid from the cerebrospinal fluid to form clumps similar to Alzheimer's plaques. There are other studies that do link a zinc deficiency with the symptoms of Alzheimer's.

In short then, we can say this: The jury is still out on the link between aluminum and zinc levels and Alzheimer's disease. We can expect investigations to continue in both of those areas in the decade to come.

A Combined Medical and Nutritional Approach to Alzheimer's Disease

Slowing the progression of Alzheimer's disease is dependent on saving the brain's acetylcholine-producing neurons from untimely deterioration and death and boosting both memory and cognitive function to improve quality of life.

Here, we describe a complete nutritional, hormonal, and medical protocol for aggressively treating patients with Alzheimer's. This protocol includes the latest recommendations for incorporating neuroimmunomodulators into your therapy.

When Should You Suspect Alzheimer's?

Both for those afflicted with the disease and for the people who care for them, Alzheimer's is one of the most heartbreaking diseases known to mankind. When untreated, the disease eventually impairs all aspects of thought, feeling, and behavior, and carries a sentence of eventual mental emptiness imposed anywhere from ten months to ten years after onset.

Not all symptoms are present consistently or concurrently. While a cardinal feature of Alzheimer's disease is memory loss, early symptoms may also include changes in personality, speech difficulty, and errors in perception and judgment.

Initially, Alzheimer's victims may become withdrawn or lose interest in activities they used to enjoy—leading some family members and physicians to believe the person is suffering from clinical depression. Indeed, the two diseases have a strong association, which we will discuss later.

Additionally, Alzheimer's patients may have trouble recalling recently acquired information, while their long-term memories remain preserved. Misplacing objects and missing appointments are two cues for this stage of the disease.

People with Alzheimer's may exhibit paranoid behavior as the disease progresses. For example, a husband might accuse his wife of cheating on him, or a grandmother who lives alone might believe someone is sneaking into her house and rearranging things. Typically, the person you know with Alzheimer's will also have sleep disturbances, waking up in the middle of the night to get dressed and carry out activities as if it were daytime.

In later stages of Alzheimer's, language difficulties may become insurmountable, beginning with difficulty in recalling the names of objects or family members, and progressing to the point where people with Alzheimer's produce completely meaningless sentences.

In advanced stages of Alzheimer's, patients may become completely bedridden, regressed, and unable to perform even life's most basic tasks, such as getting dressed or feeding themselves.

Diagnosing Alzheimer's: Seeing Behind the Masks

As with most diseases, the earlier Alzheimer's is diagnosed, the better our chances are of using aggressive therapies to slow its progress.

Because Alzheimer's mimics so many other disorders, the disease can wear many masks. It's crucial to see behind those masks in order to make a correct diagnosis. There is no single laboratory test we can perform to diagnose the disease.

We stress that anyone who suspects Alzheimer's in themselves or in a loved one because of the symptoms described above should see a qualified neurologist to rule out other common—and often treatable—causes of similar symptoms.

Some of the other disorders that may masquerade as Alzheimer's include:

Ministrokes The second most common cause of dementia, multi-infarct dementia, is a consequence of brain damage caused by a series of small strokes or injuries to blood vessels in the brain. Ministrokes are different from Alzheimer's in that the damage is localized to one side of the body and the dementia progresses in rapid steps, rather than along the steady ramp of decline experienced by those with Alzheimer's. Ministrokes can be detected by a CAT scan or MRI scan of the brain.

Visual and Hearing Impairment Because elderly patients are particularly vulnerable to declining sensory function, it's important to rule this out as a cause for your loved one's perceptual errors. Adequate hearing and visual evaluations can determine whether the person simply needs corrective lenses or a hearing aid to improve function.

Depression We will discuss the etiology of clinical depression later in this book. Here, it is important to note that depression is often referred to as "pseudodementia" because mood changes can significantly affect how a person behaves. Depression can produce poor concentration, withdrawn behavior, and forgetfulness—all of which can be addressed through nutritional therapies and antidepressants.

Drug Use As older people are often being treated with pharmacological compounds for other illnesses or injuries, it's important to rule out possible side effects of drug use before arriving at an Alzheimer's diagnosis. Compounds which most easily cause Alzheimer's-like symptoms include minor tranquilizers, certain heart drugs, and substances known as anticholinergics, all of which may cause memory problems. (**Note:** Never discontinue any medication on your own without consulting your physician.)

Vitamins B_{12} and B_1 Deficiency As we noted in earlier chapters, vitamin deficiencies have been the culprits for many a disease. We now have virtually indisputable evidence that all of the B vitamins play critical roles in brain health, but we place an added value on the benefits of thiamine (B_1) and cobalamin (B_{12}).

For people with Alzheimer's, it is essential that a vitamin B deficiency be ruled out, as many symptoms of a vitamin B deficiency mimic Alzheimer's symptoms—yet are readily treated by increasing the individual's intake of B vitamins.

In addition, there may be a relationship between Alzheimer's and vitamin B deficiency as well. Several studies, for example, have pointed to low levels of vitamin B_{12} in the cerebrospinal fluid of Alzheimer's patients. In 1990, researchers from the Yamaguchi University School of Medicine in Japan found that patients with Alzheimer's disease had significantly lower cerebrospinal fluid vitamin B_{12} levels than patients suffering multi-infarct dementia.

Researchers in various medical centers have discovered that

patients with Alzheimer's have significantly lower plasma thiamine levels than control patients. In addition, the improper metabolism of thiamine in Alzheimer's patients may result in a deficiency of the important thiamine diphosphate molecule in the brain, impairing the ability to think. In one study reported in the *Annals of Neurology,* Alzheimer's patients treated with thiamine improved their cognitive abilities.

Unfortunately, many times test results show vitamin B levels which would not automatically arouse suspicion of a deficiency. Adequate blood levels of nutrients very often do not reflect tissue stores. It is necessary to run additional tests to diagnose the problem. One specific type of blood test, known as a measurement of homocysteine, may be a much more sensitive index of subclinical B_{12} deficiency.

Sleep Disorder One of the most common but frequently overlooked contributors to memory disorder in the elderly is the fact that some people have a great deal of trouble sleeping as they age. One condition, known as sleep apnea, is associated with forgetfulness, high blood pressure, and falling asleep at odd times during the day. Sleep apnea can contribute to both dementia and hypertension. One clue to its appearance is snoring at night.

The Three R's of Managing Alzheimer's Disease: Reduce Inflammation, Raise Mitochondrial Action, and Regenerate Neurons and Neurotransmitter Levels

Once your neurologist has determined that you or your loved one is suffering from Alzheimer's, there are a number of nutritional supplements you can immediately—and safely—incorporate into your diet.

The focus of nutritional therapy for Alzheimer's patients is on improving memory, language, reasoning, and judgment by assisting with the synthesis and release of neurotransmitters, increasing blood flow, reducing the production of amyloid via interleukin-6, and slowing or stopping the progression of oxidative damage to the brain.

These goals may be accomplished through nutritional therapy in combination with medical and hormonal interventions. The nutritional therapy includes supplements, standardized herb extracts, and hormone balancing.

The nutritional compounds we have found to be of the most benefit in slowing or even halting the progress of Alzheimer's are vitamin E, ALC (acetyl-L-carnitine), PS, DHA, and Huperzine A.

Additionally, we recommend that patients consider taking antioxidants and *Ginkgo biloba* supplements. All these agents are under examination for their potential as neuroimmunomodulators, and show promise in alleviating the symptoms of memory loss and problems in cognitive thinking, thus improving the quality of life for Alzheimer's patients.

All of these nutritional agents are readily available by themselves—and are safe to take over the counter in the dosages recommended below. These compounds show no evidence of interacting with other medications in any negative way.

One more compound, CDP choline, is currently being examined worldwide for its potential neuroimmunomodulating benefits in treating Alzheimer's, and may become available by prescription in the United States pending further studies.

Anti-inflammatory Therapies and Alzheimer's Disease

• *Rationale for Use of Anti-inflammatory Therapies in Alzheimer's*

An emerging strategy for reducing inflammation in Alzheimer's disease is to inhibit the Cox-II enzyme. This can be accomplished either pharmacologically, with FDA-approved drugs like Vioxx and Celebrex, or nutraceutically, with natural compounds.

Recently, a variety of natural substances have been identified as Cox-II inhibitors. These include plant compounds derived from flavonoids, like resveratrol, urosolic acid, caffeic acid, and bupleurum. Whether natural Cox-II inhibitors or their synthetic counterparts will have benefit in Alzheimer's is still not determined. However, inhibiting the overactivity of the immune system by knocking out the Cox-II enzyme is a rational approach to the treatment of Alzheimer's disease and should be explored further in clinical studies.

Now, new studies provide additional hope for Alzheimer's patients diagnosed in the later stages of the disease. By using a form of choline called CDP (cytidine diphosphate choline), scientists have discovered that they can provoke the brain to manufacture more acetylcholine. CDP choline can also increase the amounts of phospholipids in brain membranes.

For instance, in a study published in the *Annals of the New York Academy of Sciences,* Spanish investigators reported patients with Alzheimer's disease treated with a daily dose of 1,000 mg per day of CDP for one month showed a modest improvement in mental performance. They hypothesized that CDP choline may contribute to neuron membrane repair, bestow a moderate antidepressant effect, and slow the overactive immune response by reducing serum interleukin-1B levels, particularly in patients in the early stages of Alzheimer's.

RECOMMENDED DOSE: Check with your physician to find out when CDP choline will become available in the U.S. market. Meanwhile, patients with Alzheimer's should ensure they are receiving adequate choline. We recommend taking 4 g of choline with a meal, either as phosphatidylcholine (PC) or as a combination of PC and choline bitartrate or choline chloride.

Strategies to Reduce Inflammation

• Using Antioxidants to Fight Free Radicals

As researchers understand more about how we age, one thing has become abundantly clear: One of the most significant reasons people age is our cells' increasing inability to fight off destructive oxygen free radicals.

As you already know from reading our earlier chapters, when the body's immune system mobilizes, our cells metabolize more oxygen and spin off by-products called oxygen free radicals. These free radicals destroy invaders efficiently. Unfortunately, they can also rampage through the body and attack our own cells, chewing through cellular membranes and attacking the very DNA that contains cellular genetic codes.

Alzheimer's patients suffer from higher than normal levels of free radicals. Recently, Canadian scientists discovered that samples of Alzheimer's brain tissue produced nearly 50 percent more free radicals than did controls. Studies like this one lead investigators to conclude that there is great promise for Alzheimer's patients in the potential of antioxidants to help reduce the inflammation and inadvertent cell death caused by the body's own immune system's oxidative stress on cells.

In particular, clinicians and researchers are now examining the possible protective effects of fat-soluble antioxidants against free radicals, as these are able to cross the blood-brain barrier and enter the regions of the brain where they are most desperately needed.*

Various antioxidants have been studied for use in Alzheimer's disease, including vitamin E and *Ginkgo biloba,* as well as melatonin. Each of these will be discussed separately, along with prescription and nonprescription anti-inflammatory medications.

---

*A recent study which appeared in the *New England Journal of Medicine* supports the connection between free radicals and Alzheimer's disease. Alzheimer's patients treated with high doses of vitamin E and Selegiline were demonstrated to have a significant delay in progression of cognitive impairment.

Antioxidants and Alzheimer's Disease

• *Vitamin E and Alzheimer's Disease*

Rationale for Use of Vitamin E in Alzheimer's Disease Oxidative damage due to free radical damage has been reported in numerous studies of patients with Alzheimer's disease. Free radicals exert numerous detrimental effects on brain function, including promoting the harmful effects of amyloid, damage to brain cells' mitochondria, and injury to the acetylcholine receptor sites on brain cells. Vitamin E is a potent antioxidant that has been shown to inhibit the beta amyloid–induced damage to brain cells, and to prevent free radical–medicated cell death.

Clinical Studies of Vitamin E in Alzheimer's A double-blind, placebo-controlled study was conducted in 341 patients who received either vitamin E, vitamin E and Selegiline (an antioxidant drug that is currently employed for Parkinson's disease), or placebo over a one-year period. In patients who received 2000 units of vitamin E daily, either alone or in combination with Selegiline, there were significant delays in the progression of Alzheimer's. The study was performed at Columbia Presbyterian Hospital and reported in the *New England Journal of Medicine*.

RECOMMENDED DOSE: These studies were performed using 2000 IU of vitamin E on a daily basis. Patients should discuss using this superphysiological dose with their health care providers before undertaking such a treatment.

• Ginkgo biloba *and Alzheimer's Disease*

Rationale for Use of **Ginkgo biloba** *in Alzheimer's* Ginkgo biloba extract has been widely used in Europe to treat dementia. Ginkgo may have several beneficial effects for Alzheimer's. One of those is thought to be predominantly through its activity as an antioxidant. Certain flavonoids found in ginkgo, including compounds known as terpenoids, are free radical scavengers. This free radical–scavenging activity of *Ginkgo biloba* prevents damage to brain cells.

Clinical Studies of Ginkgo biloba *in Alzheimer's* In a recent study reported in the *Journal of the American Medical Association,* 202 patients with Alzheimer's dementia received 120 mg of ginkgo over a one-year period, compared to a group who received only a placebo. Results of the study demonstrated that *Ginkgo biloba* is safe, as well as being capable of improving cognitive function and stabilizing disease progression in a significant number of patients.

> RECOMMENDED DOSE: 120–240 mg daily. There have been case reports that *Ginkgo biloba* may potentially produce bleeding abnormalities, especially in patients who are already taking prescription blood thinners, such as Coumadin, or aspirin. Speak to your doctor prior to using *Ginkgo biloba* if you are taking any of these medications.

• Melatonin and Alzheimer's Disease

Rationale for Use of Melatonin in Alzheimer's Melatonin is an effective free radical scavenger that crosses the blood-brain barrier. It stimulates two antioxidant systems, superoxide dismutase and gluthathione peroxidase, in the brain. Melatonin has also been shown to reduce the nerve damage caused by amyloid plaque, the characteristic lesions in Alzheimer's disease.

Clinical Studies of Melatonin in Alzheimer's Recently, the molecular effect of melatonin on brain cells has been more clearly elucidated. Researchers at the Indiana University School of Medicine analyzed the effects of melatonin on the production of amyloid in neurons and found that it reduces the cells' production of this destructive protein. Their finding suggests that melatonin may be protective against the amyloid-related progression of Alzheimer's disease.

In collaboration, researchers in the Netherlands measured melatonin levels in the spinal fluid of Alzheimer's patients and compared them to the levels found in age-matched controls. A dramatic decrease in melatonin levels—more than 50 percent—was found in Alzheimer's patients. This reduction in Alzheimer's disease may account for some of the characteristic symptoms of the disorder, including sleep disturbances, day/night confusion, and worsening of symptoms during the night.

RECOMMENDED DOSE: Physiological requirements of melatonin are approximately 1.5 mg per day. It is unclear if patients with Alzheimer's need much higher doses to affect the course of the disease. Clearly, more research is needed to determine the exact amount of melatonin that is required to treat Alzheimer's disease.

• Anti-inflammatory Agents and Alzheimer's Disease

Rationale for Use of Cyclo-oxygenase Inhibitors in Alzheimer's Disease Many studies now delineate specific inflammatory mechanisms that play roles in the neurodegeneration of Alzheimer's disease. Evidence that inflammation is a culprit in Alzheimer's disease came from epidemiological studies examining the use of nonsteroidal drugs (NSAIDs) and other anti-inflammatories. In these studies, patients who took NSAIDs had a lower incidence of Alzheimer's disease as well as a slower disease progression (in the cases in which Alzheimer's occurred).

We've continued to learn more about the role played by the immune system in the destruction seen in Alzheimer's disease. Various pro-inflammatory processes are implicated in causing injury to otherwise normal brain cells. These include a specific enzyme known as cyclo-oxygenase of "Cox" that acts like an "on switch" in the immune system's activity.

Cyclo-oxygenases are involved in prostanglandin synthesis. Prostaglandins are derived from a fatty-like substance, arachidonic acid, which is normally found in our cells. A specific prostaglandin, referred to as PGE2, is the predominant prostaglandin in diseases of inflammation.

In the early 1970s, it was demonstrated that nonsteroidals inhibit the cyclo-oxygenase enzyme, thus preventing the synthesis of prostaglandins and, consequently, the inflammation it generates. Recently it was discovered that cyclo-oxygenase is not one, but two enzymes, now referred to as Cox-I and Cox-II.

The now-appreciated inverse relationship between Alzheimer's and prior use of anti-inflammatories—that is, use of

NSAIDs appears to result in a reduced risk for Alzheimer's disease—has led to the search for newer agents with the same capability but with fewer side effects. With the recent discovery that the Cox-II enzyme is specifically implicated in the disease-causing aspect of prostaglandin-induced inflammation, new drugs that are selective inhibitors of the enzyme have been introduced. These drugs are currently approved for the treatment of osteoarthritis, menstrual pain, and acute pain. At the time of this writing, two FDA-approved Cox-II inhibitors are available by prescription, Vioxx (made by Merck) and Celebrex (Searle).

Several studies suggest that Cox-II inhibitors may be important potential therapies for Alzheimer's. It has been demonstrated that, not only are Cox-II levels elevated in the brains of Alzheimer's patients, but these elevated levels of Cox-II enzyme are selectively increased in the hippocampus, the specific brain region affected in Alzheimer's disease. Furthermore, the elevated levels of Cox-II correlate with amyloid plaque formation.

These studies make a compelling argument to employ Cox-II inhibitors in the treatment of Alzheimer's disease. Research is currently under way with Celebrex and/or Vioxx to determine their ability to slow disease progression. Based on the ability of Cox-II inhibitors to inhibit the inflammatory aspects of this degenerative disease, we suspect the results of these studies will be promising. Natural alternatives to the Cox-II pharmaceutical agents have been identified, and we'll examine them next.

RECOMMENDED DOSE: Vioxx and Celebrex are prescription drugs, but are not approved for treating Alzheimer's disease. Consult with your health care provider.

• Natural Cox-II Inhibitors and Alzheimer's Disease

Rationale for Use of Natural Cox-II Inhibitors in Alzheimer's Disease
Natural Cox-II inhibitors are most often derived from the flavonoid components of various fruits and herbs. These flavonoids include resveratrol, caffeic acid, and bupleurum. Each has demonstrated the ability to block the pro-inflammatory Cox-II enzyme. Because of this ability, these natural Cox-II inhibitors may be effective alternatives to the prescription drugs Celebrex

and Vioxx in treating the inflammatory component of Alzheimer's disease.

RECOMMENDED DOSE: Check with your health care practitioner regarding dosage.

• Resveratrol and Alzheimer's Disease

Rationale for Use of Resveratrol in Alzheimer's Disease There are several basic favorable effects of resveratrol which make it an exciting candidate for the treatment of Alzheimer's disease and other neurodegenerative conditions including Parkinson's disease, amytrophic lateral sclerosis, and multiple sclerosis as well. Resveratrol is a natural Cox-II enzyme inhibitor. As you may recall, Cox-II is a trigger for amplifying immune responses in every cell of our body including the brain. In fact, the Cox-II enzyme is overexpressed in the brains of Alzheimer's patients, suggesting that Alzheimer's is, in fact, a pro-inflammatory condition in the brain. Resveratrol, by inhibiting the Cox-II enzyme, may offer a way of inhibiting the excessive inflammation and prevent progression of the disease. Resveratrol also inhibits the influx of calcium into cells. Calcium influx into cells activates several destructive enzymes which break down cell membranes within a cell. By inhibiting the influx of calcium into brain cells, resveratrol may prevent these destructive enzymes from being activated. Resveratrol also is known to be a free radical scavenger at the site where most free radicals are produced, which is the mitochondria. Resveratrol also helps activate an enzyme known as mapkinase. Mapkinase is an essential enzyme fundamental to memory and learning within the brain. Based upon these favorable effects of resveratrol, it makes a natural compound found in grape skin an exciting candidate for a neuroprotective agent in Alzheimer's and other neurological diseases.

Clinical Studies Supporting the Use of Resveratrol in Alzheimer's Disease Unfortunately, there are no current studies analyzing the effects of resveratrol in Alzheimer's or other neurodegenerative conditions. Unfortunately, this is probably a matter of financing, because most drug companies will not finance a clinical study with a nutritional substance that they cannot market. However, based upon its numerous positive effects including its ability to inhibit the cyclo-oxygenase enzyme, reduce calcium influx into cells, prevent free radical production, and enhance the activity of mapkinase, it is strongly urged by the author that resveratrol be used in clinical studies for neurodegenerative diseases.

RECOMMENDED DOSE: Between 100 mg and 200 mg daily. Resveratrol also may have beneficial effects on cardiovascular health as well.

•DHEA and Alzheimer's Disease

Rationale for Use of DHEA in Alzheimer's Disease   DHEA is a natural anti-inflammatory hormone that reduces the level of cortisol and a pro-inflammatory gene known as nuclear factor kappa beta. It has been postulated that decreased levels of DHEA may contribute to the development of Alzheimer's disease. DHEA has displayed neuroprotective effects, memory enhancing effects, and antioxidant properties.

Clinical Studies of DHEA in Alzheimer's Disease   While no controlled studies employ DHEA to treat Alzheimer's disease, several laboratory evaluations have demonstrated a neuroprotective effect of DHEA in brain cells. This neuroprotective effect appears to be related to DHEA's ability to prevent oxidative stress in particular areas of the brain that are involved in memory. These data, which detail its antioxidant and anti-inflammatory effects in the brain, suggest that DHEA may be a useful treatment in preventing the progression of Alzheimer's disease.

RECOMMENDED DOSE: Check with your health care practitioner regarding dosage.

Strategies for Raising Mitochondrial Action in Alzheimer's Disease

There is a compelling body of evidence that the mitochondria, the energy-producing units of the cell, are dysfunctional in various disorders of aging, including Alzheimer's disease. Every cellular process is driven by the mitochondria. They make a high-energy compound called ATP that drives every enzymatic process in our cells. As we age, and in diseases like Alzheimer's, the mitochondria are increasingly vulnerable to injury. This damage may occur because of the effects of free radicals, which increase during aging, and in states in which the immune system is over-activated. Mitochondrial function is a target of the immune system and of free radicals, in particular. When mitochondria become impaired, the normal cellular processes are no longer energetically supported, and the cell ultimately dies. Therefore, the mitochondria have been closely associated with neurodegen-erative diseases like Alzheimer's. There are several natural agents that improve mitochondrial function and so have been suggested for use in Alzheimer's disease. These include acetyl-L-carnitine, coenzyme Q10 or its synthetic counterpart, Idebenone, and NADH.

• Acetyl-L-Carnitine (ALC) and Alzheimer's Disease

Rationale for Use of Acetyl-L-Carnitine (ALC) in Alzheimer's Disease
Acetyl-L carnitine is a natural substance derived from the amino acid L-carnitine, and works with L-carnitine to help fatty acids cross into the mitochondrial membrane.

Acetyl-L-carnitine is also speculated to be of benefit to patients with Alzheimer's disease because of its effect on the brain chemical acetylcholine, the memory neurotransmitter. Scientists and clinicians have noted that acetyl-L-carnitine is structurally similar to acetylcholine. In fact, acetyl-L-carnitine displays similar actions in the central nervous system both directly and through its supportive effects on choline acetyl transferase, the enzyme we count on for acetylcholine synthesis and release.

Acetyl-L-carnitine is an active antioxidant and protects nerve cell membranes against free radical attacks. In addition, acetyl-L-carnitine promotes phospholipid metabolism and enhances brain energy production. Since investigators have implicated abnormal energy processing as a culprit of cell death and cell membrane disruption in Alzheimer's, they theorize that acetyl-

L-carnitine's benefits may extend far beyond its ability to influence the way our brains produce acetylcholine.

Additionally, acetyl-L-carnitine counteracts the age-dependent loss of several receptors in the central nervous systems of animals, including receptors for neurotransmitters and nerve growth factor.

Clinical Studies of Acetyl-L-Carnitine in Alzheimer's Disease   In 1996, a multicenter study was conducted by researchers at the University of California, New York University, and Columbia Presbyterian Hospital with 450 Alzheimer's patients to determine the effectiveness of treating them with acetyl-L-carnitine. In this landmark investigation, researchers found that the majority of patients under age sixty-five who were taking acetyl-L-carnitine demonstrated significant reduction in their rate of mental decline when compared to patients taking a placebo substance.

In another study, 2.5 grams of acetyl-L-carnitine administered daily for three months helped Alzheimer's patients perform better on a variety of cognitive tasks. Investigators concluded that acetyl-L-carnitine may retard dementia, particularly in patients suffering only mild-to-moderate symptoms of Alzheimer's disease.

RECOMMENDED DOSE: 1.5–2.5 g daily. Precautions: none.

• Coenzyme Q10 and Alzheimer's Disease

Rationale for Use of Coenzyme Q10 in Alzheimer's Disease   As mentioned earlier, mitochondrial dysfunction is a common feature of neurodegenerative diseases like Alzheimer's, Parkinson's, and ALS. In Alzheimer's, this mitochondrial activity is thought to be caused by excessive free radical activity. Because of the link between brain energy and mitochrondrial dysfunction in Alzheimer's, clinicians have proposed strategies to enhance mitochondrial function to improve this disorder clinically (that is, improve its symptoms). One of the most effective ways to increase mitochondrial function is to administer the compound Idebenone, a synthetic coenzyme Q10 analog. It is preferable to taking coenzyme Q10, because it is more lipid-soluble, thus allowing better passage from the blood into our brains.

Clinical Studies of Idebenone in Alzheimer's Idebenone is an excellent antioxidant that protects brain mitochondria from free radical injury. Idebenone also protects the brain from ischemic damage that occurs during aging, making it a potentially useful agent in the treatment of multi-infarct dementia, as well.

In a study of 450 patients with mild-to-moderate Alzheimer's disease, those given Idebenone over a 12–24-month period demonstrated a statistically significant improvement in tests of memory. Furthermore, Idebenone appeared to slow the progression of Alzheimer's disease, making this a compound worthy of recommending to patients.

RECOMMENDED DOSE: 90–120 mg three times daily. Idebenone is currently not available in the United States, but is used in treating Alzheimer's disease in Europe and Japan. Until Idebenone is available, use coenzyme Q10, 50–200 mg per day.

• NADH and Alzheimer's Disease

Rationale for Use of NADH in Alzheimer's Disease NADH is an enzyme involved in cellular energy production, including within neurons in the brain. Decreased levels of NADH alter the ability of a cell to perform normally, with pathological consequences. Researchers have noted that NADH levels are diminished in brain cells that exhibit the characteristic abnormalities of Alzheimer's disease.

Clinical Studies of NADH in Alzheimer's In a study of 17 patients with Alzheimer's disease, NADH was administered in an open-label fashion—that is, there was no "control" group; everyone received NADH. Improvements in patients' mental status were noted, with no side effects. The authors recommend that a double-blind, placebo-controlled study be conducted to further elucidate the beneficial role of NADH in Alzheimer's.

RECOMMENDED DOSE: 5–10 mg daily. Precautions: None.

• Phosphatidylserine and Alzheimer's Disease

Rationale for Use of Phosphatidylserine in Alzheimer's Disease The first step in treating patients with Alzheimer's disease is to rebuild defective cell membranes. As you already know, neuron membranes are made up primarily of different lipids, or fats.

The brain's major phospholipids are key to providing cell membranes with "fluidity," the ability to allow various substances to pass in and out of the cell. As you can guess, this property is essential to the cell-to-cell "talk" carried on by neurotransmitters.

Our brain health depends on one major phospholipid, or fatty acid, in particular, phosphatidylserine (PS), for a number of important metabolic effects. Besides making it possible for nutrients to move freely in and out of neurons, PS is necessary for cells to metabolize energy-essential glucose. PS also helps cells protect themselves from lethal free radicals on a blitzkrieg through our bodies as a result of the overboard immune response associated with Alzheimer's.

Clinical Studies of Phosphatidylserine in Alzheimer's Disease When researchers at the Vanderbilt University School of Medicine's Memory Study studied PS in clinical trials, they found that taking PS orally helped patients with Alzheimer's improve memory, learning, and cognitive functions. Not surprisingly, differences in PS-treated groups versus the placebo groups in that study were most apparent among patients in the early stages of Alzheimer's.

In further support of the benefits of PS as a neuroimmunomodulator, investigators who conducted a multicenter study with over 140 patients found that those who took PS showed significant improvement on cognitive tests. Even after treatment stopped, the group that had received PS sustained improvement, leading those investigators to hypothesize that PS produces structural change in cell membranes rather than transient metabolic changes.

A double-blind, crossover study of phosphatidylserine in patients with early dementia of the Alzheimer's type was also reported by researchers in Munich, Germany. Thirty-three patients with mild Alzheimer's disease participated in a double-blind study using 300 mg of phosphatidylserine per day for eight weeks, compared to a placebo. Overall clinical improvement in the patients' health was noted in those who were taking phosphatidylserine compared to those taking the placebo.

Phosphatidylserine is also intimately involved in mitochondrial function. This phospholipid is located in the inner layer of the mitochondria. During exposure to free radicals, phosphatidylserine shifts from the inner layer of the mitchrondria to the outer layer. This movement within the mitochondria is associated with the induction of apoptosis, the process of cellular death in Alzheimer's and other neurodegenerative diseases. When phosphatidylserine is exposed to the outside of the mitochondrial wall, its integrity is disrupted. Mitochondrial damage results. Conversely, by preserving the integrity of phosphatidylserine, mitochondria are protected and the cell is protected from cell death.

Today, PS is available from soy lecithin extract in 100 mg softgels. It is interesting to note that the bovine extract used in the study described above may have contained other important neuronutrients, such as the omega-3 fatty acid docosahexanoic acid (DHA).

RECOMMENDED DOSE: 300 mg daily, taken with a meal. Precautions: None.

Strategies Based on Raising Neurotransmitter Levels, in Particular, Acetycholine

The fundamental defect in Alzheimer's disease is a depressed level of acetylcholine, the single most important neurotransmitter for cognition. Pharmacological and nonpharmacological agents for raising brain acetylcholine levels include the natural substances Huperzine A and CDP choline as well as the prescription drug Donepezil.

• Huperzine A and Alzheimer's Disease

Rationale for Use of Huperzine A in Alzheimer's Disease Huperzine A is a powerful extract from a rare type of Chinese moss. It has been used in traditional Chinese medicine for patients with memory impairment and Alzheimer's disease for hundreds of years. Recently, the molecular structure and action of Huperzine A have been discovered. Interestingly, it blocks an enzyme, acetylcholinesterase, that is responsible for the breakdown of acetylcholine. By inhibiting the acetylcholine enzyme, Huperzine A allows for increased acetylcholine levels in the brain and thereby enhances cognitive function. Huperzine A has also been shown to block certain types of neurotransmitter receptors that are involved in inappropriate cell death. By blocking these receptors, it may exert an additional beneficial effect other than increasing brain acetylcholine levels, i.e. protecting brain cells from premature cell death.

Clinical Studies of Huperzine A in Alzheimer's Disease   Phase II clinical studies using Huperzine A in more than 100 patients in China showed that approximately 60 percent of those treated with this herbal compound exhibited marked improvement in memory as well as cognitive and behavioral functioning. Side effects were minimal, and no toxic effects were detected on liver or kidney function.

Several other open-label and preclinical studies of Huperzine A have reported benefit in patients with Alzheimer's disease, and a double-blind study is currently being initiated. Because Huperzine A has an activity similar to Donepezil, an FDA-approved drug for use in Alzheimer's, the benefits of Huperzine A are expected to be similar to the prescription medication. However, Huperzine A may have some additional advantages to the currently approved drug, because it has a greater binding capacity to the acetylcholinesterase enzyme, thereby enhancing the activity of acetylcholine by preventing its degradation.

RECOMMENDED DOSE: 50–200 mcg daily. Speak to your health care practitioner before starting to take Huperzine A. Side effects are similar to the prescription drug Donepezil, and include nausea and cramps.

•Donepezil and Alzheimer's Disease

Rationale for Use of Donepezil in Alzheimer's Disease   Donepezil is a reversible acetylcholinesterase inhibitor. Acetylcholine esterase is an enzyme that breaks down the neurotransmitter acetyl-choline. By blocking the effects of this enzyme, Donepezil significantly increases brain acetylcholine levels.

Clinical Studies of Donepezil in Alzheimer's Disease Donepezil has improved several parameters of function in Alzheimer's disease. In an open-label study, patients (who all received Donepezil) showed a reduction in the rate of cognitive decline, compared to the expected course of the disease. In controlled studies of Donepezil, this medication improved certain neuropsychological test scores.

RECOMMENDED DOSE: Donepezil is a prescription medication. Speak to your physician about its use in Alzheimer's disease.

• CDP Choline In Alzheimer's Disease

Rationale for Use of CDP Choline in Alzheimer's Disease Phosphatidylcholine is another phospholipid that's essential for the integrity of brain cell membranes, which become increasingly vulnerable as we age and in Alzheimer's disease. The changes that occur in brain cell membranes during aging and in Alzheimer's interfere with the ability of specific neurotransmitters to interact with receptors. This diminishes a process known as "synaptic transmission." CDP choline plays a major role in the synthesis of phosphatidylcholine—thus protecting the integrity of brain cell membranes—and is crucial in membrane function and repair. CDP choline also stimulates the production of the neurotransmitter acetylcholine.

Clinical Studies on CDP in Alzheimer's Researchers at the Massachusetts Institute of Technology performed a study administering 1–2 g of CDP choline to patients who exhibited verbal memory deficits associated with aging over a five-month period. It was demonstrated that CDP choline was clearly associated with improved short- and long-term memory.

A prospective study in 1989 examined 288 patients with dementia caused either by Alzheimer's disease or by a vascular type of dementia. A particularly significant improvement in memory was seen in patients who took CDP choline, especially in patients with the vascular type of disease (called multi-infarct dementia). It was also noted that CDP choline was able to improve the brain wave activity of Alzheimer's patients, producing a trend toward normalization.

For example, in a study published in the *Annals of the New York Academy of Sciences,* Spanish investigators reported patients with Alzheimer's disease treated with a daily dose of 1000 mg per day of CDP choline for one month showed a modest improvement in mental performance. They hypothesized that CDP choline may contribute to neuron membrane repair, bestow a moderate antidepressant effect, and slow the overactive immune response by reducing serum interleukin-1B levels, particularly in patients in the early stages of Alzheimer's.

RECOMMENDED DOSE: 1–2 g daily, but check with your health care practitioner prior to use.

Strategies for Regenerating Neurotransmitters

• Estrogen and Alzheimer's Disease

Rationale for Use of Estrogen in Alzheimer's Estrogen is a hormone that has considerable effect on brain function. It stimulates the growth of new neurons and synapses, and also prevents the age-related decline in brain function. Estrogen also enhances the production of certain proteins that inhibit the death of brain cells, and it stimulates the enzymes required to manufacture acetylcholine in the brain, known as choline acetyltransferase.

Estrogen may have direct effects on the disease process in Alzheimer's, as well. In particular, estrogen has been demonstrated to inhibit the production of amyloid. Deposition of amyloid is the critical pathological change in Alzheimer's brains. Amyloid is derived from a compound known as amyloid precursor protein, APP. Recently, a major breakthrough in Alzheimer's research was the identification of an enzyme, beta secretase, that stimulates the production of amyloid from amyloid precursor protein. Estrogen inhibits beta secretase and thereby decreases the production of amyloid in the brain.

Furthermore, it has recently been observed that postmenopausal women have a much higher incidence of Alzheimer's than any other segment of the population. It has also been noted in epidemiological studies that women who use estrogen as part of hormone replacement therapy have a significantly lower incidence of Alzheimer's disease than women who do not.

Clinical Studies of Estrogen in Alzheimer's   Large-scale clinical studies are currently under way in several medical centers to define the effects of estrogen replacement therapy on the course and treatment of Alzheimer's disease.

RECOMMENDED DOSE: Ask your health care practitioner about taking estrogen. Women who have an estrogen-dependent cancer like breast cancer should not take estrogen. Furthermore, if you have a history of blood clots, estrogen therapy is contraindicated.

•*Alternatives to Estrogens in Alzheimer's Disease*

Due to the controversy surrounding estrogen replacement therapy, we strongly suggest that patients explore the possibility of alternative, natural approaches to influencing the body's estrogen production.

One of these is to add soybeans and soy-derived foods (like tofu) to the diet, since these foods contain a group of interesting compounds called isoflavones. Isoflavones are natural plant phytoestrogens and have several beneficial effects on human health, including regulating hormone balance and providing protection against cancer and heart disease.

Chemically, isoflavones look like estrogen and are converted into very weak estrogens in the body. This "weakness" is only associated with the negative effects of estrogen, however; isoflavones are potent protective compounds in the body and play an important role in estrogen replacement therapy.

• Phytoestrogens and Alzheimer's Disease

Rationale for Use of Phytoestrogens in Alzheimer's Disease It has been demonstrated that phytoestrogens possess similar effects as estrogen in various tissues of our bodies. These beneficial effects also appear in the brain. Recently, soy phytoestrogens have been shown to markedly increase a neurotrophic factor referred to as brain-derived nerve factor, or BDNF. This is a very compelling finding, because low levels of BDNF are associated with Alzheimer's disease. In fact, many researchers are actively pursuing strategies to raise BDNF in efforts to prevent the progression of Alzheimer's disease.

Clinical Studies of Phytoestrogens in Alzheimer's In a recent study published in *Neuroscience Letters* by researchers at the Wake Forest University School of Medicine, it was demonstrated that both estrogen and soy phytoestrogens significantly increase the levels of BDNF in rat brains. This finding suggests that soy phytoestrogens may act as estrogen agonists and promote the beneficial effects of estrogen on brain function.

Recently, genistein was observed to exert beneficial effects similar to those of estrogen in the aging brain. Like estrogen, genistein stimulates the enzyme acetylcholine transferase, which enhances the production of acetylcholine. Genistein also binds to growth receptors in the brain that promote the formation of new nerve cells while inhibiting the death of existing cells.

RECOMMENDED DOSE: 100 mg of isoflavone concentrate and 50 mg of genistein with a meal. Precautions: Because of its similarity to estrogen, patients should consult with their health care practitioners prior to the use of genistein, especially if there is a history of breast cancer or blood clots.

A Cocktail Approach to Treating Alzheimer's Disease

I. Reduce Inflammation

1. Antioxidants

a. Vitamin E is a potent antioxidant that inhibits the beta amyloid–induced damage to brain cells. Recommended dosage is 400–800 IU daily.

b. *Ginkgo biloba* has free radical–scavenging activity that may prevent damage to brain cells. Recommended dosage is 120–240 mg daily.

c. Melatonin is a free radical scavenger that also crosses the blood-brain barrier. Recommended dosage is 1.5 mg per day.

2. Cox-II Inhibitors

a. Celebrex and Vioxx are the two currently FDA-approved, prescription cyclo-oxygenase (Cox-II) inhibitors (which are anti-inflammatories). Both are available by prescription for treating pain and inflammation, and are currently being studied for Alzheimer's disease as well. Discuss with your health care provider.

b. Natural Cox-II inhibitors are found as plant flavonoids, and include resveratrol, caffeic acid, ursolic acid, and bupleurum. Dosage will be determined by your health care provider.

c. DHEA: This natural anti-inflammatory may turn out to be useful in Alzheimer's disease. Dosage will be determined by your health care provider.

II. Raise Mitochondrial Action

1. Acetyl-L-carnitine: This amino acid improves mitochrondrial function and has also been demonstrated to be efficacious in early to moderate stages of Alzheimer's. Recommended dose: 1.5–2.5 g daily.

2. Coenzyme Q10 or Idebenone: This synthetic coenzyme Q10 analog has been shown to be effective in Alzheimer's disease in several clinical studies. Recommended dose: 90–120 mg daily.

3. NADH: This nutritional substance improves one of the enzymes within the mitochrondria and has also been recently suggested as an effective agent for Alzheimer's disease. Recommended dose: 5–10 mg daily.

4. Phosphatidylserine protects the mitochondria. Recommended dose: 300 mg per day, taken with a meal.

III. Regenerate Neurotransmitters

1. Huperzine A: This Chinese herb blocks the enzyme that breaks down acetylcholine, and is currently being studied for Alzheimer's and mild cognitive impairment. The recommended dose is 100–200 mcg daily.

2. CDP Choline. This nutritional substance also raises brain acetylcholine levels and protects cell membranes from oxidative damage. The recommended dose is 500–1000 mg daily.

3. DHEA: DHEA appears to have a neuroprotective effect in the brain. The recommended dose is to be determined by your health care practitioner.

4. Pharmacological Drugs That Increase Acetylcholine.

  a. Donepezil (Aricept) blocks the breakdown of acetylcholine. It is a prescription medication, so speak to your physician about its use in treating Alzheimer's disease.

IV. Prevent the Production of Amyloid

1. Estrogen is a hormone that has been shown to inhibit the enzyme beta secretase, and so decrease amyloid production. Consult with your health care provider about taking prescription estrogen for Alzheimer's disease. Anyone who has had a hormone-sensitive cancer or blood clots should not take estrogen.

2. Genistein, which is a soy extract that has estrogen-like properties, has also been demonstrated to have similar effects in the brain. Consult your health care practitioner prior to taking genistein, because of the precautions mentioned earlier in this chapter.

CHAPTER 6

PARKINSON'S DISEASE

No doubt about it: The tremor in his right hand was getting worse. Mark had first noticed it almost a year ago, but because it seemed to happen only after working out at the gym, he attributed the shaking to his advancing years and to his new routine with free weights. After all, he was nearly sixty-eight years old, and how many men his age still exercised regularly?

"No pain, no gain," Mark told himself, and so he kept up his workouts, hoping to improve the muscle fatigue over time.

However, lately he felt tired all the time. His wife was always telling him to speak up, because she could hardly hear him. Another funny thing—and Mark might not have noticed this by itself—was that his skin seemed oilier, almost like when he was in his teens.

Mark, who had celebrated his sixty-fifth birthday and retirement by purchasing the sweet little two-seater car of his dreams, waited another eight months to see his physician.

By then, one of his hands shook so badly he could hardly read the newspaper. His handwriting looked like a spider had run across the page. And he felt irritable and depressed for no reason at all.

"I just want to feel better," he told his doctor. "This is the time in my life when I should really be taking advantage of my freedom and enjoying life. What's wrong with me?"

When his doctor diagnosed Parkinson's disease, Mark felt as if the floor had dropped out from under him. "So what do I do now?" he asked.

Parkinson's Disease: An Overview

Like most of us, Mark attributed his muscle fatigue and tremor to the normal aging process. However, in Mark's case—as with one out of every forty people—these were early symptoms of Parkinson's disease.

A neurological disease of late middle age, Parkinson's disease affects more than a million Americans. Up to 50,000 new cases are diagnosed each year. Some experts maintain that the disease is increasing in the population and predict it will soon affect one out of every twenty Americans over age fifty.

This slow degenerative nervous disorder most frequently attacks people in their late fifties or sixties. However, more physicians are now reporting cases of Parkinson's in younger patients. Some estimate that up to 10 percent of Parkinson's patients are now diagnosed before they turn forty.

First described in 1817 by James Parkinson, a British physician who published a medical report on "the shaking palsy," Parkinson's disease is characterized by tremor, slowness of movement, and rigidity. Although it is rarely a cause of death, Parkinson's can weaken sufferers enough to fall prey to other diseases.

While researchers have not yet fully defined its causes, range of symptoms, or a cure, we now know that Parkinson's symptoms are clearly linked to the progressive deterioration of dopamine-producing cells in the brain.

Normally, nature creates so many of these neurons that we're able to lose them every day without noticing, as these brain cells disintegrate owing to head injuries, toxins, air pollutants, and aging. In fact, we have to lose over 75 percent of our dopamine neurons before our body shows the telltale symptoms of Parkinson's.

Some people suffering from Parkinson's may end up severely handicapped after a decade or less. Others experience few symptoms even twenty-five years post-diagnosis. Recent popular figures to bring Parkinson's to the public eye include Pope John Paul II, the actor Michael J. Fox, and fighter Muhammad Ali.

Society pays an enormous price for Parkinson's disease. According to the National Parkinson's Foundation, medications cost the average patient upward of $2,500 annually. When office visits, social security payments, nursing home expenditures, and lost income are totaled for Parkinson's patients, experts estimate that the disease costs the United States more than $5.6 billion a year.

That economic cost pales in comparison to the emotional toll the disease exacts on patients, for who wants to spend their "golden" years trapped in a body that shakes uncontrollably or freezes in place, behind a face devoid of expression owing to inactive muscles?

The good news is this: Advances in treating Parkinson's represent one of the major neurological research success stories of the past decade. It is now hailed as one of the few chronic neurological diseases for which we have found effective treatments.

From the onset of symptoms to diagnosis, from treatment to hope on the horizon, in this chapter we discuss Parkinson's disease in light of what we know about the disease's effects on the brain-immune system connection on its most intricate, biochemical level. At the end of the chapter, you will find an aggressive treatment plan based on the most current information available on medications and nutritional therapies.

What Goes Wrong in Parkinson's Disease, and Why

Although no specific genes have been identified for Parkinson's, the disease most likely results from an interaction between genetics and enviroment.

• A Genetic Predisposition

While there is still more work to do in unraveling the genetic basis for Parkinson's disease, scientists today believe that genetically impaired cellular detoxification mechanisms are the key reason why certain individuals are at risk. When neurons are unable to naturally neutralize environmental toxins, the immune system mounts its forces against those invaders—and may end up killing off the body's own neurons in the process.

• Exposure to Environmental Toxins

Although all of us are exposed to environmental toxins, current epidemiological studies demonstrate that Parkinson's disease is much more prevalent in areas where individuals are more likely to be exposed to toxins like pesticides, carbon monoxide, carbon disulfide, and other environmental contaminants.

In fact, clinical researchers have identified antibodies specifically targeted to brain cells in the cerebrospinal fluid of Parkinson's patients. When the immune system is activated by a combination of impaired cellular detoxification systems and high exposure to toxins, the result is a cascade of responses that damages neurons in certain areas of the brain—in this case, the neurons responsible for producing dopamine, the neurotransmitter that conveys messages from the brain to control muscle movement and balance.

• The Death of Dopamine-Producing Neurons at the Hands of MPTP and Other Neurotoxins

Just about sixty years after James Parkinson first linked such symptoms as gait disorder, postural leaning, and tremor as a single chronic disease, Parkinson's patients were treated by medications developed by French neurologist and hypnotist Jean-Martin Charcot. Charcot, known as the "father of clinical neurology," used potions derived from jimsonweed, a North American plant. The herbal remedy brought relief from tremor and rigidity.

During the next century, patients with Parkinson's were treated with extracts from the belladonna plant, a cousin of jimsonweed, and following World War II, with extracts of belladonna-like drugs.

Real progress was finally made in the 1950s, when scientists began experimenting with tranquilizers to control high blood pressure. These investigations yielded new information about neurotransmitters, the chemical substances that transfer information between nerve cells in the brain.

By 1960, University of Vienna scientists had conducted autopsies of the brains of Parkinson's patients and found those brains strikingly short on the dopamine neurotransmitter.

Another piece of the Parkinson's puzzle fell into place in the 1980s, when illicit drug dealers made a designer drug to sell as a synthetic heroin. In an effort to boost their profits and the speed of the manufacturing process, these drug dealers inadvertently created a toxic substance known as MPTP. As reported in *Science* by neurologists at Stanford University School of Medicine, people who took the drug developed symptoms of Parkinson's within a week, puzzling physicians unaccustomed to seeing the disease in young people.

Investigators eventually linked their common use of the MPTP-containing drug to the Parkinson's symptoms. Subsequent studies with laboratory animals have revealed that administering MPTP produces Parkinson's-like symptoms.

As a result, today's researchers believe that Parkinson's disease may be acquired by individuals with a genetic predisposition for the disease if they are exposed to environmental neurotoxins with chemical properties similar to MPTP.

A number of those neurotoxins are found in agricultural pesticides and herbicides commonly used in Western countries, where the prevalence of Parkinson's is highest.

Recall that dopamine is a neurotransmitter that helps activate adrenaline to noradrenaline, thus gearing us up for "fight or flight" at times of stress. Dopamine also helps regulate our daily moods—as we explain later in our chapter on depression. More relevant for Parkinson's patients, however, is the fact that dopamine levels are directly related to our ability to move our muscles and keep our balance.

The brain cells that produce dopamine are located deep in the brain stem. Most of these are in an area called the "substantia nigra." The name, which means "black substance" in Latin, describes a darkly pigmented area of the brain that is connected to other parts of the basal ganglia by a network of long, twisting nerve fibers.

Once dopamine is manufactured in the substantia nigra, it travels along those nerve fibers, acting as a messenger for the neurological impulses that help regulate our muscular responses and overall motor functions.

Since discovering the link between Parkinson's and low brain levels of dopamine, scientists in several laboratories have been examining the distribution of dopamine receptors, the chemistry of that particular neurotransmitter, and toxin-induced damage specifically to dopamine-containing neurons.

• Mitochondrial Damage and Neuron Death

Recently, Japanese investigators who published their findings in a 1995 issue of *Biochimica et Biophysica Acta* have concluded that MPTP selectively destroys neurons in the region of the brain that makes dopamine.

In examining the pathogenesis of Parkinson's on a molecular level, these scientists and others have discovered that the cellular damage may be due to a decrease in the mitochondrial electron transfer—especially in the substantia nigra. This led them to conclude that an energy crisis—literally, the respiratory failure of mitochondria—was responsible for the neuron death.

As you may recall, mitochondria are cellular energy factories often dubbed "the powerhouses of the cell" for the way they function within cells to convert glucose into energy.

In neurons, which require large amounts of protein to perform their functional activities, the mitochondria are small slender rods and spheres located randomly throughout the cell body, but typically near nerve terminals.

Each mitochondria organelle is bounded by two membranes: a smooth outer membrane and an inner membrane, which has numerous infoldings. The matrix, the area enclosed by the inner membrane, is about half protein and contains the mitochondria's DNA, or genetic guideline.

The mitochondrial inner membrane is where oxidative phosphorylation takes place—the chemical process so fundamental to all aspects of cellular life in organisms that rely on oxygen. That's because the mitochondrial membrane is responsible for moving certain metabolites and mineral ions back and forth between the matrix and the surrounding area.

Now, scientists are finally beginning to grasp just how MPTP, the active toxic agent in that street drug we discussed earlier, damages the cellular mitochondria and produces Parkinson's symptoms, particularly in individuals whose cellular detoxification systems may already be genetically impaired in some way.

• Nitric Oxide: Good Cop, Bad Cop

Some of the most exciting research in the arena of mitochondrial injury and Parkinson's also throws the spotlight directly on the relationship of dopamine loss to neuronal nitric oxide, a neurotransmitter which also occurs naturally in skeletal muscle and which has attracted the spotlight in recent years for its multiple roles.

Once investigators linked MPTP to clinical, biochemical, and neuropathologic changes similar to those occurring in Parkinson's, subsequent studies led researchers to rapidly conclude that the tragic metabolic changes leading to Parkinson's find center stage in the very mitochondria of those cells.

How? Basically, when MPP, a metabolite of MPTP, collects within the mitochondria of the dopamine-containing neurons, it activates excitatory amino acid receptors, causing the mitochondria of those cells to vacuum up more calcium. This increase in calcium sets off heightened free radical production, activating nitric oxide synthesis within the neurons.

It is this step—the generation of free radical nitric oxide within neurons—that serves as a tragic cellular death sentence. That's because nitric oxide combines with superoxide to form peroxynitrite, the most highly toxic free radical in the body. Peroxynitrite essentially leads to cell death by energy deprivation.

According to Professor P. Jenner, DSc of the Neurodegenerative Disease Research Centre at King's College, London, there is solid evidence for increased lipid peroxidation in the substantia nigra of people with Parkinson's disease. This suggests that free radical production in their bodies is on the rampage. Jenner also concludes that Parkinson's patients have a weakened protective antioxidant defense, and that their bodies' natural repair systems for mending free radical damage are not operating efficiently.

In a 1994 issue of the *Annals of the New York Academy of Sciences,* other investigators concurred with this finding, correlating oxidative stress and the activation of the nitric oxide pathway in the context of cytokine activation. Thus, as with so many neurological disorders, we find that the breakdown of the body's brain-immune system connection and of the immune system itself play an enormous role in causing the disease.

Not only do the brains of Parkinson's patients show a loss of dopamine-producing neurons, they also demonstrate an increase in the number of macrophages that appear to gulp down degenerating neurons. For the immune system's foot soldier macrophages, nitric oxide serves as a signal to step up superoxide production. This cuts back on essential mitochondrial oxidative phosphorylation and increases the spin-off of toxic free radicals—ultimately leading to oxidative stress and cellular death.

Fortunately, the evidence is so compelling that nitric oxide mediates Parkinson's, we can now make use of medications and nutritional compounds to turn that process around.

In simplest terms, if we can prevent neurons from oversynthesizing nitric oxide in the first place, peroxynitrite won't be around to kill off the brain's dopamine-producing neurons.

Neurologist M. Flint Beal at Massachusetts General Hospital and his associates in the United States and France have done exactly that. In studies with baboons, they administered MPTP and discovered that the drug produced a dopamine depletion of up to 98 percent in certain parts of the brain, causing the primates to suffer Parkinson's symptoms.

Then, by administering a drug called 7NI (7-nitroindazole), the researchers discovered that they could counter the effect of the neurotoxin by inhibiting nitric acid production, successfully protecting the animals against MPTP-induced dopamine depletion.

• *The Devastating Effects of Lowered Glutathione Levels*

One of the body's free radical terminators, glutathione is a naturally occurring amino acid produced in all cells of the body as part of your body's natural detoxification system. Glutathione is particularly effective when it comes to neutralizing free radical attacks on fat.

Because cellular mitochondria churn out so many free radicals in the course of their work on the body's behalf, glutathione deficiency can lead to widespread mitochondrial damage.

Now, scientists have discovered yet another link between lowered glutathione levels and Parkinson's disease. In a study published in 1994 by the *Annals of Neurology,* researchers measured glutathione and oxidized glutathione levels in various areas of the brain in patients dying from Parkinson's. Not surprisingly, these investigators also discovered that the glutathione levels were reduced.

Since glutathione is one of the body's most important naturally occurring antioxidants, this finding is consistent with the concept of oxidative stress as a major component in the death of dopamine-producing neurons.

A Combined Medical and Nutritional Approach to Parkinson's Disease

If you or a loved one is diagnosed with Parkinson's disease, the first question to ask is whether Parkinson's is impeding function and quality of life.

If the answer is no, then we recommend avoiding medication until symptoms worsen. In our experience, the longer a patient with Parkinson's is able to get by comfortably without taking medication, the less chance there is of the medication losing efficacy in later stages of the disease.

However, we do believe that patients with Parkinson's should immediately begin a nutritional therapy that combines a low-protein diet with neuroimmunomodulating nutritional sub-

TABLE **4**

A CASCADE OF BRAIN CELL DAMAGE

1. Genetic defects impair the natural ability of dopamine-producing brain cells to naturally cleanse themselves of toxins.

2. The susceptible individual is exposed to environmental toxins (pesticides, viruses, heavy metals).

3. There is trauma to the head.

4. The immune system is called into action as a result of 1, 2, 3, or a combination of those factors.

5. Cells are subjected to oxidative stress via free radicals.

6. Cellular mitochondria are damaged and unable to convert energy needed for healthy cellular reactions.

7. Dopamine-producing neurons are damaged or die.

stances that have proved to be of benefit in mending the brain-immune connection for people with this disease.

Why this particular protocol? Remember that, with Parkinson's disease, patients may suffer from excessive free radical damage caused by a combination of (1) impaired cellular detoxification systems, (2) exposure to toxins, (3) an immune system gone haywire, and (4) lowered levels of naturally cleansing antioxidants such as glutathione.

Thus, our neuroimmunomodulating therapy for Parkinson's disease consists of boosting the body's own antioxidants through nutritional substances. Additionally, we ask patients to modify their intake of protein, calories, fiber, and fluids to maximize the benefits of therapy while avoiding constipation and dehydration—common complaints of people with Parkinson's.

The earlier this nutritional therapy is begun, the earlier we can help ameliorate or even halt the relentless progress of this disease, as the neuroprotective nutrients we recommend will help preserve the remaining dopamine-producing neurons.

When Should You Suspect Parkinson's Disease?

Parkinson's disease strikes men and women in almost equal numbers. Early symptoms of the disease are subtle and occur gradually. Not everyone is affected the same way. In some individuals, the disease rampages through the body, causing early disability, while others experience only minor motor disruptions.

Parkinson's may involve one or both sides of the body with anywhere from mild postural imbalance to critical instability. Patients afflicted with severe Parkinson's may eventually be restricted to a bed or chair. Some patients indicate that their early symptoms appeared during periods of stress, then subsided, only to reappear several years later on a more consistent basis.

Tremor is the major symptom for some Parkinson's patients, while for others tremor is only a minor complaint and different symptoms pose more problems. The tremor associated with Parkinson's takes on a characteristic appearance that physicians call "pill rolling."

Typically, tremor begins in a hand, and takes the form of a rhythmic back-and-forth motion of forefinger and thumb. It is most obvious when someone is under stress. Tremor may also affect a foot or jaw first. In most patients, the tremor affects only one side or one part of the body during early stages of the disease.

The second symptom common to most Parkinson's patients is rigidity, or resistance to movement. A major principle of body movement is that all muscles have an opposing muscle. In other words, you are able to move a muscle not just because it becomes more active, but because the opposing muscle relaxes.

Parkinson's patients experience rigidity because communication between the brain and the muscles is disturbed. Instead of relaxing, the opposing muscles remain constantly tensed to the point of aching. The rigidity becomes obvious when another person tries to move the patient's arm and is able to do so only in jerky, ratchetlike movements.

The third symptom, bradykinesia, is often the most frustrating. The term describes the slowing down of spontaneous and automatic muscle movement—like the movements you use to wash or dress—so that common daily activities take hours instead of minutes.

In the advanced stages of Parkinson's, patients experience postural instability which may cause them to lean and fall over easily. As the disease progresses, Parkinson's patients may halt in mid-stride and "freeze" in place, possibly even tipping over. Or they may walk with quick, tiny steps to keep their balance as they move forward.

Various other symptoms may accompany Parkinson's as well, such as depression and emotional changes. Many patients lose their motivation and become dependent on family members. About a third of Parkinson's patients also suffer memory loss.

Diagnosing Parkinson's: A Complex Masquerade

One of the difficulties in finding ways to inhibit or reverse the neurological deterioration in Parkinson's disease is the long delay in diagnosis. Too often, patients are not diagnosed until full-blown symptoms develop—which means they have already experienced at least a 70–80 percent decrease in the neurons we rely on to make dopamine, the neurotransmitter so essential for muscle control. To effectively treat Parkinson's patients, an early diagnosis is imperative.

However, even for an experienced neurologist, it is sometimes difficult to make an accurate diagnosis in the early stages of Parkinson's, as there is no sophisticated blood or laboratory test available to date.

Complicating things further is the fact that Parkinson's can masquerade as other conditions, including:

- Neurological disorders resulting from stroke, tumors, and head traumas
- Metabolic conditions, such as hypoparathyroidism
- Symptoms brought on by major tranquilizers and antinausea drugs
- Benign essential tremor

To ensure a correct early diagnosis of Parkinson's, the physician may need to observe you or your loved one for some time, until it is apparent that a tremor is present and one or more of the other classic symptoms are also manifest. Another potentially promising laboratory marker for the diagnosis of Parkinson's disease involves measuring the amount of free radical activity in white blood cells, which appears higher than normal in Parkinson's patients.

The First Step to Take: Begin a Low-Protein Diet

It is sometimes difficult for investigators to determine the effects of disease progression in Parkinson's patients, because there are some patients with Parkinson's who reveal only one or two symptoms for many years, while others worsen rapidly after diagnosis. However, there is a solid, scientific foundation for using a low-protein diet and taking the neuroimmunomodulating nutritional supplements we recommend below as a means of preserving the remaining healthy dopamine-producing neurons.

Because the human body converts protein to amino acids, a low-protein diet may help Parkinson's patients by allowing more dopamine to become available in the brain.

This is a simple matter of competition: the precursors of dopamine include the amino acid tyrosine, which is converted in the body in a series of steps first to dopa and then to dopamine. Dopa ends up competing with other amino acids to enter through the blood-brain barrier. If fewer amino acids are available, then more dopa can be rushed past the border guards and into the brain, where it can be converted to dopamine.

In addition, some researchers have found that high-protein diets may actually increase the risk of dying from Parkinson's disease. For example, physicians at Georgetown University's School of Medicine have conducted comparative studies of Parkinson's patients in countries as diverse as the United States, Mexico, and Japan. They found a striking correlation between high levels of dietary protein and death from Parkinson's. Low-protein diets therefore may offer more than just symptomatic relief to Parkinson's patients.

In summary, then, because the large, neutral amino acids derived from dietary proteins compete with dopa—an essential natural precursor to dopamine synthesis—we recommend that patients take just 10 percent of their allotted daily protein during the day, with the bulk of dietary protein to be consumed at night. That allows dopa to make its way to the brain with as little competition from other amino acids as possible. Studies have demonstrated that patients who restrict their protein intake to the evening meal show greater improvement than those who do not.

It's important to note, in adjusting the diet to better manage Parkinson's, that many patients with the disease are at risk for malnutrition owing to a variety of factors, including low income, social isolation, impaired appetite, depression, dementia, inactivity, and increased metabolic requirements.

Therefore, in addition to restricting protein intake, we urge Parkinson's patients to maintain an ideal body weight through adequate caloric intake (between 12 and 16 calories per pound of body weight).

Other Dietary Suggestions for Managing Parkinson's

• Enhance Fluid and Fiber Intake

Studies have demonstrated that a diet rich in insoluble fiber lessens constipation while increasing the availability of dopa for uptake by the brain's neurons.

We suggest incorporating insoluble types of fiber into your diet throughout the day with such foods as wheat bran, rice bran, whole wheat breads, crackers, and cereals. In addition, we ask patients to drink a minimum of eight glasses of water daily to avoid constipation. Another route we recommend is to take miller's bran and psyllium fiber supplements as directed by your nutritionist or physician. Lastly, the use of "friendly" bacteria is crucial in maintaining normal bowel flora and regulation. Look for a combination product that contains both lactobaccilli and bifido organisms.

•Ensure Adequate Antioxidant Foods

The hallmark of Parkinson's disease is a lowered level of glutathione, the detoxifying free radical scavenger that is especially important to protecting brain cells. Our neuroprotective therapy is based on boosting deficiencies in antioxidants and important antioxidant enzyme systems such as glutathione peroxidase.

Patients with insufficient intake of antioxidants such as vitamins C and E, tocotrienols, selenium, carotenoids, N-acetyl-cysteine, and glutathione run the risk of free radicals rampaging through the body and causing further damage to already weakened cells.

Dr. Stanley Fahn, a professor of neurology at Columbia Presbyterian Hospital and a world-renowned researcher in Parkinson's disease, has presented a considerable body of evidence in both human and animal models to support the concept of oxidative stress heightening the pathology of Parkinson's.

Among the evidence supporting this concept is the fact that the brains of patients with Parkinson's have increased lipid peroxidation, reduced levels of glutathione, increased iron, and by-products of oxidant stress, such as abnormal enzyme activity. As a result of this evidence, clinicians are now recommending that patients with Parkinson's receive aggressive antioxidant treatment.

•Avoid Certain Supplements

In a 1995 issue of *Toxicology,* University of Arizona College of Medicine researcher Dr. Erwin Montgomery reviewed the role of heavy metals such as iron and manganese in Parkinson's disease. According to his report, the combination of high iron and the nerve transmitter dopamine may result in free radical damage to the brain's substantia nigra. Also, dopamine may break down and produce free radicals in the presence of iron and other heavy metals, such as manganese and copper.

A number of other investigators concur with this finding, while still others have ferreted out evidence of elevated iron levels and enhanced oxidative damage in the substantia nigra of Parkinson's disease patients.

Based on these and other findings, we recommend that patients with Parkinson's should not only step up their intake of antioxidants, but also steer away from supplements of iron, copper, and manganese—all of which have been shown to worsen the progression of Parkinson's or to be correlated with developing the disease in the first place.

The Three R's of Managing Parkinson's Disease: Reduce Inflammation, Raise Mitochondrial Action, and Regenerate Dopamine Production

The most effective strategy for managing Parkinson's disease is three-pronged: reducing inflammation, raising mitochondrial action, and regenerating dopamine production. Let's examine the pharmaceutical drugs and nutritional substances that are most effective in achieving each of these three objectives.

Strategies to Reduce Inflammation

How is inflammation tied to Parkinson's disease? As we discussed earlier, it appears that an aggravating factor in the development of Parkinson's is an inflammatory reaction produced by specific neurological-immune cells. The neurological-immune cells are called glial cells; they damage the area of the brain where dopamine is produced, the substantia nigra. When activated, glial cells produce pro-inflammatory molecules, including certain cytokines and free radicals, especially nitric oxide. Nitric oxide may, in turn, alter the iron balance in the brain, and result in damage to the mitochondria. Neuroprotective strategies involve adressing these issues, including nitric oxide production, free radical inhibition, and compounds that buffer excessive iron. The principle antioxidant in protecting the brain from free radicals is a sulfur-based molecule, glutathione. A rational approach to treating Parkinson's disease would include not only glutathione but also other antioxidants that combat inflammation.

•Antioxidants That Increase Glutathione

Reducing inflammation in Parkinson's disease involves employing antioxidants that control excessive free radical activity (some of which also bind excessive iron). Antioxidants that raise cellular glutathione levels include: a super pronutritional, selenium-based protein known as "ebselen"; lipoic acid in its preferred form, dihydrolipoic acid; certain teas and pine bark extracts, which contain antioxidant polyphenols; NAC; and glutathione itself. Another class of antioxidants currently under development, the isothiocyanates, potentially have great promise in the treatment of Parkinson's disease because they increase glutathione levels.

Rationale for Use of Antioxidants in Parkinson's Disease When the body's immune system mobilizes, the white blood cells release free radicals to protect against foreign invaders like bacteria, viruses, and toxic compounds. These free radicals destroy invaders efficiently by attacking their very biological components and mechanisms. Unfortunately, they can also terrorize our own cells, if they misidentify their target. Subsequently, they release free radicals, damaging various components of the cells; cell membranes, cell receptors in the brain, vital proteins that control enzymes, and the DNA that contains cellular genetic codes.

In Parkinson's, we know that the free radical nitric oxide, which is released by white blood cells, is detrimental to dopamine-producing neurons and combines with superoxide to form peroxynitrite, the most highly toxic free radical in the body. Peroxynitrite leads to cell death by inhibiting the mitochondria within the cell, resulting in energy deprivation.

Studies have shown that Parkinson's disease is exacerbated by a chronic antioxidant deficiency state. As we previously discussed, drug therapy for Parkinson's may add to the free radical damage to neurons.

Today, a significant body of evidence links excessive free radical activity to Parkinson's disease. Researchers have detected increased markers of lipid peroxidation—which signals free radical damage—in selective brain regions in Parkinson's patients, specifically in the dopamine-manufacturing area of the brain, the substantia nigra.

In particular, glutathione, an essential intracellular antioxidant, has been found at reduced levels in the substantia nigra of Parkinson's patients. Furthermore, increased levels of iron, a metal that catalyzes the production of free radical activity, has been reported to be elevated in Parkinson's patients. It's suspected that both of these parameters—decreased levels of the antioxidant glutathione and increased levels of the free radical–producer iron—may contribute to the development of Parkinson's disease. It's also suspected that if the concentration of antioxidants (like glutathione) were higher in the brains of Parkinson's patients, they might suffer less free radical damage and the progression of this disorder might be prevented.

Let's discuss each antioxidant individually, along with its potentially supportive role as a neuroprotective agent in Parkinson's disease: vitamin E, ebselen, lipoic acid, green tea extract, glutathione, and the isothiocyanates.

• Vitamin E and Parkinson's Disease

Rationale for Use of Vitamin E in Parkinson's Disease Vitamin E is a lipid-soluble antioxidant that prevents the peroxidation (breakdown) of brain cell membranes, which are composed of lipid. Therefore, its use in Parkinson's disease has been suggested. Vitamin E also protects against free radical damage.

Clinical Studies of Vitamin E in Parkinson's Disease A negative study using vitamin E in Parkinson's disease was recently reported, but its results were questioned because oral vitamin E may not raise antioxidant levels in the brain sufficiently to affect the progression of the illness. Nevertheless, keep in mind that antioxidants work synergistically—that is, they work better together than they do individually. Therefore, it is not surprising that a clinical trial assessing vitamin E alone would not show a positive effect on the symptoms of Parkinson's disease. However, a study examining numerous antioxidants employed simultaneously might show that, used together, they alleviate Parkinson's symptoms.

RECOMMENDED DOSE: 800 IU (international units) daily.

• Increasing Glutathione: Ebselen and Parkinson's Disease

Rationale for Use of Ebselen in Parkinson's Disease Ebselen is a selenium-like compound with antioxidant activity. It enhances the enzyme glutathione peroxidase and, thus, raises glutathione levels in the brain. It also inhibits the free radical nitric oxide, and has been suggested as a useful anti-inflammatory agent.

Although this compound has never been formally studied in Parkinson's patients, its mechanisms of action make it a leading candidate for use as a possible neuroprotective agent. Ebselen stimulates the enzyme glutathione peroxidase, an important step in glutathione production. It protects cells from a form of death known as "apoptosis." Ebselen has also been shown to be efficacious in arthritic conditions (where it helps rebuild cartilage) and in helping people recover from stroke damage. Interestingly, ebselen works best in conjunction with dihydrolipoic acid, an antioxidant commonly known as "lipoic acid" (or "alpha lipoic acid"), which also raises brain glutathione levels. Ebselen is currently the subject of intense scientific scrutiny in clinical studies as an agent that will help inflammatory conditions like arthritis, as well as stroke. Its use in Parkinson's disease is based upon its profound antioxidant activity and in particular by raising glutathione levels in the brain.

RECOMMENDED DOSE: To be recommended by your health care practitioner.

• Lipoic Acid and Parkinson's Disease

Rationale for Use of Lipoic Acid in Parkinson's Disease Lipoic acid is a pro-glutathione dietary supplement that enhances the production of glutathione, prevents oxidative damage, and improves mitochondrial function. The preferred form of lipoic acid in Parkinson's disease may be dihydrolipoic acid, although neither compound has been extensively studied for efficacy in Parkinson's.

In a study performed by the renowned Dr. Lester Packer at the University of California, Berkeley, it was demonstrated that lipoic acid supplementation significantly lowers oxidative stress by helping to restore normal cellular glutathione levels. The antioxidant properties of lipoic acid also include its ability to bind iron and copper, two metals implicated in neurodegenerative disease. An additional protective mechanism of lipoic acid is its ability to inhibit dopamine's potential to generate free radicals. Dopamine is the neurotransmitter deficient in Parkinson's disease, which is restored by drugs like Sinemet. There is some concern about the use of Sinemet because its dopamine component has the potential to accelerate cell death in Parkinson's brains, an effect that appears related to the oxidation of dopamine, which generates highly toxic free radical substances. This effect can be inhibited by dihydrolipoic acid, the preferred form of lipoic acid.

RECOMMENDED DOSE: 300–600 mg, or as recommended by your health care practitioner.

• Green Tea Extract and Parkinson's Disease

Rationale for Use of Green Tea Extract in Parkinson's Disease Green tea extract possesses a potent antioxidant compound known as epigallocatechingallate (or EGCG, for short). EGCG is a polyphenol that possesses cellular protective effects as well as anticancer effects. EGCG increases the activity of natural antioxidant and detoxifying enzymes, including glutathione peroxidase. It suppresses the activation of free radicals, and prevents lipid peroxidation. It has better antioxidant activity than vitamin E and vitamin C. These properties make EGCG an excellent candidate as a neuroprotective agent in Parkinson's disease.

RECOMMENDED DOSE: 60–120 mg of standardized green tea daily.

• Pycnogenol® and Parkinson's Disease

Rationale for Use of Pycnogenol® in Parkinson's Disease Pycnogenol® is a standardized extract of a French pine bark. It contains a mixture of certain flavonoids known as proanthocyanidines. The potential therapeutic effect of Pycnogenol® is related to its powerful free radical–scavenging activity. Pycnogenol® helps to maintain glutathione levels in various tissues, including the brain, as well as the immune and circulatory systems. It inhibits the generation of the free radical nitric oxide, which has been implicated as a detrimental agent in Parkinson's disease.

RECOMMENDED DOSE: 100–200 mg daily.

• Glutathione and Parkinson's Disease

Rationale for Use of Glutathione in Parkinson's Disease A significant aspect of Parkinson's disease is the loss of the antioxidant glutathione in the brain's substantia nigra. Glutathione works to protect cells and their mitochondria, in particular, from free radical damage. Defects in glutathione synthesis in Parkinson's patients may account for their increased susceptibility to environmental toxins and pesticides. It may, in fact, explain the still-mysterious relationship of these noxious environmental agents to the onset of Parkinson's disease.

Clinical Studies of Glutathione in Parkinson's Disease Oral glutathione is not well absorbed; however, intravenous glutathione has been studied in Parkinson's disease.

Nine patients with untreated Parkinson's disease received intravenous glutathione, 600 mg twice daily for 30 days, in an open-label study (that is, the doctors and patients both knew that the patients were receiving glutathione; there was no "control group"). All of the patients improved significantly after glutathione therapy, showing an estimated 40 percent decline in disability scores. The authors of the study concluded that intravenous glutathione improves symptoms and may even retard the progression of Parkinson's disease.

RECOMMENDED DOSE: IV glutathione can only be given under the supervision of a health care practitioner. Oral glutathione is not readily absorbed; however, certain natural and synthetic compounds raise the levels of glutathione in the bloodstream and in the brain and have been suggested for use in Parkinson's disease.

• Isothiocyanates and Parkinson's Disease

Rationale for Use of Isothiocyanates in Parkinson's Disease New antioxidants that possess the ability to cross the blood-brain barrier, and so potentially be more effective for Parkinson's patients, are under development. These include compounds called "isothiocyanates," naturally occurring substances found in cruciferous vegetables (like broccoli, cauliflower, and Brussels sprouts). Isothiocyanates increase antioxidant defenses, raise glutathione levels, cross the blood-brain barrier, and inhibit specific proteins that initiate cell death in neurons. Their use in Parkinson's and other neurodegenerative diseases characterized by excessive free radical activity is currently under investigation.

The protective effects of isothiocyanates are due to their ability to induce cellular antioxidant defense systems, including the enzyme glutathione peroxidase. It's advantageous to increase glutathione peroxidase, since it's the rate-limiting factor in the brain's production of glutathione. Therefore, isothiocyanates enhance both the production of glutathione peroxidase and of glutathione in the brain. In addition, isothiocyanates have the ability to cross the blood-brain barrier, which gives them a clear advantage over many existing antioxidants that lack this ability.

RECOMMENDED DOSE: Daily intake of the cruciferous vegetables is recommended. At present, since isothiocyanates are unstable compounds, efficacious supplements are unavailable.

• NAC (N-acetyl-cysteine) and Parkinson's Disease

Rationale for Use of NAC in Parkinson's Disease NAC serves as a cysteine donor, contributing to the synthesis of glutathione in brain cells and other tissues. Some investigators have suggested using NAC as a part of the neuroprotective strategy in Parkinson's disease, and many clinicians now employ it for this purpose. However, some studies have cast doubt on NAC's use, suggesting that one particular conjugation on N-acetyl-cysteine with dopamine is toxic to cells in the area of the brain where dopamine is deficient, the substantia nigra. Further studies on the use of N-acetyl-cysteine in Parkinson's are certainly required.

Buffering Iron in Parkinson's Disease

Iron enhances the free radical activity of destructive compounds within the brain, and it's suspected that overexposure to iron may contribute to the development of Parkinson's disease. Numerous treatments that buffer iron, including the supplement lactoferrin, have been suggested as treatments for Parkinson's disease.

• *Lactoferrin and Parkinson's Disease*

Rationale for Use of Lactoferrin in Parkinson's Disease Iron has been implicated in the development of Parkinson's disease because it generates free radical activity, and excessive iron is found in the brains of people who have Parkinson's. Therefore, to halt the progression of Parkinson's, we need to bind the excessive iron found in the brains of these patients. Various treatment strategies have been suggested to buffer excessive iron, including a compound known as lactoferrin, which is available in health food stores. Currently, there is little support among physicians for the use of lactoferrin in treating Parkinson's; however, increased lactoferrin receptors are found in the brains of Parkinson's patients, suggesting that a decreased iron-binding capacity allows free iron to contribute to the physiological cascade of Parkinson's disease. Therefore, lactoferrin may be beneficial in Parkinson's disease by binding this excessive iron, hopefully preventing free radical formation.

RECOMMENDED DOSE: To be recommended by your health care practitioner.

Detoxifying the Liver

The liver detoxifies the entire body; when it isn't working optimally, it becomes saturated with toxic substances it can't process, and so detoxifies the body less and less. Some Parkinson's disease patients have liver enzyme problems, and it's suspected that a genetic liver problem is present in the hereditary form of Parkinson's. Milk thistle contains active ingredients that help the liver detoxify itself and the entire body, and so may be useful to people with Parkinson's disease.

• Milk Thistle and Parkinson's Disease

Rationale for Use of Milk Thistle in Parkinson's As we discussed earlier in this chapter, neurotoxins—both those from the external enviroment and those we produce in our own bodies, i.e., free radicals—are likely to play roles in causing Parkinson's disease. Several studies have demonstrated that the livers of Parkinson's patients don't work properly. For example, some Parkinson's patients have abnormal liver enzymes that may hamper the liver's ability to cleanse the body's tissues of toxins. In particular, it appears that a specific process that detoxifies environmental toxins, called the "Phase II biotransformation process," is impaired in Parkinson's patients.

Recent research supports the notion that Parkinson's patients may have a genetic defect that renders their livers particularly susceptible to enviromental toxins, including pesticides. The liver normally processes these toxins in a two-step process known as Phase 1 and Phase 2 detoxification. Phase 1, the "activation" phase, employs an enzyme known as CYP2D6. Phase 2, the "conjugation" phase of liver detoxification, utilizes an enzyme named GSTM. Researchers have found that people in whom these enzymes are defective have a ten- to fourteen-fold increase in risk of developing Parkinson's disease.

Based upon these observations, increasing the activity of liver enzymes involved in detoxification has been suggested as a treatment strategy for Parkinson's disease. Milk thistle, with its active ingredient silymarin, is a natural herb that has been shown to increase glutathione levels and improve the liver's ability to detoxify compounds. Silymarin administration markedly increases the activity of Phase 2 liver detoxification systems, making it an excellent candidate to use as a detoxifying agent in Parkinson's disease. Milk thistle has not been studied in Parkinson's disease, but it is a logical candidate for future studies.

RECOMMENDED DOSE: 150–300 mg of standardized extract daily.

Strategies to Raise Mitochondrial Activity

Substances That Raise Mitochondrial Activity Free radicals are known to damage mitochondria, the body's energy producers. Mitochondrial damage and reduced activity can result in the death of cells, including brain cells, which don't receive enough energy. Parkinson's patients suffer from free radical damage, and some have been found to have defective mitochondria. The defect in mitochondria may be the determining factor in the gradual decline in dopamine-producing cells in Parkinson's disease. Therefore, it's important to support the mitochondria and raise their activity levels. Two compounds are known to enhance mitochondrial function: coenzyme Q10 and NADH.

• Coenzyme Q10 and Parkinson's Disease

Rationale for Use of Coenzyme Q10 in Parkinson's Disease Parkinson's disease has been speculated to be caused, in part, by mitochondrial damage, in particular by damage to an enzyme called Complex 1. Coenzyme Q10 increases Complex 1 activity, a mechanism of action that may be helpful in Parkinson's patients who have a defective mitochondrial system. Coenzyme Q10 also protects the mitochondria from free radical activity. Oral coenzyme Q10 has been found to be protective to dopamine-manufacturing neurons in the brain, and is also protective against Parkinson's disease in the animal models studied by researchers.

Clinical Studies of Coenzyme Q10 in Parkinson's Disease Coenzyme Q10 has not proved beneficial in improving disability scores in studies with Parkinson's disease patients. However, coenzyme Q10 is more likely to exert a neuroprotective effect rather than to affect symptoms, which would account for these results. There-fore, no conclusions can be drawn about the utility of coenzyme Q10 in preventing the progression of Parkinson's disease until large-scale studies are performed. Multicenter studies are cur-rently being conducted by the Parkinson's Study Group (associ-ated with the National Parkinson's Disease Foundation) to evaluate the usefulness of coenzyme Q10 in Parkinson's disease.

RECOMMENDED DOSE: 50–200 mg daily. Precautions: None.

• NADH (Nicotinamide Adenine Dinucleotide) and Parkinson's Disease

Rationale for Use of NADH in Parkinson's Disease If we traveled along the brain's assembly line that produces the essential neuro-transmitter dopamine, we'd find that one of the earliest work stations adds an enzyme called tyrosine hydroxylase, which helps to synthesize dopa, the precursor to dopamine. This reaction requires a compound called BH4, which is produced in the brain with the help of NADH. In other words, to produce dopamine—and thereby stave off the development of Parkinson's disease—we absolutely require adequate levels of NADH.

Tyrosine hydroxylase, as you can see, is also required for dopamine manufacture. However, various studies have shown that this enzyme is reduced in Parkinson's patients, possibly pro-viding a clue about why these patients do not produce enough dopamine. The same studies have also shown that NADH can increase tyrosine hydroxylase levels and, therefore, increase dopa-mine production.

Clinical Studies of NADH in Parkinson's Disease One study using intravenous NADH (reported in the *Journal of Neural Transmis-sion*) showed that Parkinson's patients experienced a significant beneficial response from seven days of treatment with NADH.

Follow-up studies of NADH use in Parkinson's have been equivocal, however, including a study performed by neurological researchers in Sweden that found no significant benefit from treating five patients with 25 mg of intravenous NADH. However, interpretation of these studies is limited, because each study treated a very small number of patients.

In contrast, studies performed by Dr. George Birkmayer at the Birkmayer Institute of Parkinson's Therapy in Vienna showed that Parkinson's disease patients who were treated with intravenous NADH significantly improved their abilities to walk, push, stand upright, and speak. When the NADH treatment stopped, however, their disabling symptoms returned within three weeks.

RECOMMENDED DOSE: 10 mg daily, divided into two 5 mg doses. Precautions: There are no precautions against using NADH. It is a safe, natural compound which will probably be studied in more detail in the next few years.

Strategies to Regenerate Dopamine-Producing Cells in the Brain

• *Substances That Regenerate Dopamine-Producing Cells*

The best solution for stopping or slowing the progression of Parkinson's disease, of course, is to restore functioning to the cells that produce dopamine. While that is not always possible, it is certainly a goal in every case. We are fortunate to have now identified several substances that help to regenerate dopamine-producing cells. One such substance is gangliosides, a sugar-and-fat complex found at high levels in our brains. Additionally, several pharmaceutical drugs that interact with dopamine receptors in the brain have been developed. One of the exciting new developments in Parkinson's disease research is that these drugs may be able to regenerate dopamine-producing neurons.

• *Dopamine-Stimulating Drugs, Dopamine Agonists, and Parkinson's Disease*

Rationale for Use of Pharmaceutical Agents in Parkinson's Disease If the symptoms of Parkinson's worsen to the point that they impair function and cause a decline in quality of life, we suggest that patients discuss the possibility of combining medication with nutritional substances in neuroimmunomodulating therapy.

Parkinson's disease medications act on the dopamine receptors in the brain. Some stimulate the release of dopamine; these are called "dopamine agonists." These drugs may also have symptomatic and neuroprotective effects. These drugs include pergolide (or Permax), as well as two new drugs, Mirapex and Requip.

• Pharmacological Dopamine Agonists

An "agonist" is a chemical with the ability to work together with a neurotransmitter and enhance its action. Pergolide or Permax is a dopamine agonist proved to be beneficial in slowing the rate of Parkinson's and in treating symptoms.

In a seven-year follow-up study conducted with Parkinson's patients who took pergolide, for example, researchers in Rochester, New York, discovered that the subgroup of participants who had received pergolide for up to seven years had no clinical progression in their Parkinson's disease; in other words, their symptoms did not worsen over the seven years of the study while they took pergolide. In related studies, investigators have found that constant administration of pergolide to rats slowed the age-related loss of dopamine-containing neurons. Similar findings have also been observed with Mirapex and Requip, two newly developed dopamine-agonist drugs. These medications are only available by prescription.

RECOMMENDED DOSE: These drugs are available by prescription only; consult with your health care provider.

Gangliosides and Parkinson's Disease

Rationale for Use of Gangliosides in Parkinson's Disease Gangliosides are a particular mixture of sugars and fats that are found in high concentrations in our nervous systems. Administration of gangliosides stimulates the activity of dopamine-producing cells and repairs them after injury. Gangliosides also help in the maintenance and integrity of brain axons, as well as in rebuilding myelin in the brain.

Interestingly, milk from different species contains different proportions of gangliosides, and human milk has a high concentration of a beneficial ganglioside known as GM1. Investigators have studied GM1 for its beneficial effect in Parkinson's disease.

Clinical Studies of GM1 in Parkinson's Disease Forty-five patients with mild to moderate Parkinson's disease were treated with 200 mg of GM1 daily for 16 weeks. They were examined monthly by neurologists trained to evaluate motor disability in Parkinson's patients. At the end of the study, there was a significant improvement in the Parkinson's patients treated with GM1, which was well tolerated (no adverse effects were reported by patients).

RECOMMENDED DOSE: Studies were done on Parkinson's patients who were using subcutaneous injections of GM1. Abbott Laboratories in Spain has produced a ganglioside which is supplemented in infant formulas and may be available for adult use in oral form.

Symptomatic Compounds

While medications that treat symptoms don't get to the root of what is causing a disease, we should control symptoms as much as possible in diseases like Parkinson's. Unfortunately, many patients develop tolerance, over time, to the drugs that control the symptoms of Parkinson's disease—Deprenyl and Sinemet— and Sinemet, in particular, can produce major side effects.

• Deprenyl

A number of studies have shown that Deprenyl can decrease the symptoms of Parkinson's in some patients by blocking the enzyme that controls how much dopamine is broken down.

By putting the brakes on this enzyme, which is called monoamine oxidase B, dopamine supplies are allowed to accumulate in the brain. A multicenter study reported in the *New England Journal of Medicine* showed that Deprenyl slowed the progression of Parkinson's disease and delayed the need for symptomatic treatment with Sinemet. Deprenyl is available only by prescription.

> *RECOMMENDED DOSE:* Deprenyl is available only by prescription. Consult your health care professional about using Deprenyl.

• Sinemet

Sinemet, a drug that combines L-dopa with carbi-dopa, is unquestionably the best symptomatic treatment for Parkinson's today. However, since some studies show that treatment with L-dopa hastens the appearance of adverse side effects and eventually results in an intolerance of this drug, we recommend treating Parkinson's symptoms with this agent only when the disease is causing a functional disability. The decision to use Sinemet should be based on the patient's individual needs. Common side effects include nausea, vomiting, and sometimes hallucinations. Sinemet is available only by prescription.

> *RECOMMENDED DOSE:* Sinemet is available only by prescription. Consult your health care professional about using Sinemet.

A Cocktail Approach to Treating Parkinson's Disease

I. Block excessive immune system activity, especially nitric oxide.

1. Vitamin E is an antioxidant that increases glutathione. Recommended dosage of vitamin E is 800 IU daily.

2. Ebselen: This selenium-like compound acts as an antioxidant, enhancing glutathione peroxidase and raising glutathione levels in the brain. It's currently under study.

3. Lipoic acid: This dietary supplement enhances glutathione production, prevents oxidative damage, and improves mitochondrial function. Recommended dosage: 300–600 mg daily.

4. Green tea extract: This powerful antioxidant increases

glutathione levels and possesses anticancer properties. Dosage: 60–120 mg standardized extract daily.

5. Pycnogenol®: This extract of French pine bark maintains glutathione levels in the brain, immune, and circulatory systems, as well as inhibiting the free radical nitric oxide. Dosage: 100–200 mg daily.

6. Glutathione itself protects cells and their mitochondria from free radical damage. Parkinson's patients are deficient in glutathione, and IV gluthathione may improve symptoms and retard the progression of Parkinson's disease. It should be used only under the supervision of a health care provider.

7. Isothiocyanates, a new type of antioxidant that can cross the blood-brain barrier, promise to be neuroprotective and increase glutathione levels.

8. Lactoferrin: This compound, available in health food stores, binds excessive iron and prevents its absorption. It should not be used except under the care of a health care practitioner.

9. Milk thistle is a natural herb that detoxifies the liver and increases glutathione levels. Dosage: 150–300 mg of standardized extract daily.

II. Enhance mitochondrial function in Parkinson's patients.

1. Coenzyme Q10 protects the mitochondria from free radical damage. Recommended dosage is 200 mg daily with food. Idebenone is a coenzyme Q10 analog that may also be beneficial for Parkinson's patients, but it is not available in the United States.

2. NADH is a natural compound that contributes to the production of dopamine. Recommended dosage of NADH is 10 mg daily, divided into two 5 mg doses.

III. Regenerate dopamine-producing cells.

1. Dopamine agonist drugs stimulate the production of dopamine.

a. Pergolide (Permax) slows the loss of dopamine-producing neurons. It is available only by prescription; check with your health care provider.

b. Mirapex slows the loss of dopamine-producing neurons. It is available only by prescription; check with your health care provider.

    c. Requip slows the loss of dopamine-producing neurons. It is available only by prescription; check with your health care provider.

    2. Gangliosides: This mixture of sugars and fats found in high concentrations in the brain stimulates dopamine-producing cells and repairs them after injury. Gangliosides are not currently available as supplements in the United States.

    IV. Provide symptomatic relief.

    1. Deprenyl: This prescription medication appears to slow the progression of Parkinson's disease. Deprenyl is available only by prescription; speak to your health care provider about its use.

    2. Sinemet: This drug has excellent symptomatic benefit, but its use in early Parkinson's disease is controversial because of its potential to stimulate free radical production and its side effects. Sinemet is available only by prescription.

CHAPTER 7

MULTIPLE SCLEROSIS

Regina was just twenty-eight years old when she first started experiencing numbness and tingling in her left foot. She ignored the sensation, since it wasn't painful, and soon enough the symptoms went away.

It was during her divorce nearly two years later, after a bad bout with the flu, that the numbness returned. However, this time she felt the strange feeling in both feet. She was anxious these days, and having a lot of trouble sleeping, but she attributed all her symptoms to the increased stress in her life. After all, here she was, suddenly a single mother of two young children and working full-time besides.

Her doctor found nothing wrong and prescribed antidepressants. The symptoms receded, and she didn't think much more about them—other than to be thankful that she was feeling good again. Then, just a year later, she suddenly lost the vision in one eye while reading the newspaper.

That's when her family doctor sent Regina to a neurologist. An MRI scan of her brain revealed the classic plaques of multiple sclerosis on the nerve fibers in her brain, confirming the neurologist's suspicions.

Multiple Sclerosis: An Overview

In recent decades, investigators have been relentless in their search for understanding the causes of multiple sclerosis and the development of new treatment protocols aimed at throwing a stumbling block in its path. They have succeeded in ferreting out a great deal of information. Yet, many practitioners still catalogue multiple sclerosis as a chronic disease for which there is no known cause or cure.

In fact, multiple sclerosis affects about 300,000 Americans in ways as various as the individuals whose lives it strikes. For some, the disease is relatively mild. Others experience severe disability. Although there are no magic bullets for curing multiple sclerosis, it is now possible to aggressively—and successfully—treat the disease.

Multiple sclerosis typically affects women of childbearing age and almost always strikes adults between the ages of thirty and fifty. The term "multiple sclerosis" literally means "many scars," and refers to the scarring on the nerve fibers—or plaques—caused by the disease.

The plaques, which are readily seen with today's MRI techniques, represent areas on nerve cell fibers in the brain and spinal cord where the myelin—the fatty insulation covering the fibers—has worn away. These gaps in myelin sheathing interfere with the high-speed transmission of electrical messages between the central nervous system and the rest of the body.

Although multiple sclerosis is categorized as a neurological disease, it is also a disease of the immune system. For patients with multiple sclerosis, the immune system turns against the body instead of defending it—thus putting multiple sclerosis in the broader category of autoimmune diseases. In other words, multiple sclerosis is a good example of the interrelatedness of our body systems.

In the case of multiple sclerosis, myelin is clearly the target of the immune system's attack. More specifically, the bull's-eye of the target is a myelin basic protein.

You'll read about myelin basic protein later in this chapter. We will also discuss the controversial link between certain dietary fats and multiple sclerosis, and point out the value of nutritional supplements in preventing myelin degeneration.

From the onset of symptoms to diagnosis, from treatment to hope on the horizon, in this chapter we discuss multiple sclerosis in the light of what we know about how the disease affects the brain-immune system at its most intricate biochemical level. At the end of the chapter, you will find an aggressive treatment plan based on the most current information available on medications and nutritional therapies.

What Goes Wrong in Multiple Sclerosis, and Why

In multiple sclerosis, normal immunological reactions become damaging because immune cells target the body's own cellular structures—in other words, the immune system loses its capacity to recognize its own body. Our new grasp of what makes otherwise protective immune mechanisms tailspin out of control is the basis for treating the disease today.

As we know, the immune system is normally capable of identifying invaders such as viruses and bacteria by "reading" molecular codes found on cell surfaces. These molecular codes are like the flags of different armies. The immune system will not attack an invader if it sees a flag belonging to its own army.

However, various types of viruses and bacteria successfully camouflage themselves against attack by the immune system with molecular codes on their cell surfaces identical to the components in your own body. Several viruses can play hide-and-seek with the immune system by changing their flag colors to look like the colors sported by its host. These foxy viruses include measles, herpes simplex 6, and the Epstein-Barr virus.

Viruses have been implicated by various researchers as being the initiating event in multiple sclerosis. The evidence supporting a viral etiology of multiple sclerosis includes geographic clustering of multiple sclerosis cases, animal models in which a viral infection mimics the effects of multiple sclerosis, and high levels of antibodies to certain viral infections in multiple sclerosis patients.

Recently, a human herpesvirus (human herpesvirus 6 or HHV-6) has been reported to be found at high levels in the plaques of multiple sclerosis patients. Furthermore, an elevated antibody response to HHV-6 has also been detected in patients with relapsing-remitting types of multiple sclerosis.

When this happens, the immune system becomes confused and may either ignore the invader completely or go on the offensive against parts of itself. This "molecular mimicry" is especially relevant to multiple sclerosis. Although the mechanism is still not completely understood, scientists now believe that previous exposure to one of these mimicking viruses causes the immune system to create antibodies to that virus. When the virus is no longer around, something prompts the immune system to create antibodies to the body's own brain myelin—which has molecular components bearing an uncanny resemblance to that virus.

Myelin is the fatty insulating substance surrounding nerve sheaths in the brain and spinal cord much the same way we coat electrical wires with protective rubber to ensure effective transmissions. Made up of fats, it is white in appearance and serves to conduct nerve impulses between various regions of the nervous system.

Disruption of myelin, or demyelination, impairs the ability of nerve fibers to transmit impulses and is responsible for many symptoms of multiple sclerosis, including weakness, sensory loss, and visual disturbances. How severely multiple sclerosis affects patients may be directly related to the profusion and locations of the scarring, or plaques, on the brain and spinal cord.

In multiple sclerosis patients, all of the immune system's components are involved in one way or another in this inadvertent attack on the brain's myelin. These components include B cells, T cells, macrophages, and all of the associated cytokines, the chemical mediators serving in this biological warfare.

B cells, as you may recall, are the immune system components responsible for manufacturing immunoglobulins such as IgG, large protein molecules designed to specifically recognize and bind to invading substances—also called the "antigens"—in order to transform them into targets for future attack by other immune system warriors, including T cells and macrophages.

People with multiple sclerosis have elevated levels of the IgG immunoglobulin in their cerebrospinal fluid, as well as in the brain. Tragically, these IgG protein molecules have chosen to target the myelin basic protein.

Why does this happen? To put it in simplest terms, myelin is made up of lipids, complex fats, and proteins. The immune system can misidentify the myelin basic protein as a foreign substance because it has a similar molecular code as a virus that the multiple sclerosis patient was exposed to earlier in life, such as measles.

Once the B cells go on the attack, warrior T cells and foot soldier macrophages are automatically called into action, further damaging the wrongly victimized brain tissue. T cells perpetuate the biological error, signaling further reserves when they release their cytokines, the chemical mediators of the immune system.

Many studies reveal a clear association between one particular cytokine, called tumor necrosis factor (TNF), and multiple sclerosis attacks. In a two-year study conducted with multiple sclerosis patients between twenty and fifty years old, Dr. Romain Hentges and his colleagues measured the levels of TNF in the cerebrospinal fluid and serum and correlated those levels with the way the disease progressed in each patient.

Their results, which they published in the *New England Journal of Medicine,* demonstrated that over half of the patients with chronic progressive multiple sclerosis had elevated TNF levels. Not one of the patients with stable multiple sclerosis had the same escalating levels of this busy cytokine.

Why would patients with elevated TNF levels suffer more from multiple sclerosis attacks?

When your immune system is working properly, the body's own blood-brain barrier—the cellular and chemical guards that select which substances are granted permission to pass into the brain from the blood capillaries—keeps out invaders.

However, one function of the TNF cytokine is to create passages for other components of the immune system to cross the blood-brain barrier and enter into the battle zone, much the way army engineers build roads and bridges to allow further reserve troops to enter a war zone.

Without the help of TNF, the hand-to-hand combatants of our immune system—our macrophages—could never make it into the front line trenches of the brain. This breakdown of the blood-brain barrier is the first rung on the ladder to multiple sclerosis attacks, for it is followed by inflammation, the breakdown of myelin, and the formation of hard fibrous material (the scars, or sclerosis) on the nerve fibers.

How do the macrophages carry out their assault once they successfully cross the blood-brain barrier? Recall that macrophages are mobile white blood cells which can literally chew off pieces of invaders and engulf them. They damage the brain's myelin by secreting enzymes that break down the molecular components of the sheathing.

The macrophage-produced agents include arachidonic acid, free radicals, and other inflammatory substances which cause most of the damage to myelin in the immune system attacks common to multiple sclerosis. Gamma interferon, typically produced as a result of viral infections or nonspecific inflammation, joins in to amplify the immune response against myelin.

Other chemical mediators of inflammation, cytokines, are abnormally released in MS as well. In particular, a cytokine known as IL-12 (interleukin-12) has been implicated in multiple sclerosis. IL-12 can be stimulated by certain viruses (including the *Herpes simplex* virus), bacteria, and intracellular parasites.

IL-12 enhances the immune system response, but in the process, it can also produce considerable damage to the body. Plaques of multiple sclerosis patients contain high levels of IL-12, and most beneficial therapies for multiple sclerosis share the common feature of suppressing IL-12 activity.

Knowledge about the association of IL-12 with multiple sclerosis will allow the development of better therapies in the near future. For instance, increasing the anti-inflammatory regulatory cytokine IL-10 can reduce the harmful effects of IL-12 and may provide novel therapies for multiple sclerosis patients. They will be discussed in detail later in this chapter.

Why Does Multiple Sclerosis Affect More Women Than Men?

The estrogen hormone appears to play a role in a number of autoimmune diseases. This is supported by the fact that all autoimmune diseases are far more common in women than in men, particularly during childbearing years when estrogen levels are greatest.

At least part of the reason is that estrogen plays a role in autoimmune diseases is because estrogen stimulates the production of gamma interferon in the immune system. Gamma interferon, which is also found in the ovaries and may be manufactured there as well as in the immune system, activates macrophages and enhances the ability of T cells to target foreign substances—immune responses which are particularly detrimental in multiple sclerosis.

This does not mean that estrogen in and of itself is always bad in multiple sclerosis. In fact, the opposite may be true. It has been noted that the severity of symptoms in multiple sclerosis patients is lowest in pregnant women during their third trimester, when estrogen levels are highest. Furthermore, estriol (a low-potency estrogen compound) significantly reduces disease activity in animal models of multiple sclerosis. Estrogen appears to increase the anti-inflammatory cytokine IL-10. Levels of IL-10 are significantly lower during acute stages of multiple sclerosis. Thus, estriol may be of benefit by restoring levels of this immune compound to their normal range.

Why Are Multiple Sclerosis Attacks Often Linked to Stress?

Stress is interpreted by the body as a danger signal and results in the "fight or flight" response which affects both the brain and the immune system. On a biochemical level, the fight or flight system involves the brain's production of hormones and their influence on the adrenal glands and immune cells. This triad is known as the brain-adrenal-immune axis.

Today, we know that the brain regions involved in the fight or flight response include the hypothalamus, which releases corticotropin-releasing factor (CRF) and the pituitary, which releases ACTH. These two hormones directly influence the adrenal glands to increase the manufacture and release of cortisol, which in turn allows the muscles, brain, and heart to metabolize more glucose and have the energy at hand to respond to threatening events.

According to researchers at the National Institute of Mental Health, immune cytokines not only activate immune function when you're under stress, they also recruit the neurotransmitters essential in modulating your immune response and activating behaviors that may be important during injury or inflammation.

These investigators suggest that diseases characterized by both inflammation and emotional stress—like multiple sclerosis—may be the result of common alterations in the brain–immune system connection. Cytokines produced by immune-inflammatory cells such as interleukin and TNF (tumor necrosis factor) stimulate parts of the brain, including the hypothalamus, to secrete cortico-tropin-releasing hormone and cause a chemical domino effect. The last domino down is the release of corticosteroids.

Corticosteroids function to suppress inflammation and the immune response. To understand why your body's primary response to stress, in essence, is to produce larger amounts of cortisol, think of it this way: The effect of heightened cortisol production is to suppress the immune system's responses. And that's only logical, for why should your body care about fighting an infection when you need extra energy to combat a more immediate danger?

This suppressive effect is typically short-lived. Once the immediate danger is removed, your immune system should recover. In other words, during periods of acute stress, your body produces heightened levels of cortisol and a decrease in inflammation.

However, during periods of chronic stress, this sustained increase in cortisol is capable of derailing the immune system in ways that persist far beyond immediate goals. This derailment is analogous to "the boy who cried wolf," in that the danger signals are ignored because of their persistence. The inflammation continues, because the cortisol receptors have blunted the immuno-suppressant response.

Clinicians typically define stress as life events that require significant changes in behavior to readjust to them. Since research into a possible relationship between stress and illness began half a century ago, a number of studies have linked emotional stress to illnesses as varied as tuberculosis, ulcers, heart attacks, leukemia, juvenile diabetes, and a general susceptibility

TABLE **5**

MULTIPLE SCLEROSIS: A CASCADE OF MYELIN DAMAGE

1. The body is exposed early to a virus which mimics myelin basic protein, such as herpes simplex 6, Epstein-Barr virus, adenovirus, or measles.

2. The immune system calls B cells into action, making IgG.

3. IgG binds to myelin basic protein, further identifying it as a foreign invader.

4. T cells respond to the IgG signal, starting the next phase of immune response: the production of tumor necrosis factor and gamma interferon cytokines.

5. Tumor necrosis factor paves the way for macrophages to begin devouring "invaders."

6. Macrophages use toxic biological weaponry, such as arachidonic acid and free radicals, to chew off neuron myelin and impair electrical transmission between the central nervous system and muscles.

to illness. Now researchers believe that stress can be one of the components of any disease.

In patients with multiple sclerosis, stress unleashes destructive immune processes from their normal regulatory constraints. As we saw in Regina's case, a multiple sclerosis attack is often preceded by a stressful life event such as a divorce. A number of researchers have examined the lives of multiple sclerosis patients and discovered relationships between the disease and emotional stress.

Infections: Another Kind of Stress

As we saw in Chapter 1, infections provoke the immune system into action. Common viral, urinary tract, and yeast infections can all prod the immune system and result in a relapse for multiple sclerosis patients when the foreign invader produces a state of heightened alertness by the immune system.

A Combined Medical and Nutritional Approach to Multiple Sclerosis

In the section below, we outline a complete guideline for care of patients with multiple sclerosis. This plan combines the latest information on the benefits of low-fat diets and neuroimmuno-modulating substances you can add to your diet right away.

Perhaps more than any other neurological illness described in these pages, the severity of multiple sclerosis attacks has been clearly linked to stress. Therefore, all patients diagnosed with multiple sclerosis should consider including such support as psychotherapy or counseling groups, meditation, and biofeedback as a first step toward treating the disease.

In addition to modulating stress, multiple sclerosis patients can immediately begin decreasing the number of pro-inflammatory immune cells and increasing anti-inflammatory immune cells by adopting a low-fat diet and adding nutritional supplements that are readily available at your health food store. These neuroimmunomodulating agents include PS (phosphatidylserine) and antioxidants.

When Should You Suspect Multiple Sclerosis?

There are three types of multiple sclerosis. The first, and most common, is the "relapse-remitting" form of the disease, where an attack with full-blown symptoms is followed by a period of remission when the body returns to its former state or to a slightly worsened state.

In some individuals, however, the disease can take a more chronic, progressive path with very few instances of remission. Rarer still is the case of "galloping" multiple sclerosis, where the disease moves quickly through the body and causes rapid debilitation.

Early signs of multiple sclerosis include the following:

- A tingling sensation in the extremities
- Dragging either foot while walking
- Loss of sensation and coordination

- Blurred or double vision
- Problems urinating
- Abnormal fatigue, to the point where even common daily activities are too tiring

Diagnosing Multiple Sclerosis

Over the past decade, physicians have armed themselves with a number of tests to diagnose multiple sclerosis. Early tests involved drawing blood samples and analyzing it for the presence of abnormal amounts of IgG or red cell mobility. Today's neurologists rely on CAT (computed axial tomography) scans, MRI (magnetic resonance imaging), and analysis of immunological markers in cerebrospinal fluid. These scanning devices all help pinpoint specific tissue damage such as plaques, atrophy, and inflammation.

Multiple sclerosis symptoms mimic those of other disorders, including Lyme disease, certain viral infections, other autoimmune diseases such as lupus, and B_{12} deficiency. It is essential to rule these disorders out during diagnosis, as many of them are easily treatable.

• *Lyme Disease*

Endemic to certain areas of the United States, Lyme disease is spread by ticks. It may be characterized by a bull's-eye-shaped rash, fever, and swollen, painful joints. However, these symptoms are not inevitable, and Lyme disease may produce a clinical state that is very similar to multiple sclerosis, including demyelination of the brain. Unfortunately, the routine blood test for Lyme disease may not be specific or sensitive enough to give an accurate result. To adequately determine whether the symptoms are caused by Lyme or multiple sclerosis, the physician may order a spinal tap with analysis of Lyme in the cerebrospinal fluid.

• *Lupus, Sjogren's Syndrome and Other Autoimmune Diseases*

All autoimmune diseases require blood testing to determine the presence of certain antibodies that serve as biological markers.

• B_{12} Deficiency

A deficiency of the B_{12} vitamin can cause demyelination, as normal B_{12} levels are required for adequate myelin synthesis. Patients with multiple sclerosis should be screened for B_{12} deficiency, as such a deficiency requires treatment.

Dietary Suggestions for Patients with Multiple Sclerosis

• Begin a Low-Fat Diet

As in the case of so many other chronic diseases, saturated fats do terrible damage to blood vessel walls in multiple sclerosis patients. A diet high in saturated fats causes platelets in the blood to bunch together and stretch blood vessel walls. When the blood-brain barrier breaks down, toxic materials seep through the blood into the brain and a cascade of immune responses begins, resulting in the myelin breakdown and scarring of nerve fibers so characteristic of multiple sclerosis.

Investigators now believe that a diet low in saturated fat is one of the best tools in the fight against multiple sclerosis. Shifting to certain polyunsaturated (omega-3) fats may also strengthen blood vessel walls, as these are the fats that make up the lipids in the brain and myelin sheathing.

Since 1948, clinicians have been employing diets low in saturated fats when treating multiple sclerosis patients, while researchers strive to find the biochemical links between fat and the disease's pathway.

Researchers attempting to unearth the causes of multiple sclerosis have pinpointed a number of dietary factors based simply on the disease's prevalence around the world.

For example, more cases of multiple sclerosis show up in populations living in higher latitudes, and the highest risk areas include the northern United States and Canada, Great Britain, Scandinavia, northern Europe, New Zealand, and Tasmania. In other words, multiple sclerosis is far more common among people who rely on diets high in saturated fat.

Comparing inland farming communities in Norway to seacoast villages in that country, for instance, has led investigators to conclude that the inland farmers suffered a higher incidence of multiple sclerosis at least partly because they ate greater quantities of saturated animal fat than their seacoast neighbors.

Dr. Roy Swank, professor of neurology at the University of Oregon Medical School, has provided the most successful dietary programs designed to treat multiple sclerosis. As early as 1950, he proposed an association between high levels of dietary fat and the incidence of multiple sclerosis.

In Swank's studies, which were conducted over a period of more than fifteen years, he has found that patients who ate low-fat diets (less than 20 grams a day) are less likely to be disabled by multiple sclerosis attacks. In particular, minimally disabled patients who followed his dietary recommendations deteriorated little if at all.

Some investigators are currently studying whether a deficient intake in certain polyunsaturated fatty acids—so crucial for cell metabolism and healthy cell membranes—might also be an essential link between fats and multiple sclerosis. For example, in a trial using polyunsaturated fatty acids in treating multiple sclerosis, researchers at the Royal Victoria Infirmary of Newcastle, England, have confirmed earlier studies demonstrating that manipulating and supplementing dietary intake of "good" fats—the omega-3 and omega-6 polyunsaturated fatty acids—can alter the percentages of fatty acids in the blood serum of multiple sclerosis patients.

In light of the research conducted so far on using nutrition to manage multiple sclerosis, we recommend the following:

- Decrease your saturated fat intake to no more than 5–10 grams per day by opting for vegetarian protein from beans, grains, and vegetables.
- Increase your omega-3 and GLA omega-6 fats to 50 grams a day by eating more fish and fish oils, particularly those containing EPA and DHA, flaxseed oil, and borage oil.
- Follow the basic nutritional principles outlined earlier in this book.

The Three R's of Managing Multiple Sclerosis: Reduce Inflammation, Raise Mitochondrial Action, and Regenerate Myelin

The most effective strategy for managing multiple sclerosis is to reduce inflammation, raise mitochondrial action, and regenerate the myelin sheaths that protect our nerves, including the spinal cord (or at the very least, slow the destruction of those myelin sheaths). Let's examine the pharmaceutical drugs and nutritional substances that help to accomplish each of these objectives.

Strategies to Reduce Inflammation

• *Vitamin Therapy and Multiple Sclerosis*

The most-studied nutritional substances in the treatment of multiple sclerosis are essential vitamin D, antioxidants, and fatty acids. We will discuss each one separately.

• *Vitamin D and Multiple Sclerosis*

Rationale for Use of Vitamin D in Multiple Sclerosis It has been speculated that sunlight plays a protective role in multiple sclerosis. Epidemiological studies have demonstrated that people in northern climates are more commonly affected with multiple sclerosis than those in southern climates. The protective effect of sunlight against multiple sclerosis may have to do with the fact that vitamin D is capable of suppressing an overactive immune system by inhibiting the activity of the pro-inflammatory cytokine IL-12 and enhancing production of the anti-inflammatory cytokine IL-10.

Clinical Studies of Vitamin D in Multiple Sclerosis Vitamin D deficiency has been reported commonly in multiple sclerosis patients. Although no human studies have been performed to date, administration of vitamin D has shown a beneficial effect on various animal models of the disease. Vitamin D increases IL-10, the cytokine responsible for suppressing multiple sclerosis disease activity.

> RECOMMENDED DOSE: The RDA of vitamin D is 400 international units (IU) a day, but researchers studying the effects of vitamin D in multiple sclerosis believe that much higher doses are necessary to inhibit excess immune system activity. Doses up to 3200 units a day have been suggested, but consult with your health care practitioner prior to using this higher dose of vitamin D. This vitamin produces high calcium levels and should be used with caution when using higher-than-RDA doses.

•Antioxidants and Multiple Sclerosis

Protecting Cells Subjected to Oxidative Stress Recall that one of the major mechanisms of injury in cells is oxidative stress, and that oxidative stress is increased when the immune system mobilizes and causes our cells to metabolize more oxygen and spin off greater numbers of oxygen free radicals desperately searching for electrons. While these free radicals accomplish their goal of destroying invaders, they may also damage healthy cells in the process, tearing apart cell membranes and dissolving valuable genetic material.

Cell membrane destruction may result in cellular death. This oxidative stress death warrant may have a greater impact on brain cells because of their constant high rate of oxygen consumption and high numbers of mitochondria, the cellular energy factories our bodies depend on to convert glucose into energy.

A number of studies with multiple sclerosis patients have demonstrated that they experience higher levels of lipid oxidation during attacks. For instance, French researchers reporting in a 1996 *Journal of Neuroimmunology* article tested multiple sclerosis patients for antibodies directed against ten fatty acids and found that these patients had significantly elevated levels of antibodies to those fatty acids. They concluded that, in multiple sclerosis, the cell membranes are being attacked by the immune system, a factor that may arise because the membranes have already been battered by oxidative processes.

In short, then, patients with multiple sclerosis may suffer from increased lipid oxidation that is potentially damaging to the myelin sheath so essential to conducting messages along nerve cells. Basically, free radicals amplify injury to myelin by disrupting its fatty acid components.

Evidence of direct free radical damage in multiple sclerosis patients has recently been reported by researchers in the *Journal of Neurology*. Multiple sclerosis patients have significantly increased levels of lipid peroxidation during exacerbation of attacks, as well as lower vitamin E levels. In particular, the free radical nitric oxide appears to wreak havoc on the myelin of patients with multiple sclerosis. Nitric acid is released by macrophages, the foot soldiers of the immune system, during immune system attack. Nitric oxide is a very profound free radical that performs its activities as a gas. Antioxidants that inhibit nitric oxide production and therefore its attack on myelin may be of benefit in multiple sclerosis patients. Certain antioxidants, including proanthocyanidins, are known to inhibit nitric oxide. Nitric oxide is also inhibited by the cholesterol-lowering drug Lovastatin.

Clinical Studies of Use of Antioxidants in Multiple Sclerosis While no clinical studies have demonstrated the beneficial effects of antioxidants in multiple sclerosis patients, based on the experimental data mentioned above, it seems worthwhile to recommend that multiple sclerosis patients take a balanced, complete antioxidant formula, as outlined in earlier chapters of this book.

Furthermore, specifically targeting free radical activity appears to be especially important. This includes targeting the compound nitric oxide. As we mentioned earlier, nitric oxide is released by macrophages during immune system activity and is a known cause of injury to myelin during multiple sclerosis attacks. Nitric oxide inhibitors are currently under study for the treatment of multiple sclerosis. These include the dietary supplements Pycnogenol® and green tea extract, and the cholesterol-lowering drug Lovastatin.

• Pycnogenol® and Multiple Sclerosis

Rationale for Use of Pycnogenol® in Multiple Sclerosis Pycnogenol® is an extract of French pine bark. It contains a specific mixture of flavonoids, and Pycnogenol®'s therapeutic effects are due to its strong free radical–scavenging ability. In particular, Pycnogenol® is able to inhibit free radical production of nitric oxide from macrophages. This is likely to be important in multiple sclerosis since, as we've discussed, macrophage-generated nitric oxide is particularly destructive to the myelin sheath.

There are no clinical studies utilizing Pycnogenol® in multiple sclerosis, but it is strongly suggested, based on its mechanism of action.

RECOMMENDED DOSE: 100–200 mg daily.

• Epigallocatechin, a Green Tea Extract, and Multiple Sclerosis

Rationale for Use of Epigallocatechin in Multiple Sclerosis As mentioned above, the free radical nitric oxide participates in the inflammatory cascade that ultimately results in myelin damage. Epigallocatechin inhibits nitric oxide production by reducing the activity of a gene known as nuclear factor kappa beta. By reducing nuclear factor kappa beta, epigallocatechin protects our brains from excessive immune system activity.

While there are no clinical data supporting the use of epigallocatechin in multiple sclerosis, its ability to turn off pro-inflammatory genes like nuclear factor kappa beta and reduce nitric oxide make it a strong candidate for potential use in multiple sclerosis.

RECOMMENDED DOSE: 60–120 mg of standardized green tea extract.

• Lovastatin and Multiple Sclerosis

Rationale for Use of Lovastatin in Multiple Sclerosis Lovastatin is an anticholesterol medication that has been demonstrated to decrease the production of the free radical nitric oxide. By preventing the release of nitric oxide, Lovastatin may prevent this free radical from injuring myelin sheaths in multiple sclerosis. Lovastatin also reduces the proinflammatory cytokines TNF and gamma interferon.

Clinical Studies of Lovastatin in Multiple Sclerosis In a recent study reported in *Neuroscience Letters,* researchers at the University of South Carolina demonstrated that administration of Lovastatin to animals with an experimental form of multiple sclerosis significantly lessened the severity of the disease. This beneficial effect of Lovastatin in the animal model of multiple sclerosis appears to be mediated by its ability to inhibit the production of the free radical nitric oxide.

More studies are certainly required to support this observation, but patients with multiple sclerosis as well as elevated cholesterol should discuss the use of Lovastatin therapy with their health care practitioners.

RECOMMENDED DOSE: The dose of this prescription medication should be determined by your physician.

• Tumor Necrosis Factor Blockers and Multiple Sclerosis

Rationale for Use of Tumor Necrosis Factor Blockers in Multiple Sclerosis Tumor necrosis factor is a pro-inflammatory cytokine produced by white blood cells, and it has been implicated in the pathogenesis of multiple sclerosis. Tumor necrosis factor contributes to the inflammatory process by enhancing the ability of white blood cells to penetrate the blood-brain barrier, as well as upregulating the inflammatory cells of the immune system. Several drugs that block tumor necrosis factor have recently been developed. They are currently indicated and marketed for treating rheumatoid arthritis. Two classes of natural compounds, which are also tumor necrosis factor blockers, potentially have usefulness in multiple sclerosis. These include a phospholipid known as phosphatidylserine, and other substances called phosphodiesterase inhibitors.

• Phosphatidylserine (PS) and Multiple Sclerosis

Rationale for Use of Phosphatidylserine in Multiple Sclerosis As we mentioned earlier, TNF (tumor necrosis factor) is a potent cytokine, one of the most tireless advance soldiers of the immune system. As a pro-inflammatory substance, it plays a crucial role in the development and debilitating progress of multiple sclerosis by creating passageways for crusading macrophages to barge across the blood-brain barrier and attack myelin. Multiple sclerosis patients have elevated levels of TNF in various organs of their bodies during acute attacks, and higher levels of TNF overall than people who do not have the disease.

Today, researchers are using this information to investigate the potential benefits of a variety of substances heralded for their anti-TNF activity. These include the phospholipid phosphatidylserine.

One of the essential lipids in cell membranes, phosphatidylserine is a safe, over-the-counter substance that definitely reduces levels of the TNF cytokine. Animal studies conducted by Dr. Cedric Raine and his colleagues at Albert Einstein College of Medicine reveal that this phospholipid protects against "experimental autoimmune encephalomyelitis," or EAE, an animal model for multiple sclerosis. EAE models multiple sclerosis because it, too, is an acute inflammatory disease of the central nervous system induced by sensitization to the molecular components of myelin.

In EAE, as in multiple sclerosis, the cytokine mediator TNF charges to battle, causing inflammation and paving the way for macrophages to reach the brain. Recent experiments show that administering extra doses of phosphatidylserine, the phospholipid normally present in cell membranes, can actually reduce the levels of TNF in mice.

In addition, phosphatidylserine may also inhibit the overzealous production of fighter T cells that can contribute to the progression of diseases like EAE and multiple sclerosis. We recommend that all multiple sclerosis patients incorporate a PS supplement into their diets.

Clinical Studies of Phosphatidylserine in Multiple Sclerosis In an animal model of multiple sclerosis, researchers at the Albert Einstein College of Medicine tested phosphatidylserine's ability to inhibit tumor necrosis factor and affect disease activity in experimental mice with the disease. Animals treated with phosphatidylserine did not relapse, while untreated mice developed severe clinical demyelination. Furthermore, in the phosphatidylserine-treated animals, tumor necrosis factor was inhibited by up to 80–90 percent.

To date, there are no human studies to support a role for phosphatidylserine in treating multiple sclerosis. However, based upon the above data, phosphatidylserine seems worthy of clinical studies, and has been employed in many clinicians' practices as an adjunctive treatment for multiple sclerosis.

RECOMMENDED DOSE: 300 mg daily. Precautions: None.

• PD4 Inhibitors and Multiple Sclerosis

Rationale for Use of PD4 Inhibitors in Multiple Sclerosis Phosphodiesterase, or PD4, inhibitors are compounds that increase an intracellular compound known as cyclic AMP. By increasing AMP, these compounds act as an anti-inflammatory agent. PD4 inhibitors are currently under study for possible benefit in multiple sclerosis. Researchers at the National Institute of Neurological Disorders observed that PD4 inhibitors suppressed the induction of multiple sclerosis in animal models of the disease. It is speculated that the beneficial effects of PD4 inhibitors are due to their ability to suppress tumor necrosis factor.

Certain flavonoids found in nature are also PD4 inhibitors. These include the compound genistein and sculteria, two dietary supplements. While there are no studies examining the effects of these flavonoids on multiple sclerosis and their activity as PD4 inhibitors (and, therefore, also as tumor necrosis factor blockers), these properties make them excellent candidates for adjunctive treatment for multiple sclerosis patients. Furthermore, with regard to genistein, an additional benefit in multiple sclerosis may be due to its estrogen-mimicking effect. As you may recall, estrogen has been demonstrated to suppress multiple sclerosis by acting as an anti-inflammatory and increasing the anti-inflammatory cytokine interleukin-10. Genistein, by sharing those properties with estrogen, may provide additional support against multiple sclerosis by this mechanism.

RECOMMENDED DOSE: 50 mg of genistein daily; 200 mg of quercetin daily.

•Estrogen and Multiple Sclerosis

Rationale for Use of Estrogen in Multiple Sclerosis Estriol is a natural estrogen compound that has favorable effects on the immune system in MS patients. It has been noted that MS severity is reduced during late pregnancy, when estrogen levels are highest. Estriol increases the anti-inflammatory cytokine IL-10. Subsequently, increased IL-10 levels are associated with decreased severity of MS disease.

Clinical Studies of Estriol in Multiple Sclerosis In experimental models of multiple sclerosis, estriol significantly reduced the severity of multiple sclerosis symptoms. This finding was recently reported in the journal *Neurology* by researchers at the University of California-Los Angeles.

RECOMMENDED DOSE: 2 mg per day. Precautions: All people considering use of estriol or estrogen should consult with their health care practitioners before use. Absolute contraindications include breast cancer, breast masses, uterine cancer, and blood clots.

•Phytoestrogens in Multiple Sclerosis

Rationale for Use of Phytoestrogens in Multiple Sclerosis Phytoestrogens, plant-derived estrogen-like compounds, are alternatives to the use of estrogen or estriol. The phytoestrogen genistein mimics estrogen's effects on estrogen receptors, and also has an anti-inflammatory activity. As we discussed previously, genistein acts as an anti-inflammatory by blocking the phosphodiesterase enzyme.

RECOMMENDED DOSE: 50 mg daily.

•Omega-3 Fatty Acids as Anti-inflammatory Agents in Multiple Sclerosis

Rationale for Use of Omega-3 Fatty Acids in Multiple Sclerosis Remember that the important omega-3 fatty acid DHA is involved in a number of cellular functions and is essential to good communication between nerve cells. In addition, omega-3 fatty acids are important ingredients for your body's production of prostaglandins, some of which serve to tone down immune response.

Certainly, additional research needs to be completed before we can be certain of the role fatty acids play in protecting against multiple sclerosis. However, there is ample evidence now to suggest that omega-3 fatty acids such as DHA should get top billing for their contributions to building up central nervous system lipids and discouraging the formation of certain prostaglandins capable of triggering inflammatory processes and overall cellular malfunction.

Some fatty acids have the potential to build up damaged myelin and help bring the immune system back under control. In addition, studies designed to examine the role that fatty acids play in modulating immune system responses demonstrate that omega-3 fatty acids have a significant modulating effect on the immune system.

We therefore recommend that multiple sclerosis patients supplement their intake of fatty acids with DHA, flaxseed oil, and primrose or borage oils.

RECOMMENDED DOSE:

DHA	300 mg, with a meal.
Flaxseed oil	1 tbsp with a meal.
Primrose or borage oil	2 g with a meal.

Medications for Multiple Sclerosis

• Copaxone and Multiple Sclerosis

Rationale for Use of Copaxone in Multiple Sclerosis Our new understanding of the biochemical processes involved in multiple sclerosis has led to a number of new treatment strategies. One strategy has been to flag the myelin so it doesn't fall under friendly fire from the immune system.

In other studies, physicians have discovered that copolymer-1 is also effective in reversing the process of molecular mimicry that results in myelin breakdown. The copolymer-1 compound was developed at the Weissman Institute in Israel. It is composed of four amino acids with the same sequence and length as myelin basic protein.

The principle in using copolymer-1 to treat multiple sclerosis is simple: When the immune system identifies copolymer-1 as a myelin basic protein, its warriors are distracted from attacking the myelin itself. The drug resembles myelin basic protein so much, in fact, that it may actually inhibit that activation of certain types of warrior T cells in the immune system.

Clinical Studies of Copaxone in Multiple Sclerosis When physicians treated over 250 multiple sclerosis patients with copolymer-1 in a trial involving researchers and patients from eleven different universities, they found that this drug reduced the relapse rate. In fact, over half of the patients taking copolymer-1 were relapse-free, and few patients suffered side effects.

Copaxone is FDA approved for use in multiple sclerosis. It is currently administered by injection. Recently, however, an oral form of Copaxone has been shown to be as effective as the injectible formulation. Copaxone acts to reduce pro-inflammatory cells that attack myelin in the nervous system, and is available only by prescription.

RECOMMENDED DOSE: Copaxone is available only by prescription. Consult with your health care practitioner about use of Copaxone to treat multiple sclerosis.

• Beta Serones and Multiple Sclerosis

Rationale for Betaserones in Multiple Sclerosis Betaserones are currently approved by the FDA for use in multiple sclerosis, but their exact mechanism is unclear. It has recently been proposed that the beneficial activity seen with betaserone treatment is related to increasing levels of interleukin-10, the anti-inflammatory cytokine that is depleted in multiple sclerosis patients.

Interferons are naturally occurring proteins produced by the immune system. Beta interferon has been advocated for use in treating multiple sclerosis because of its antiviral activity and its ability to boost the immune system. In fact, it is produced within the human body naturally in cases of inflammation.

Avonex, a genetically produced beta interferon identical to human interferon, has been approved by the FDA to treat relapsing multiple sclerosis. Recently, a multicenter study showed that Avonex decreases the frequency and extent of attacks in patients with multiple sclerosis.

The drawback to treating multiple sclerosis with interferons lies in the significant side effects that some patients experience, including severe flu symptoms and depression.

However, Avonex, a natural betaserone as opposed to the synthetic ones, has a significantly lesser occurrence of these side effects.

Strategies for Raising Mitochondrial Activity

As we have discussed throughout this book, mitochondrial dysfunction is intimately related to neurological disease. Impairments of mitochondrial activity have been implicated in the pathogenesis of Alzheimer's disease, Parkinson's disease, ALS, and autism.

The role of mitochondrial dysfunction in multiple sclerosis has also recently been suggested. The mitochondria are the workhorses of our cells, including the neurons in our brains. They generate ATP, the biochemical energy that drives all our cells' activities. When mitochondria are injured, cells lose the ability to manufacture ATP, and eventually they die.

Mitochondria are particularly vulnerable to the free radical nitric oxide. As we've discussed, nitric oxide levels are increased in multiple sclerosis patients, and they directly injure myelin sheaths. But nitric oxide is also detrimental to mitochondria; it is toxic to certain enzymes found in the mitochondria, producing cellular energy deficiency. The depletion of cellular energy by nitric oxide may lead to neuronal cell death in multiple sclerosis.

• Mitochondrial Protective Agents and Multiple Sclerosis

Rationale for Use of Mitochondrial-Protective Agents in Multiple Sclerosis Nitric oxide–mediated damage to mitochondrial enzymes can be inhibited by drugs and nutritional compounds that block the production of this destructive free radical. These compounds include Pycnogenol®, green tea extract, and Lovastatin, which we discussed earlier in this chapter. Currently, researchers are developing specific inhibitors of the enzyme that produces nitric oxide. These compounds are promising therapeutic agents in managing multiple sclerosis. Until these drugs become available, we recommend that the specific antioxidants that block nitric oxide production mentioned earlier in this chapter should be employed as part of the cocktail approach to multiple sclerosis.

Strategies for Regenerating Myelin

Rationale for Use of Substances that Regenerate Myelin in Multiple Sclerosis The conventional thinking about the possibility of regenerating myelin in the central nervous system is that it is impossible. While myelin regenerates in our peripheral nerves, myelin had not been thought to be able to regenerate in the central nervous system. However, myelin regeneration in the central nervous system has now been shown in scientific studies. Specific interventions, including drugs under development and experimental treatment with fetal stem cells, have shown the ability to increase myelin in the central nervous system.

• Eliprodil and Multiple Sclerosis

Rationale for Use of Eliprodil in Multiple Sclerosis Eliprodil is a drug currently under study in Europe as a neuroprotective agent. It has two functions: First, it blocks NMDA receptors, while simultaneously increasing the activity of sigma receptors. NMDA receptors, as you may recall from our earlier discussion, potentiate the neurotoxic effects of the amino acid glutamate, resulting in the death of neurons. Like other NMDA blockers, Eliprodil protects cells from excitotoxic death. Second, Eliprodil acts on opiate receptors in the cell. This effect appears to stimulate remyelination in the central nervous system.

Clinical Studies of Eliprodil in Multiple Sclerosis In a recent study, Eliprodil was reported to increase myelin in cell cultures. Further studies in animals and humans are required before widespread use of this compound becomes feasible.

RECOMMENDED DOSE: This drug is being tested in Europe, but is not currently available in the United States.

• Fetal Stem Cells and Multiple Sclerosis

Rationale for Use of Stem Cells in Multiple Sclerosis Stem cells are pluripotent cells; that is, they can grow in any area in the body and replace damaged tissue. Recent data suggest that stem cells have the potential to repair and regenerate myelin sheaths. Currently, researchers are actively studying the use of fetal stem cells as a multiple sclerosis treatment, based on this potential.

RECOMMENDED DOSE: Stem cell treatment is currently experimental.

Putting It All Together

One of the first steps we took in treating Regina was to start her on a low-fat diet and encourage her to begin incorporating vegetarian protein from beans, grains, and vegetables. We also boosted Regina's intake of essential fatty acids with supplements of 300 mg PS and 400 mg DHA, as well as upping her antioxidant activity with a complete antioxidant supplement.

Probably just as important to Regina's health was her ability to manage stress in her life—an essential step in preventing further multiple sclerosis attacks and in getting herself back on her feet following her divorce. Regina joined a support group for single parents at her church, and she is now practicing biofeedback and meditation after a series of stress reduction classes at the hospital. After more than two years, Regina has not experienced another multiple sclerosis attack.

Now that you have an overview of multiple sclerosis and how it affects the very structure, function, and biochemical metabolism of the brain–immune system connection, you are probably eager to get started—or to help someone you love begin—investigating a complete treatment protocol.

Here is our summary guideline for treatment.

A Cocktail Approach to Treating Multiple Sclerosis

I. Reduce inflammation.

1. Vitamin D: Suppresses an overactive immune system. Recommended dosage: 400–3,200 IU, but consult with your health care provider before taking high levels of vitamin D.

2. Take antioxidants that reduce nitric oxide, a free radical.

a. Pycnogenol® inhibits the free radical nitric oxide. Recommended dosage: 100–200 mg.

b. Green tea extract inhibits the free radical nitric oxide. Recommended dosage: 60–120 mg.

c. Lovastatin: This cholesterol-lowering drug is available by prescription only. Consult with your health care provider about taking Lovastatin for MS.

3. Reduce tumor necrosis factor.

a. Phosphatidylserine inhibits tumor necrosis factor. Recommended dose: 300 mg daily.

4. Inhibit the pro-inflammatory PD4 enzyme.

a. Genistein: This phytoestrogen inhibits tumor necrosis factor. Recommended dosage: 50 mg.

b. Quercetin: This dietary supplement inhibits tumor necrosis factor. Recommended dosage: 200 mg.

5. Estriol, a form of estrogen, is available only by prescription. People who have had blood-clotting problems or hormone-sensitive cancers should not take estriol. Your health care provider will determine the dose of estriol that is right for you.

6. Phytoestrogens: These plant-derived substances mimic the effects of estrogen, without its side effects. Recommended dosage: 75–100 mg.

7. Omega-3 fatty acids build up lipids in the central nervous system, and contribute to the production of anti-inflammatory prostaglandins.

a. DHA: Recommended dose: 300 mg with a meal.

b. Primrose oil: Recommended dose: 1 tbsp with a meal.

c. Borage oil: Take 2 g daily with a meal.

8. Medications

a. Copaxone reduces pro-inflammatory cells that attack myelin in the nervous system, and is available only by prescription. Consult with your physician.

b. Betaserones appear to increase levels of interleukin-10, the anti-inflammatory cytokine that is depleted in multiple sclerosis patients. This treatment is available only by prescription. Consult with your health care provider.

II. Raise mitochondrial action.

1. Pyconogenol® protects the mitochondria by inhibiting the free radical nitric oxide. Recommended dosage: 100–200 mg.

2. Green tea extract protects the mitochondria by inhibiting the free radical nitric oxide. Recommended dosage: 60–120 mg of standardized extract.

3. Lovastatin: This cholesterol-lowering drug is available by prescription only. Consult with your health care provider about taking Lovastatin for MS.

III. Regenerate myelin.

1. Eliprodil is an experimental treatment being studied in Europe. It is not approved for use in the United States.

2. Fetal stem cells are being studied for use in treating a number of neurodegenerative diseases, but are still experimental at this time.

CHAPTER 8

AMYOTROPHIC LATERAL SCLEROSIS
(LOU GEHRIG'S DISEASE)

Leonard, an avid golfer, usually left his dental practice early on Wednesdays to get in a round with his partner at the public course just outside of town. It was there, one fine May afternoon, that he noticed he couldn't flex his ankle properly. Leonard attributed this symptom to an old sprain which sometimes acted up in damp weather.

However, Leonard's ankle was no less stiff by Christmas, and he was beginning to notice that his hands, too, were so lame that he had trouble buttoning his shirts. What's more, he felt tired all the time.

"You're too young to act so old," Leonard's wife teased, until he finally relented and saw their family physician.

Leonard's doctor was more concerned than Leonard had expected him to be. He immediately referred Leonard to a neurologist, who performed a complete physical exam and discovered that Leonard showed brisk, abnormal reflexes in his lower extremities.

The neurologist asked Leonard to come in to the hospital for several laboratory and radiographic tests, including a spinal fluid test, a blood test, a magnetic resonance imaging (MRI) test on his brain and spinal cord, and an EMG (electromyogram) to measure the electrical activity in Leonard's nerves and muscles.

These tests confirmed the neurologist's suspicions. He diagnosed amyotrophic lateral sclerosis (ALS), and set up an appointment with Leonard and his wife to discuss treatment options.

Amyotrophic Lateral Sclerosis: An Overview

A progressive neuromuscular disease, amyotrophic lateral sclerosis (ALS) is sometimes referrred to as "Lou Gehrig's disease" for the famous baseball star afflicted with this condition. Other celebrities to be diagnosed with ALS include the musician Charles Mingus and astrophysicist Stephen Hawking.

Nearly 1 out of every 50,000 people worldwide is diagnosed with ALS each year, with over 5,000 new cases reported in the United States annually. Of the U.S. population living today, about 300,000 will die from ALS, with 35,000 Americans suffering from the disease at any one time.

Nearly twice as many men are affected by ALS as women. While most people are diagnosed with the disease in their mid-fifties, ALS has been reported in teenagers and in much older patients.

The incidence of ALS is about equal to that of multiple sclerosis. However, people diagnosed with multiple sclerosis may live for decades with the disease, while those with ALS typically die of the disease between two and five years after diagnosis. ALS places a great financial burden on families, as all people with ALS eventually become bedridden. Care can amount to more than $200,000 annually.

Thankfully, the outlook for people with ALS is now brighter than ever before. Research conducted over the past decades has finally begun to shed light on the actual mechanisms involved in ALS, which was first described in 1869 by the noted French neurologist Jean-Martin Charcot. In fact, in 1996 the first drug ever to prove effective in treating ALS was approved by the FDA.

More promising ALS treatments are in the offing as we continue to develop our understanding of the disease's pathways and mechanisms. Now, up to 10 percent of those with ALS can be expected to survive more than ten years after diagnosis.

While researchers have not yet fully defined the causes or

pathways of ALS, we now know that the disease attacks specific motor neurons in the brain and spinal cord. These nerve cells are among the body's largest and extend from the brain to the spinal cord, and from the spinal cord to muscles throughout the body.

In patients with ALS, the motor neurons die and the brain's ability to control muscle movement dies with them. Hence the name "amyotrophic," which comes from the Greek for "no muscle nourishment." The word "lateral" refers to the fact that most of these nerve cells die in the spinal cord of ALS patients, leading to "sclerosis," or scarring.

As a result of losing so many motor neurons, ALS patients eventually become totally paralyzed, though their minds remain unaffected by the disease. Both experimental animal and clinical studies suggest that the key causes of ALS are an overabundance of glutamate, the neurotransmitter that nerve cells rely on to transmit signals, and excessive oxidative damage to cells.

In essence, then, it seems that ALS, like Alzheimer's, Parkinson's, and many other neurological illnesses, may in large part be caused by a series of biochemical events leading to excessive free radical damage to healthy brain cells.

In this chapter, we discuss ALS from the onset of symptoms to diagnosis, beginning with what we know about the disease's effects on motor neurons at the most basic, molecular level.

At our chapter's conclusion, we offer a complete treatment plan for ALS based on the most current information available on diet, nutritional supplements, and medications.

What Goes Wrong in ALS, and Why

Essentially, ALS is characterized by dying motor nerve cells in the brain—called the "upper motor neurons"—and in the spine, where the "lower motor neurons" are located. As the disease progresses, the long nerve cells that go from the top of the skull to the spinal cord and from the spinal cord to the limbs progressively deteriorate, eventually leaving the patient completely paralyzed.

At present, scientists can predict no specific similarities of all people diagnosed with ALS, so the cause remains unknown. Physicians currently classify ALS according to how nerve damage progresses and whether or not it is inherited. The categories of ALS include:

1. Classic ALS, which affects over two-thirds of all people with ALS and is characterized by the deterioration of both upper and lower motor nerve cells.
2. Primary lateral sclerosis, which causes only the upper motor neurons to deteriorate.
3. Progressive muscular atrophy, in which only the lower motor neurons degenerate.
4. Progressive bulbar palsy, a condition that begins with difficulties in chewing, swallowing, and speech.
5. Familial ALS, so named because it affects more than one member in the same family.

• Families with ALS Provide a Genetic Clue

There are two ways of developing ALS. One way is inherited. The other is random. In the genetic form, each child of a parent with ALS has a 50 percent chance of inheriting the ALS gene. Everyone who inherits the gene is eventually diagnosed with the disease. Although only 5–10 percent of patients with ALS inherited the disease, familial ALS has led scientists to uncover genetic clues that may prove useful in detailing the disease's pathways in all types of ALS.

In 1991, for example, a team of researchers linked ALS to chromosome 21. Just two years later, this same group of investigators identified a defective SOD1 (superoxide dismutase enzyme) gene on that chromosome as the culprit responsible for many cases of familial ALS.

Why is the SOD enzyme so important to your body that a defective version of it could lead to this devastating illness?

In healthy brains, this enzyme performs a crucial maintenance task by mopping up peroxynitrite, the highly toxic free radical produced as a result of excessive levels of the glutamate neurotransmitter (see below).

Peroxynitrite is normally released in abundance by white

blood cells during the course of immune system battles—as in viral or bacterial infections—and plays a powerful role in immune system inflammation. If the SOD enzyme is ineffective in clearing the brain of that toxic free radical, however, the destructive effect to healthy cells is equivalent to turning a herd of bulls loose in a china shop, with free radicals causing rampant destruction.

In one recent study, for example, the brains of patients with ALS were analyzed for glutathione peroxidase and superoxide dismutase, two of the enzymes so critical for inhibiting free radical destruction. This study demonstrated that the brains of patients who died of ALS had significantly reduced amounts of these enzymes, suggesting that they had less protection against free radical attacks on healthy brain cells. Meanwhile, researchers at the University of California have concluded that oxidative reactions in the brains of patients with a defective SOD gene initiates the domino effect of neuropathologic changes among those with ALS.

Although SOD1 mutations have been discovered in only a minority of all patients—about 30 percent of the patients among those with familial ALS—this landmark discovery is certain to lead to a clearer understanding of the disease. That's because ALS progresses in essentially the same manner even in the 98 percent of the patients without the mutation.

• Too Much Glutamate Causes Too Much Excitement

Some natural substances stimulate brain cells. Glutamate, the amino acid neurotransmitter responsible for exciting neurons to fire off messages, is one of them. Glutamate's normal interactions with specific membrane receptors in brain cells are responsible for driving many important neurological functions. These include cognition, memory, movement, and sensation, as Harvard researchers have reported in *Mechanisms of Disease.*

However, as in the case of so many neurotransmitters, just a little too much of a good thing can throw the brain's complex communication network completely off kilter. When too much glutamate lingers outside cells and binds with neuron receptors, neurotransmitters are triggered to fire more than they should.

Essentially, the brain cells then wear themselves out and die from exhaustion as a result.

Glutamate has been implicated in a variety of brain diseases. This is because excessive activation of glutamate receptors—called "excitotoxicity"—serves as a final common pathway leading to neuron death.

Researchers at Baylor College of Medicine and other institutions are attempting to identify exactly what happens to cause extracellular glutamate to build up toxic levels, and what governs selective motor neuron death in ALS. (Several other studies have demonstrated that patients have elevated glutamate in their cerebral spinal fluid.) This indicates that they are unable to metabolize glutamate normally.

•What Could Cause Patients with ALS to Have Too Much Glutamate in the First Place?

As we have discussed, patients with ALS suffer from high levels of glutamate. In fact, research has uncovered evidence revealing that glutamate levels are higher in the blood serum and cerebrospinal fluid of people with ALS than in those without the disease.

The leading theory about why patients with ALS suffer from toxic levels of glutamate throws the spotlight on astrocytes, the brain's star-shaped cells that normally sop up extra neurotransmitter molecules around neurons to protect them from overstimulation.

Much as unwanted garbage collects if a city's trash collectors go on strike, patients with ALS may suffer when astrocytes fail to adequately pick up glutamate and transport it away from neurons. The question, then, is why should the astrocytes go on strike and fail to perform their clean-up duties in the brain?

As with anyone who goes on strike, astrocytes may be reacting to poor working conditions or low "pay." Glutamate uptake by astrocytes requires an enormous amount of energy expenditure, as well as a key enzyme known as GLT-1. A careful analysis of the glutamate transport system in patients with ALS has demonstrated a selective loss of GLT-1.

According to a number of studies performed by leading ALS researcher Dr. Jeffrey Rothstein and his colleagues at Johns Hopkins University, this is probably due to damage by free radicals or environmental toxins. Currently, scientists at the University of British Columbia, UCLA, and the University of California, Irvine, are among those investigating further the reasons for astrocytes falling down on the job of glutamate cleanup.

Besides a deficiency in GLT-1, astrocytes may be subjected to poor working conditions as a result of being exposed to methylmercury and other toxic metals. Methylmercury is a common contaminant in industrial society that can be highly hazardous to brain cells—principally because it inhibits the uptake of glutamate by astrocyte cleanup cells. It may be one of the poisons causing the destruction of the GLT-1 protein.

Does heavy metal accumulation in neurons automatically mark those cells for eventual degeneration?

The answer seems to be that it does, and that motor neurons, in particular, possess a selective affinity for certain toxic metals.

The concept that toxic metals may be linked to ALS has been extensively studied, with continuing reports of ALS-like syndromes associated with toxic metal intake and exposure. Some toxic metals, such as mercury, lead, and aluminum, are such ubiquitous environmental pollutants that the stage is set for long-term, low-level exposure for many of us, as the half-lives for most toxic metals in the body are very long.

For example, chronic dietary deficiencies of calcium and magnesium, when combined with excess intake of aluminum and manganese, have been implicated in the high incidence of ALS among people living in the Western Pacific. This is most likely because poor metabolism of calcium and magnesium is implicated in the inability to displace aluminum out of body tissue among ALS patients.

Japanese studies have revealed that ALS patients suffered from low serum selenium and mercury levels. While a low serum mercury level may seem to be desirable, it reflects greater stores in body tissue, where it exerts its toxic effect. Additionally, it is well known that selenium can decrease mercury toxicity because of selenium's role in promoting glutathione enzyme detoxification. Therefore, mercury exposure and adequate selenium intake should both be assessed in patients with ALS.

Other Western Pacific studies have demonstrated that chronic dietary deficiencies of calcium and magnesium, with excess intakes of aluminum and manganese, are also associated with a high incidence of ALS. Additional studies detecting elevated aluminum levels in the CNS tissue of people with ALS also reveal increased calcified material, similar to calcium.

To date, investigators are honing in on various antioxidants with the potential to act as free radical scavengers able to confer protection against heavy metal toxicity. These include lipoic acid, glutathione, selenium, and n-acetyl-cysteine, which we will discuss in the nutritional section at the end of this chapter.

•What Actually Causes Cells to Die If They Are Overstimulated by Too Much Glutamate?

In recent years, researchers around the world have been investigating this puzzling paradox: Why have our brains evolved with such extraordinary vulnerability to our own neurotransmitters? And what events actually lead to the abnormal accumulation of such neurotransmitters?

In the case of glutamate, neurons swell and die just a few hours after exposure. Glutamate-related neuron death goes something like this: The excess of glutamate causes neurons to fire too often. This excessive neuron stimulation provokes a rise in intracellular calcium, which in turn interferes with the cell's necessary energy stores of glucose and oxygen.

In addition, the brain cells caused to fire too often by the presence of an overabundance of glutamate end up allowing too much calcium to cross into the cell through membrane channels. While intracellular calcium is essential for a number of processes, too much calcium inside a cell can trigger harmful reactions, including the activation of various cell-busting enzymes. One of these enzymes can even lead to the production of arachidonic acid, the deadly substance discussed earlier in this book.

In the case of ALS, arachidonic acid perpetuates cell damage by further inhibiting the uptake of glutamate by the brain's astrocytes. Free radicals formed as a result of arachidonic acid metabolism can inflict further damage on cells.

What's more, when receptors are stimulated because too much

glutamate is hammering on brain cell membranes, nitric oxide and superoxide may be produced. Together, these substances may react to form one of the free radicals that serves a death warrant to cells: peroxynitrite.

In essence, then, excessive glutamate in the brain actually causes motor neurons to self-destruct through a combination of sodium and calcium imbalances, protein breakdown, and free radical damage.

Now, researchers are looking into ways to stop this biochemical domino effect before it starts.

Because the glutamate neurotransmitter must "match up" with certain receptors on receiving neurons to succeed in stimulating those neurons, investigators are now exploring ways to block those receptors. If those receptors can be prevented from receiving glutamate stimulation, then we may one day successfully protect cells against death by exhaustion.

Another protective strategy is to block the release of excitatory glutamate from brain cells in the first place. Riluzole, the first drug approved for patients with ALS, has proven effective in doing just that. We will discuss this drug later, in our section on ALS medications.

•Why Are More Men Diagnosed with ALS than Women?

Investigators are currently investigating possible reasons to explain why more men are diagnosed with ALS than women. One theory concerns DHEA.

DHEA (dehydroepiandrosterone), a natural hormone produced by the brain, has been closely scrutinized by scientists in recent years for its potential for everything from restoring memory to delaying aging, and has been shown to reduce body fat and to protect against cardiovascular mortality among men.

In fact, DHEA is naturally abundant in the brain, and is important for its "neurotrophic" factor. That is, DHEA is one of the nourishing agents that neurons depend on for growth and survival. Other important neuron growth factors, as we will see in our section on nutrition, include brain-derived nerve growth factor and insulin-like growth factor. All of these serve as "fertilizer" for brain cells, allowing them to grow strong and communicate efficiently.

The higher incidence of ALS in men may reflect the fact that DHEA levels in men start out much higher than in women. DHEA levels peak in adolescence, however, and decline with age among most men, so that production of that hormone at age sixty-five is just 10–20 percent of what it was at age twenty.

Researchers reporting in a 1995 issue of *Muscle and Nerve* postulate that the rapid decline of this hormone among men may be an important factor in causing more men to be diagnosed with ALS than women. It may be that men need more DHEA than women do, and the age related decline affects them more adversely.

A Combined Medical and Nutritional Approach to ALS

If you or a loved one is diagnosed with ALS, the most important step you can take is to work with your physician to discuss both standard and research treatment protocols. Because of the disease's rapid progress, it is essential to take action immediately toward preventing neuron degeneration and maintaining the highest quality of life possible.

Patients with ALS suffer from inefficient glutamate metabolism resulting in a state of neuron excitotoxicity and excessive free radical damage to motor neurons.

Here, we present an aggressive protocol of nutritional neuroimmunomodulators with the potential to address these conditions. Our treatment strategies include adding growth factors, antioxidants, and other substances tailored to nourish motor neuron growth, inhibit glutamate release from cells, block neuron receptors from binding with glutamate, and stop free radicals in their tracks.

As the disease progresses, we offer patients a combination of counseling, medications, speech therapy, and assistive devices as necessary.

TABLE 6

ALS: THE STEPS LEADING TO MOTOR NEURON DEATH

1. In the case of familial ALS, a defective form of the SOD1 gene impairs the brain's natural ability to cleanse itself of toxic superoxide free radicals, causing nerve cells to rapidly degenerate.

2. For some patients with ALS, exposure to toxins such as methylmercury may lead to the brain's inability to properly metabolize glutamate, the brain's key excitatory neurotransmitter.

3. For all patients with ALS, the brain's ability to metabolize glutamate is faulty, possibly as a result of astrocyte cells being unable to successfully clean up the brain.

4. Because it is an excitatory neurotransmitter with the ability to trigger cells to fire, an excessive amount of glutamate in the brain can cause cells to fire too often and die.

5. Motor neurons die off progressively, causing eventual paralysis and death.

When Should You Suspect ALS?

ALS is a difficult disease to diagnose, as it affects everyone differently. However, some of the most common early symptoms of the disease include muscle twitches and cramping, especially in the hands and feet.

Patients in the early stages of ALS may also notice generalized muscle weakness and fatigue, and may discover that it is difficult to project their voices. Their speech, too, may be affected, and sound "thick" or slurred.

As the disease becomes more severe—over the course of anywhere from just a few months to several years, depending on the individual—patients may have difficulty chewing and swallowing, as the nerves degenerate, resulting in weight loss. They will also have trouble breathing.

Severe pain is not a typical symptom of ALS, nor is there any impairment in thinking or memory.

Diagnosing ALS: No Single Test

In diagnosing ALS, your neurologist will perform a complete physical exam and take a medical history. Two of the diseases most commonly misdiagnosed as ALS include:

- *Cervical spondylosis,* a degeneration of the spinal cord due to chronic arthritis. Typically, the diagnosis can be confirmed through an MRI.
- *Multifocal motor neuropathy,* a disease that specifically strikes lower motor neurons without upper motor neuron symptoms. In this case, the diagnosis can be clarified with an EMG (see below) and with a test for antibodies to motor neurons.

It is essential to rule out these two ALS-mimicking diseases, as they each require unique treatments.

In completing a lab workup to diagnose ALS definitively, your neurologist should request blood tests, a spinal fluid test, an EMG (electromyogram) to measure the electrical activity in your nerves and muscles, and an MRI (magnetic resonance imaging) to produce a complete image of the body without using X rays.

• Check for Heavy Metal Toxicity

Based on studies we cited earlier in this chapter on the possible detrimental effects to motor neurons of heavy metals such as mercury, iron, and aluminum, we recommend that all patients diagnosed with ALS consider being tested for heavy metal toxicity.

Some physicians will recommend blood testing to do this. However, if blood tests are normal and metal toxicity is still suspected, your health care practitioner may recommend a urine test performed before and after chelation. (Chelation involves administering an oral agent to increase urinary excretion of a metal.)

If such toxicity exists, certain nutritional agents can be incorporated into the daily regimen to alleviate the metal burden in the body (see below).

The First Step to Take: Ensure a Nutritious Diet

In research conducted at the University of Chicago Hospital's ALS Outpatient Clinic, clinicians discovered the following:

- About 70 percent of the patients suffered from calorie intake that fell below RDA guidelines, leading to a loss in body weight among a quarter of the patients.
- At least 25 percent of the patients suffered from moderate to severe malnutrition.
- Fifteen percent of the patients had elevated serum glucose.
- About 20 percent showed elevated cholesterol levels.

Since not all patients with ALS lose weight, we can conclude that weight loss is not just due to a loss in muscle mass. Rather, patients with ALS should be examined with an eye toward proper caloric intake, a physical ability to prepare food and feed oneself, and psychological well-being, as all of these factors contribute to the state of nourishment.

While no specific diet exists for those diagnosed with ALS, patients can help maintain quality of life by following our recommendations in the two-step Brain Wellness Plan presented earlier in this book. Good nutrition can provide patients with more energy and a better sense of well-being, as well as strengthen the immune system.

Therefore, one of the first steps we recommend is determining early on whether any nutritional problems are present so that your nutritionist or health care provider can institute appropriate nutritional interventions. Patients with ALS may need special help with swallowing problems, either through formulas or blenderized foods, for example.

• *Ease Constipation with Fluids and Dietary Fiber*

ALS patients typically have problems with constipation owing to weakened gastrointestinal muscle control. In addition to incorporating insoluble types of fiber into the diet by eating rice bran and whole grain breads, crackers, and cereals, we suggest that patients with ALS drink a minimum of eight glasses of water daily. Patients should also consider adding supplements of Miller's bran and psyllium fiber as directed by a nutritionist. Additionally, individuals with ALS should add sufficient fruits and vegetables to their diets as outlined in *The Brain Wellness Plan* dietary guidelines.

• Avoid Glutamine

As we have seen, the amino acid glutamate is a potentially potent central nervous system toxin in ALS. Now, animal studies conducted by researchers at the Arkansas National Center for Toxicological Research have demonstrated that glutamine, which can serve as an important source of nitrogen and energy for most healthy individuals, has the undesirable effect of enhancing the release of glutamate from brain cells.

This study has important implications for patients with ALS, naturally, since motor neurons are already compromised by excessive levels of glutamate. We therefore strongly discourage patients from taking any glutamine supplements.

• Avoid Iron

University of Kentucky researchers investigating the roles of aluminum, calcium, and iron have discovered that individuals with ALS had consistently elevated iron levels in their spinal neurons. These investigators concluded that the elevation of iron in the CNS was significant in the pathogenesis of motor neuron degeneration primarily because high iron levels may enhance the spinoff of deadly free radicals within specific cells.

Based on these and other studies examining iron levels in ALS patients, we recommend that individuals with ALS avoid any nutritional supplements that contain iron.

• What about Branched Chain Amino Acids?

The branched chain amino acids (BCAA) leucine, isoleucine, and valine are essential amino acids primarily involved in stress, energy, and muscle metabolism. With respect to muscle, the BCAAs are directly used as energy sources to stimulate protein synthesis.

In the past decade, researchers have been examining the association between BCAAs and the muscle wasting that is a hallmark of ALS. For example, in a study published in *Lancet*, one researcher showed that supplementing the diets of ALS patients with BCAAs resulted in a significant improvement in muscle strength.

Unfortunately, other studies have not duplicated these successful results. In fact, one study had to be discontinued when researchers noted that subjects taking BCAA experienced excess mortality. What's more, another investigation—this one conducted in a Denmark hospital by researchers O. Gredal and S. E. Moller—revealed that BCAA supplements actually elevated plasma glutamate within forty-five minutes of taking them.

For these reasons, we do not recommend supplementing the diets of ALS individuals with BCAAs, owing to potentially negative effects.

The Three R's of Managing ALS: Reduce Glutamate and Free Radical Activity as Well as Heavy Metal Concentrations, Raise Mitochondrial Activity, and Regenerate Damaged Neurons

The most effective strategies for managing ALS disease are to reduce both glutamate and free radical activity, increase mitochondrial activity, and regenerate the neurons that are damaged. Let's examine the nutritional substances, pharmaceutical drugs, and current experimental techniques that address these objectives.

Strategies to Reduce Glutamate Activity and Inflammation

• Antiglutamate Therapies and ALS

Rationale for Use of Antiglutamate Therapies in ALS Identifying drugs or vitamins that block the ill effects of glutamate is the major strategy currently used in treating ALS. Glutamate is an excitatory neurotransmitter. When glutamate binds to a receptor, it induces activation of the cell membrane. The effect of excessive glutamate on the nerve cells is known as "excitotoxicity," and is implicated as a cause of nerve damage in ALS. The reason for excessive glutamate is currently unknown, but it is thought to be due to an inability of particular cells in the brain to remove and sequester glutamate, thereby preventing it from causing harm. Therefore, current treatment strategies for ALS involve blocking glutamate production or, alternatively, blocking the interaction of glutamate with receptors. Two FDA-approved drugs achieve these goals. One is Rilutek, the only drug approved by the FDA specifically to treat ALS. The second is Topamax (or topiramate), a drug approved by the FDA for epilepsy but currently under study for ALS as well.

• Rilutek and ALS

Rationale for Use of Rilutek in ALS Glutamate stimulates receptors on motor neurons that initiate a process called "excitotoxic cell death." Rilutek blocks glutamate transmission, making it a useful compound in treating ALS. By blocking glutamate transmission, Rilutek helps reduce excitotoxicity to motor neurons and, therefore, can potentially slow or stop the progression of ALS.

Clinical Studies of Rilutek in ALS Two multicenter, randomized, double-blind studies have been performed using Rilutek to treat ALS. Results demonstrated a modest but statistically significant increase in survival time. The FDA has approved Rilutek specifically for the treatment of ALS.

RECOMMENDED DOSE: 50 mg twice daily. Rilutek is available only by prescription.

• Topamax and ALS

Rationale for Use of Topamax in ALS Topamax or topiramate is a new antiepileptic drug derived from monosaccharide (a carbohydrate). It exerts its effects on the brain by increasing the activity of GABA receptors and blocking specific types of glutamate receptors called AMPA receptors. It has been suggested that blocking AMPA receptors may be of value in the treatment of ALS.

Clinical Studies of Topamax in ALS Patients are currently being enrolled in studies taking place at multiple medical centers to determine whether Topamax is effective in the treatment of ALS.

RECOMMENDED DOSE: 200 mg daily of Topamax or Topiramate. This is an experimental treatment in ALS.

• THC Derivatives and ALS

Rationale for Use of THC in ALS The neuroprotective effect of cannabinoids has recently been discovered and reported by the National Institute of Mental Health. Glutamate, the neurotransmitter involved in neurotoxicity, is blocked by several nonpsychotic derivatives of THC including cannabinoids. Cannabinoids block NMDA receptors and AMPA receptors, which are important targets in the treatment of ALS. In particular, blocking AMPA receptors may be the most significant target in the treatment of ALS. Cannabinoids demonstrate specific blockage of these receptors. Cannabinoids also block the influx of calcium and are better antioxidants than vitamin C and vitamin E.

Clinical Studies for Use of THC Derivatives in ALS There are currently no studies examining the effects of cannabinoids in ALS. An initial requirement before clinical studies would be the confirmation that cannabinoids do, indeed, block excitotoxic receptors and, in particular, the AMPA receptor. Furthermore, it needs to be demonstrated that cannabinoids are neuroprotective in mouse models of ALS. However, we urge that research with cannabinoids be accelerated and we encourage others to join us in actively lobbying against current laws which prevent compassionate use of these compounds in humans with otherwise incurable disease.

Antioxidants and ALS

Rationale for Use of Antioxidants in ALS Many researchers now agree that the death of motor neurons in ALS is due, either directly or indirectly, to free radical–induced oxidative damage. Potentially effective therapy for ALS would likely include compounds that protect against free radical–mediated injury, i.e., antioxidants.

Various antioxidants are available over the counter, and synthetic antioxidants are also in the research pipeline. In order for an antioxidant to be effective in a disease like ALS, it has to cross the blood-brain barrier and protect against the specific injury that is occurring. In ALS, hydrogen peroxide appears to be a free radical worthy of targeting. Several compounds protect against hydrogen peroxide–induced injury to motor neurons. These include melatonin, green tea extract, and a compound known as PUT-CAT.

• Melatonin and ALS

Rationale for Use of Melatonin in ALS Melatonin has not been clinically studied in ALS, but several important physiological effects it produces may support its role in reducing motor neuron injury in ALS. Melatonin protects cells against hydrogen peroxide toxicity, and it also suppresses glutamate activity in the brain. Pharmacological concentrations of melatonin are much higher than the physiological doses, and therefore, the effective dose of melatonin is currently unknown. It is currently recommended that 1–3 mg be administered to patients wtih ALS under a health care worker's supervision.

RECOMMENDED DOSE: 1–3 mg daily. The efficacy of melatonin in ALS has not yet been demonstrated. Consult your health care provider.

•Green Tea Extract and ALS

Rationale for Use of Green Tea Extract in ALS Green (and black) tea extracts contain excellent free radical scavenger activity. In addition, they are potent inhibitors of hydrogen peroxide. A particular extract of green tea, epigallocatechin, substantially enhances hydrogen peroxide–scavenging activity. Green tea extract has not been studied in the treatment of ALS, but because of its ability to suppress the free radical hydrogen peroxide, it is worthy of future study.

RECOMMENDED DOSE: 60–120 mg of standardized extract. Precautions: None.

•PUT-CAT and ALS

Rationale for Use of PUT-CAT in ALS PUT-CAT is an antioxidant under study at the Mayo Clinic. Like epigallocatechin, PUT-CAT removes hydrogen peroxide. It is also capable of crossing the blood-brain barrier. Studies of PUT-CAT in animal models of ALS demonstrated that the compound significantly delayed the onset of ALS and increased the survival of affected mice. Further studies with PUT-CAT are required to determine its clinical utility in humans. Presently, PUT-CAT is not available as a dietary supplement.

Reducing Heavy Metal Concentrations in ALS

Rationale for Use of Metal Chelators in ALS Epidemiological studies have suggested that certain metals may be involved in the pathogenesis of ALS, including lead compounds, mercury, and copper. Abnormal calcium levels are also a factor.

Lead poisoning can cause ALS-like symptoms. Additionally, increased levels of lead have been reported in the nerves and spinal cords of ALS patients, as well as in their cerebral spinal fluid.

Mercury has also been implicated in the development of ALS. Increased urine mercury levels have been found in a proportion of ALS patients. Mercury may interfere with certain cells' ability to remove the neurotransmitter glutamate from the synapse, resulting in a prolonged excitatory effect. However, a recent study in the Netherlands that measured heavy metals, including mercury, in 53 patients suffering from ALS did not identify an increased excretion of heavy metals in these patients, throwing doubt on the relationship of mercury to ALS.

Abnormal calcium processing by cells has also been implicated as a causal factor in Lou Gehrig's disease. Increased calcium levels increase brain glutamate transmission, and glutamate is clearly associated with ALS. Calcium activates degradative processes in cells, including enzymes known as "caspases" that dissolve intracellular proteins. Furthermore, a buffering system for calcium in motor neurons, "calbindin," is markedly lower in nerve cells of patients that have died in ALS patients. This lack of calbindin in cells that die in ALS suggest that unchecked calcium is potentially destructive to cells.

Copper is a metal found in the superoxide dismutase (SOD) enzyme complex. This enzyme is abnormal in the hereditary form of ALS. The inherited abnormality in copper SOD leads to an abnormal exposure of the cells to copper, which results in excessive free radical damage.

Clinical Studies of Mercury and Lead Chelators in ALS Neither mercury nor lead chelators have been successful in treating ALS in previous clinical trials.

• Copper Chelators and ALS

Clinical Studies of Copper Chelators in ALS In a study performed by researchers in Japan, a specific genetic line of mice that possess the abnormal SOD gene were examined using a copper chelator known as trientine. In mice that received trientine in combination with ascorbic acid, there was a significant delay in the time it took for mice to reach paralysis, and treatment with this combination therapy prolonged the survival of these mice. The copper chelator Trientine is available only by prescription for patients with abnormal copper metabolism.

RECOMMENDED DOSE: This drug is available only by prescription, and is not currently approved for treatment of
ALS.

• Calcium Chelators and ALS

Clinical Studies of Calcium Chelators in ALS Vitamin D, which
binds calcium very effectively, has been suggested as a possible
therapy for ALS. It increases calbindin, the enzyme system in
every cell in the nervous system used to bind calcium, thereby
providing a buffering effect for excessive intracellular calcium.
Further clinical studies are required before dosage recommendations can be given for use in Vitamin D in ALS. However, 400–800
IU may be used daily.

RECOMMENDED DOSE: 400–800 mg daily as directed by your
health care practitioner.

Strategies to Raise Mitochondrial Activity

As mentioned in other chapters in this book, mitochondrial
dysfunction is thought to play a critical role in neurodegenerative
diseases and, specifically, in motor neuron cell death in ALS.
Mitochondrial dysfunction may be caused by free radicals or
oxidative stress, or may be part of a preprogrammed cell death
called apoptosis. Creatine is the mitochondria-stimulating substance that has been studied in ALS.

• Creatine and ALS

Rationale for Use of Creatine in ALS Creatine plays a role in
the chemical reaction during which mitochondria generate ATP,
which provides energy to all of our cells. Creatine exerts a protective effect on nerve cells by increasing mitochondrial ATP
production, preventing oxidative damage to mitochondria, and
buffering mitochondria membranes from excessive calcium accumulation.

Clinical Studies of Creatine in ALS Oral administration of creatine was recently shown to improve motor function in an animal model of ALS. Creatine was also noted to extend survival in a mouse model of ALS. In human studies, it has been demonstrated that oral creatine increases concentrations of creatine in our brains, where it exerts its beneficial effects.

A potentially improved creatine formulation may soon become available. This synthetic analog of creatine, "cyclocreatine," enhances mitochondrial function even more than creatine by boosting cellular levels of ATP. Most of the studies examining the effects of cyclocreatine have been performed by looking at heart muscle, and the compound appears to protect the heart from damage during conditions when it doesn't get enough blood (i.e., during a heart attack). However, a recent study also demonstrated that cyclocreatine protects brain cells from excitatory amino acids like glutamate.

> *RECOMMENDED DOSE:* 5–10 g a day. Precautions: Treatment should only proceed under a physician's supervision, since kidney function must be monitored during creatine therapy.

Strategies to Regenerate Damaged Neurons

Regenerating damaged neurons in the brains of patients with ALS could help to delay the progression of this paralytic disease. Our knowledge about nerve cell growth and regeneration is now progressing at an astonishing rate, and our understanding of how to stop nerve death and replace already-damaged neurons will certainly continue to increase rapidly over the next few years. Currently, we can employ various substances to help regenerate nerves, including the hormones estrogen and DHEA. Use of gene therapy and fetal cell transplantation to replace damaged or dead neurons is under study, and will probably become standard therapy in the very near future.

• Estrogen and ALS

Rationale for Use of Estrogen in ALS Estrogen and other steroid hormones possess nerve growth factor–stimulating effects. Estrogen induces specific metabolic changes within a cell that simultaneously enhance its survival and inhibit key proteins that may promote cell death. The brain and spinal cord are particularly responsive to the reparative capacity of estrogen.

The male-to-female ratio of ALS patients is estimated to be between 2:1 and 3:1, and disease severity is worse in men than in women. It is suggested that these differences are due to estrogen, which may act as a protective factor against ALS because of its ability to enhance nerve growth factor production. There are currently no studies using estrogen in ALS patients. However, genistein, a "phytoestrogen" derived from soy products, has been used in animal models of ALS. Genistein appears to have estrogen-stimulating effects, and in a recent study reported in *Biochemical and Biophysical Research Communications,* genistein was demonstrated to be protective in animal studies. Whether estrogen or genistein will be part of the regimen of ALS therapy certainly needs to be further elucidated. Precautions against using estrogen or genistein include women with a history of an estrogen-dependent cancer, or of abnormal bleeding disorders (including blood clots). Discuss your overall health picture with your health care practitioner if you are considering using estrogen or genistein therapy in treating ALS. Since estrogen therapy is so individualized, it's not possible to provide a dose recommendation here.

> **RECOMMENDED DOSES:** Dosages for estrogen and genistein are completely individual; consult with your health care practitioner. Precautions: Women with a history of an estrogen-dependent cancer or of abnormal bleeding disorders (including blood clots) should not take these substances.

• DHEA and ALS

Rationale for Use of DHEA in ALS DHEA is a steroid hormone that also protects the brain, through inhibiting cortisol (which is known to aggravate and decrease the survival of brain cells), buffering against the harmful effects of calcium within cells, and stimulating certain growth factors. Among the growth factors stimulated by DHEA is insulin-like growth factor (ILGF). ILGF is currently under study as a treatment for ALS because of its activity in promoting motor neuron survival. Furthermore, DHEA levels are reportedly lower in ALS patients.

Clinical Studies of DHEA in ALS Unfortunately, there are no studies to determine the effects of DHEA in ALS. Patients who have ALS should ask their health care practitioners to measure both DHEA and DHEA-sulfate levels. If there are no contraindications to therapy, dosage recommendations are between 50 and 200 mg per day, but should be administered only under a health care practitioner's supervision.

> RECOMMENDED DOSE: 50–200 mg per day. Precautions: DHEA should only be administered under a health care practitioner's supervision.

• Fetal Stem Cells and ALS

Rationale for Use of Fetal Stem Cells in ALS Fetal stem cells are extracted from human embryos. They represent life at a very early stage of development. These cells have not yet committed to becoming a particular cell type, and thus, they are capable of evolving into a multitude of different kinds of cells, including motor neurons. In fact, stem cells ultimately give rise to every single cell in our bodies. They also have the ability to grow in the lab, providing an indefinite source of future cells without having to obtain them from other embryos or fetuses.

Stem cells have enormous regenerative potential. They act as the building blocks of the human brain and spinal cord. Researchers have essentially harnessed the body's capacity to regenerate itself, and are now quite excited by the potential of fetal stem cells to be an effective intervention in ALS and other neurodegenerative diseases. Transplants of neural stem cells into mice replace missing or damaged cells. Stem cells, when injected into the brain, can also be used as carriers for introducing new genes into a malfunctioning brain to allow it to make proteins required for normal brain function.

Clinical Use of Stem Cells in ALS There are currently no clinical studies involving fetal stem cells in ALS. However, researchers are quite busy studying the use of stem cells in animal models of ALS, and preliminary data support their use in a variety of neurological conditions. Once the efficacy of fetal stem cells is demonstrated in animal models of diseases like ALS, human studies are expected to begin. There are two hurdles that must be overcome in the use of stem cells in human disease:

1. Researchers must determine how stem cells differentiate into the desired type of cell. For instance, what determines that a stem cell becomes a motor neuron as opposed to some other cell in the body? In an almost mystical fashion, when fetal cells are injected into a particular area of the body, the surrounding mature cells appear to emit specific signals that help coax the stem cells into becoming that type of cell. If a stem cell is injected into the liver, for example, it develops into a mature liver cell— it doesn't become a brain cell sitting in the middle of the liver. In the brain, certain chemical signals appear both to protect the brain and direct stem cells to become new nerve cells. This process is called "spontaneous differentiation."

2. The other concern is that stem cells will be rejected by the host (a problem in other types of tissue transplantation). However, it may be that stem cells, which are still in their infancy, do not possess the capacity to elicit a specific rejection response by the host, thus bypassing the need for the immunosuppressant therapies that are normally required for transplant therapy.

RECOMMENDED DOSE: This treatment is still in the experimental stages.

• Gene Therapy and ALS

Rationale for Use of Gene Therapy in ALS Over the next several years, gene therapy is likely to change the way medicine is practiced. Gene therapy is the process of transferring a particular gene into cells to treat a disease. Genes are portions of DNA that direct the manufacture of certain proteins. Proteins are critical for normal cellular function, including the thousands of enzymes that are required for cellular processes. If a genetic code is defective, proteins will malfunction in turn, leading to a particular disease. In gene therapy, new genes are inserted into cells to correct the gene defect that caused the disease in the first place.

In Lou Gehrig's disease, discovering which genes are responsible for producing the disease and replacing them has proved to be a daunting task. However, a leading candidate in ALS is the GLT-1 gene. GLT-1 encodes for the protein that is involved in the transportation of glutamate. A defect in this gene has been reported in ALS, which may explain why excessive glutamate levels contribute to the excitotoxic damage in motor neurons. Preliminary research in laboratory animals suggests that insertion of the GLT-1 gene in affected mice with ALS results in a significant delay of progression of symptoms.

A second strategy in ALS gene therapy research involves inserting genes that signal the production of certain growth factors. Growth factors are like fertilizer for cells, in that they maintain and preserve the necessary milieu for cell survival. Several growth factors are currently under study, including insulin-like growth factor, glial cell derived neurotrophic factor, and brain-derived neurotrophic factor (BDNF). BDNF promotes the survival of motor neurons. It appears to play a role in the survival of motor neurons by providing cells with the nutrients necessary for survival. Currently, some patients are actually being given BDNF directly into the spinal cord. Results of these studies are not yet known. However, there is concern among some researchers and clinicians that growth factors will eventually produce cell death. The mechanism by which they cause nerve cell death may be growth factor–induced oxidative stress; therefore, if nerve growth factors prove to be beneficial, patients should also use an antioxidant strategy to protect against oxidative stress.

While most of these treatments are experimental and currently unavailable to patients with ALS except in large medical centers performing research, an alternative strategy is to provide ALS patients with the precursors to growth factors. The precursors, including hormones like estrogen and DHEA, stimulate growth factors without the patient having to take the growth factor directly.

RECOMMENDED DOSE: Gene therapy is still in the experimental stages.

A Cocktail Approach to Treating ALS

I. Reduce glutamate and free radical activity.

    1. Reduce glutamate.

        a. Rilutek, an antiglutamate drug currently approved by the FDA for treatment of ALS. Available only by prescription. Recommended dose: 50 mg two times a day.

        b. Topamax or Topiramate, currently under study. This is an experimental treatment. Recommended dose is approximatley 200 mg a day.

    2. Reduce free radical activity.

        a. Melatonin inhibits hydrogen peroxide and dampens the effects of glutamate. Therapeutic doses are currently unknown; the physiological dose of melatonin is 1–3 mg per day.

        b. Green and black tea extracts, currently available at health food stores, acts as antioxidants. Recommended dose is 60–120 mg of standardized extract.

        c. PUT-CAT, currently under study at the Mayo Clinic, removes free radical hydrogen peroxide and crosses the blood-brain barrier.

    3. Reduce heavy metal concentrations.

        a. The copper chelator Trientine is available only by prescription for patients with abnormal copper metabolism, and is not approved for the treatment of ALS.

        b. Vitamin D helps to bind excessive levels of calcium. Recommended dose is 400–800 IU.

II. Raise mitochondrial activity.

    1. Creatine increases mitochondrial ATP production, prevents oxidative damage to mitochondria, and buffers mitochondrial membranes from excessive calcium accumulation. Recommended dosage is 5–10 g daily.

2. Cyclocreatine, a synthetic analog of creatine, is currently under testing. It should be used only under a doctor's supervision, and kidney function should be monitored.

III. Regenerate damaged neurons.

1. Estrogen and genistein (a phytoestrogen) both possess neurotrophic or nerve growth factor–stimulating effects, but they should be used only under a physician's supervision. Speak to your health care practitioner about using these compounds.

2. DHEA, another nerve growth factor, stimulates the effects of insulin-like growth factor. Again, speak to your health care practitioner prior to using.

3. BDNF, a nerve growth factor, is currently under intense clinical investigation (as are other experimental nerve growth factors). This is an experimental treatment.

4. Fetal stem cell therapy is currently being studied in animal models. If fetal stem cells demonstrate a beneficial effect, human studies may soon be under way as well. This is an experimental treatment.

5. GLT-1 gene therapy, also experimental, is currently under study for ALS.

ATTENTION DEFICIT HYPERACTIVITY DISORDER

From his first few months of life, Clarissa and Ray knew there was something different about their son Jon. For one thing, he never slept. When other babies his age were sleeping a good ten to twelve hours a night and taking at least one nap every day, Jon was wide awake by 5 A.M. and simply screamed if they tried to get him to rest anytime during the day.

By the time he was two, Jon was a whirling dervish, or as Ray called him, "the human destructo machine," practically climbing the walls. Preschool didn't seem to help. In fact, just getting Jon to sit in the car long enough to buckle his seat belt required all of Clarissa's patience and strength. Once, Jon even managed to wriggle free and jump out of the car before she closed the door, hitting his head on the paved drive. As usual, though, Jon didn't cry. He seemed heedless of danger, no matter how they cautioned him or how many scrapes he bore on his skinny knees and elbows.

In elementary school, Jon's behavior actually worsened. When the teacher tried to read a story, he constantly interrupted. If another child competed with him for a toy, Jon was likely to solve the disagreement with a slap. Clarissa and Ray were worried. If Jon was this out of control now, what would he be like as a teenager?

Jon's preschool teacher recommended that he be evaluated for attention deficit hyperactivity disorder (ADHD). The pediatrician conducted a thorough physical exam, and then referred the family to a child psychiatrist. A battery of behavioral assessment tests confirmed the ADHD diagnosis, and the psychiatrist prescribed Ritalin. However, unconvinced that this was the best solution, Clarissa and Ray sought our opinion.

"There must be other things we can do," they told us. "We really don't want our kid on medication unless there is absolutely no other choice."

Attention Deficit Hyperactivity Disorder: An Overview

ADHD ranks among the most common neurological disorders among American children, affecting up to 5 percent, or as many as 2 million, U.S. children at any one time.

In fact, in every classroom in the United States you can expect to find at least one child with ADHD. While it is not itself a specific learning disability, ADHD can interfere with concentration and attention, making it difficult for a child to do well in school and in social situations.

A syndrome usually characterized by inattention, hyperactivity, and impulsive behavior, ADHD is a close relative to attention deficit disorder (ADD), which affects the attention and impulse control of individuals but is not characterized by hyperactive behavior. Both syndromes run in families, and boys with ADHD tend to outnumber girls by at least 3 to 1.

For people with ADHD, life is like a fast-moving carousel where sounds, smells, sights, and thoughts are constantly stopping and starting, or even spinning out of control. Although many children seem to outgrow the disorder, at least 30 percent are affected throughout adulthood. However, many adults with the disorder remain unaware that they have it unless one of their children is diagnosed with ADHD. These adults may simply think of themselves as disorganized and unable to stay on task; they may consequently suffer in both personal relationships and careers as a result.

ADHD is a disorder that may require a combination of behavioral counseling, special education, nutritional intervention, and medications over many years. In the last decade, scientists have learned a great deal about the disorder and are now in the process of pinpointing its biological basis—a process certain to lead us to more effective preventive strategies and treatments.

No single cause has yet been identified for ADHD. In fact, ADHD will probably one day prove to be an umbrella term for a number of associated disorders. However, researchers around the world have come a long way in identifying environmental and biochemical links to the disease, and in tracking just how the disorder affects the brain's metabolism and function.

Leading investigators are currently exploring the association between ADHD and factors such as genetic influences, prenatal alcohol consumption, environmental toxins, brain damage, food allergies, fatty acid deficiency, faulty glucose metabolism in the brain, and thyroid abnormalities. All these studies promise us a better understanding of the syndrome, based on what we are rapidly learning about how ADHD affects the brain's biochemistry.

Although clinicians currently differ on the best treatment for ADHD, all agree that a multimodal approach—one that incorporates dietary measures, counseling, special academic strategies, and possibly medication—is best.

In this chapter, we present ADHD from the onset of symptoms to diagnosis, discussing the full range of treatments based on what we know today about the syndrome's impact on the brain's biochemistry. Finally, we offer an aggressive treatment plan incorporating the most current studies available on nutritional therapies and medications.

What Goes Wrong in ADHD, and Why

Research concerning the possible causes of ADHD revolves around this key concept: Our ability to pay attention is an active process, not a passive one.

In order to selectively sort out stimuli from our environment—as a child must do in a classroom, or a manager must accomplish at work—certain brain regions must kick into gear while others are inhibited. In other words, the act of paying attention requires the integrated input and coordination of several brain regions.

The most important of these is the tiny brain stem area known as the "locus ceruleus." This brain region is responsible for sending messages to the front of the brain to alert us to the tasks at hand.

In essence, you can't pay attention if you aren't awake, and the brain's locus ceruleus acts as a coach on the sidelines, yelling at his players on the field to rally together. The chemical messenger that the locus ceruleus relies on most to send those messages is norepinephrine, the "revving up" neurotransmitter. Two things have to happen for proper signaling: the levels of norepinephrine must be finely regulated, and the receptors for that neurotransmitter must be ready to receive messages.

If the locus ceruleus is damaged—through injury, stroke, or infection—higher brain systems receive inadequate signals and lose track of what's happening on the playing field. A number of studies worldwide have demonstrated that damage to the brain regions that control our ability to pay attention produces symptoms of impulsiveness, compulsivity, and short attention span.

While there is no structural derangement of these important brain regions in people with ADHD, scientists are now unearthing clues that point to functional derangements of these same brain structures. One of the most important tools used in recent years to perform those studies is PET scanning, a sophisticated radiological device that measures brain metabolism.

Quite simply, when your brain is at work, its cells demand glucose as a primary energy source. PET scans allow scientists to measure brain activity by determining the amount of glucose being used by certain brain regions. As you would expect, areas of high glucose metabolism show that the brain is working harder, while lowered glucose demands are equated with diminished brain metabolism. These PET scans actually produce visual images of brains at work.

In examining the brains of people with ADHD, scientists have used PET scans to demonstrate that certain areas of their brains show a decreased use of glucose and diminished brain metabolism. The results were not a surprise: People with ADHD suffer most from impaired glucose use and lowered activity in those areas of the brain controlling our ability to pay attention.

Currently, scientists are striving to determine the genetic, prenatal, physical, and biochemical factors that may lead to decreased glucose metabolism in people with ADHD. They are also searching for other differences between people with the disorder and those who are not affected. Soon, we hope to have new protocols for treating ADHD that may successfully increase activity in the parts of the brain so crucial to our ability to pay attention.

•A Genetic Predisposition

In diagnosing ADHD in you or your child, a health care practitioner should take a complete family history to determine whether any other members in the family show signs of being affected by the disorder. This is because ADHD and other attention disorders run in families. Children diagnosed with ADHD generally have at least one close relative with ADHD, the majority of identical twins share the trait, and about a third of all fathers who had ADHD as children go on to bear children with the disorder. Scientists are currently tracking a gene that may be the culprit involved in transmitting ADHD in some families.

•Fetal Alcohol Syndrome and ADHD

Research on the brains of developing fetuses have offered scientists a number of clues about neurological disorders. A human brain begins its growth from a few cells and develops into a complex, three-pound organ comprised of a billion specialized cells. Now, research reveals that mothers who indulge in heavy alcohol consumption during pregnancy put their unborn infants at risk for fetal alcohol syndrome (FAS), a disorder characterized in children by low birth weight, an impaired intellect, and certain physical defects. Children born with FAS often show the same hyperactivity, low impulse control, and inability to pay attention as those children who are diagnosed with ADHD.

•Lead Exposure May Impair Brain Development

According to the *Cecil Textbook of Medicine*, we are all lead poisoned. Our current lead burden is about 200 times greater than what it was in preindustrial times, and that exposure can have disastrous effects on the brain.

Lead is found in dust, soil, and flaking paint in areas where leaded paint and gasoline were once used, and is even in some of our drinking water pipes. Sadly, over 400,000 U.S. babies are diagnosed with toxic blood lead levels annually.

We have known for some time that lead is toxic enough to lead to miscarriage or brain damage, as it interferes with normal brain development and function by accumulating in the mitochondria of brain cells, causing them to swell and perform abnormally.

Other studies have revealed that chronic lead poisoning can cause problems in the digestive tract and nervous system. Now, researchers tracking behavioral symptoms in young children who show evidence of lead poisoning have discovered that those symptoms include irritability, sleep disturbances, difficulties concentrating, motor incoordination, and symptoms of ADHD.

A number of recent studies support the argument that children who suffer from overexposure to lead are at risk for ADHD. For example, when researchers at the University of Massachusetts School of Public Health evaluated the relationship between lead levels and ADHD by testing for this toxic metal in the tissues of children via hair analysis, they found a striking correlation between ADHD and high lead levels.

In addition, New York researchers from a number of institutions collaborated in comparing the blood and urine lead levels of hyperactive children to those of youngsters who showed no signs of hyperactivity. They found a clear association between hyperactivity and raised lead levels.

Further studies have demonstrated that children with the highest level of lead in their bones are more likely to suffer from behavioral problems and attention disorders. In an investigation performed at the University of Pittsburgh School of Medicine, researchers discovered that many of the children tested who showed high bone lead levels were also diagnosed with ADHD—although these children actually had normal blood lead levels.

Since even low levels of lead exposure are associated with hyperactivity, attention deficit disorder and development failure, the American Academy of Child and Adolescent Psychiatry recommends that any child with behavioral disorders or learning disabilities be tested for lead exposure.

In addition, as you will see in our "Combined Medical and Nutritional Approach" section of this chapter, clinicians are now exploring ways to help mend lead-induced, impaired brain function with nutritional agents such as zinc and NAC. These supplements have proven beneficial in alleviating lead toxicity and the symptoms of ADHD.

Additionally, dietary deficiencies of calcium, iron, and zinc can enhance the negative effects of lead on cognitive and behavioral development by increasing lead absorption and not being able to compete for lead in many biochemical processes in the body.

• The Relationship Between Thyroid Dysfunction and ADHD

Your thyroid gland is located at the base of your neck and, appropriately enough, wraps around your windpipe and is shaped like a bow tie.

This important gland produces hormones with a profound impact on brain and body metabolism because they regulate the rates at which various cells consume oxygen. One of those hormones is thyroxine, which regulates the pace of chemical activity in your body. In other words, the more thyroxine you have in your bloodstream, the more chemical reactions occur.

A variety of recent observations has now led investigators to conclude that a relationship exists between thyroid dysfunction and ADHD. For instance, up to 70 percent of all children with a condition known as "generalized thyroid resistance" to thyroid hormones also demonstrate ADHD symptoms.

Thyroid resistance refers to the decreased ability of body tissues to respond to those important pace-setting thyroid hormones. Patients with thyroid resistance suffer from altered glucose uptake by cells—a feature that we now know impairs brain metabolism. Altered glucose uptake is linked to ADHD if that diminished brain activity happens to be in the brain regions responsible for our ability to pay attention and control our behavior.

In addition, thyroid hormones are important in regulating the "coaching" neurotransmitter, norepinephrine. That's because thyroid hormone augments the ability of brain cell receptors to bind with norepinephrine, promoting the effect of that neurotransmitter on neurons (see below).

• What Causes Impaired Thyroid Function and ADHD?

Scientists are currently investigating possible reasons for impaired thyroid function and the subsequent inability of the locus ceruleus to produce appropriate levels of norepinephrine.

Synthetic chemicals like PCBs, phenols, thiols, and excessive histamines are possibly at fault. According to recent investigations, these environmental toxins can lead to thyroid dysfunction and brain damage, especially in the attention-governing region of the locus ceruleus.

As we mentioned earlier, thyroid hormones help regulate body chemistry by assisting neurotransmitters in their mission to attach to cell membrane receptors. Remember that, when a neurotransmitter like norepinephrine attaches to a membrane receptor, it causes a particular chain of chemical reactions in that cell. So, it is only logical that anything that interferes with that crucial neurotransmitter binding process is going to alter brain chemistry.

Now, animal studies have demonstrated that certain toxins may actually block normal thyroid hormone action because they successfully mimic the hormones and are transported to brain cells in their stead. For example, mice fed low doses of PCBs develop a "spinning syndrome" which causes them to circle their cage incessantly, and the most common neurological damage found in lab animals exposed to PCBs early in life is hyperactivity.

Our brain cells are primed to receive hormonal messages— so much so that they readily accept synthetic imposters in their stead. Luckily, our bodies have devised an elaborate detoxification mechanism to cleanse the body of these interfering imposters. This mechanism, which we call "methylation," depends largely on a powerful enzyme known as SAMe (s-adenosyl methionine), which studies now show to be an effective nutritional supplement in treating adults with ADD.

• Fatty Acids, Thyroid Function, and ADHD

As you already know, the brain is composed mostly of fats. Up to 25 percent of the brain's white matter consists of phospholipids derived from essential fatty acids, which play an important role in forming cell membranes. Fatty acids are also essential precursors to making the substances that brain cells use to communicate with one another.

Clinicians have associated fatty acid deficiency with a variety of skin problems and increased allergies—symptoms that typically affect hyperactive children. Now, a number of studies have gone one step further to identify an essential fatty acid deficiency in many hyperactive children. For example, a 1995 study published in *The American Journal of Clinical Nutrition* showed a correlation between low omega-3 blood levels and ADHD in young boys.

Why should a fatty acid deficiency lead to thyroid dysfunction and ADHD?

As you learned earlier, when a neurotransmitter binds to its cell membrane receptor, it triggers the formation of second messengers responsible for translating the event into a proper cellular response. Essential fatty acids act as these second messengers. They belong to a family of chemical compounds known as "eicosanoids," which are necessary for cell-to-cell communication by receiving the neurotransmitter's signal and ensuring that the next chemical step takes place inside the brain cell. Therefore, a deficiency in fatty acids can lead to inappropriate neurotransmitter effects and altered brain chemistry.

In particular, essential fatty acids play a role in maintaining normal sleep-wake cycles and in stimulating the growth of myelin, the insulating substance on nerve cell fibers that makes better electrical communication possible. Later on in this chapter, we will offer specific recomendations for adding fatty acids to the diet to ease the symptoms of ADHD.

• Dietary Factors: Food Additives, Allergies, and Sugar

In 1973, Dr. Benjamin Feingold first proposed that artificial flavors and artificial colors cause hyperactivity. These include benzoic acid, BHA, BHT, MSG, butylene glycol, potassium bisulfate, potassium and sodium nitrate, sulfites, tartrazines, dyes, and flavorings. In addition, Feingold recommended that hyperactive children avoid salicylates, derivatives of salicylic acid, which is commonly used as a preservative or in the manufacture of aspirin. In addition, salicylates are found in almonds, apples, cherries, pickles, grapes, raisins, oranges, peaches, plums, strawberries, tomatoes, vinegar, and phenolic compounds added to foods.

In a 1994 study at the North Shore Hospital-Cornell Medical Center, researchers M. Boris and F. S. Mandel discovered that eliminating reactive foods—those foods apt to cause a reaction in a sensitive individual—and artificial colors from the diet may actually be of benefit in treating some children with ADHD. This is only one of many such studies equating food additives with increased irritability, restlessness, sleep disturbances, and other negative behaviors among people with ADHD.

Another study, this one published in *Pediatrics,* also reported on sugar as a possible instigator of aggressive behavior, hyperactivity, and attention problems exhibited by children with ADHD. In that investigation, children with ADHD who consumed large amounts of sugar showed greater inattention in performing tasks. However, they demonstrated no more aggressive behavior than usual.

Meanwhile, investigators reporting in *The Journal of Autism and Developmental Disorders* revealed that children with ADHD experienced abnormal rhythms in the stress hormone cortisol—an abnormality frequently associated with problems in metabolizing carbohydrates. Yale researchers have confirmed that children with ADD may have a problem in metabolizing glucose, in that offering children doses of oral glucose significantly diminished their ability to concentrate.

While conflicting data exist regarding food allergies, sugar, and ADHD, clinicians generally recommmend modifying the diet to eliminate possible allergenic foods, dietary chemical preservatives, and sugar to determine whether a particular individual with ADHD or ADD is affected by any of those factors. We will discuss this procedure in greater detail below.

TABLE 7

WHAT CAUSES ADHD?

1. A genetic predisposition.

2. Overexposure to lead, PCBs, or other environmental toxins.

3. Mother's prenatal cocaine or alcohol consumption, especially if fetal alcohol syndrome is also present.

4. Brain damage by physical trauma before, after, or during birth.

5. Thyroid dysfunction.

6. Fatty acid deficiency.

7. Faulty glucose metabolism in certain brain areas that regulate the ability to pay attention.

8. Food allergies and an inability to process refined sugars.

• *Why Are More Boys Affected with ADHD than Girls?*

As we mentioned earlier, the key neurotransmitter involved in coaching the brain to pay attention is norepinephrine. Inadequate norepinephrine levels may result in the inattentiveness experienced by people with either ADD or ADHD. The hyperactivity component of ADHD—which is evidenced by far more boys than girls—is most likely related to inappropriate levels of another neurotransmitter we have discussed earlier in this book: dopamine. Girls may be more likely to have ADD instead of ADHD because estrogen inhibits the reception of dopamine by neurons.

A Combined Medical and Nutritional Approach to ADHD

When Should You Suspect ADHD or ADD?

Like so many neurological illnesses, attention disorders such as ADD and ADHD offer no definitive physical symptoms that can be clearly determined through X rays or blood tests. In general, clinicians must examine a wide range of characteristic behaviors over a period of time in order to diagnose ADD or ADHD. Professionals will determine whether these behaviors are excessive, have lasted a long time, and are a continuous problem rather than a temporary response to surroundings or stimuli.

In general, people with ADHD are diagnosed on the basis of these three characteristic behaviors:

• Hyperactivity

The person with ADHD will always be in motion. Unable to remain at rest for long periods of time, these individuals bounce and twitch in their seats, touch everything, and noisily tap their pens or chew their fingernails. They often try to do several things at once, as they are unable to focus on just one. People with ADD do not exhibit this hyperactive behavior.

• Poor Impulse Control

People with either ADD or ADHD are likely to find it impossible to stop themselves from blurting out inappropriate statements or responding immediately to stimuli. Children with ADHD or ADD are apt to sock a child in anger, for example, and are oblivious to dangers inherent in their actions. These children might jump from high places or cross the street without looking, for example, because they fail to stop and think about possible outcomes.

• Inability to Pay Attention

Everyone daydreams, and most small children have trouble paying attention for long stretches at a time. However, people who are inattentive as a result of ADD or ADHD truly cannot keep their minds on any one thing and find it difficult to pay attention long enough to learn something new. They are easily distracted by irrelevant sights and sounds, fail to pay attention to details, and find it difficult to follow instructions or keep track of personal belongings.

Diagnosing ADHD/ADD: Ensure the Right Diagnosis

A number of specialists are qualified to diagnose ADHD. These include psychiatrists, psychologists, family physicians, pediatricians, and neurologists. The specialist will begin by gathering information as a way of ruling out other possible causes for the individual's inattention and behavior at home, at school, and at work.

Monitoring tools for ADHD/ADD include the Conners Teacher/Parents Rating Scales, ADD-H Comprehensive Teacher Rating Scale, Child Attention Problems Rating Scale, Yale Children's Inventory, DSM-III-R, Wechsler Intelligence Scales for Children, Child Behavior Checklist, Attention Battery, Test of Variables of Attention, the Wide Range Achievement Test, Developmental Test of Visual Motor Integration, and the Learning Efficiency Test II.

Basically, ensuring the right diagnosis means ruling out the following possible causes for inattention, poor impulse control, or hyperactivity:

• Childhood Depression

Symptoms of childhood depression can also include irritability, poor concentration, and acting-out behavior, all of which may be inappropriately attributed to ADHD. A qualified health care professional should evaluate the child for depression as well as ADHD.

• Petit Mal Seizures

Symptoms of petit mal seizures include frequent staring episodes, which may be misinterpreted as poor concentration and hyperactivity. Petit mal seizures may also be associated with eye-blinking movements. Diagnosing petit mal seizures requires an EEG.

• Lead Toxicity

Clinical lead poisoning has been associated with an increased incidence of hyperactivity in children. It is important to test children exhibiting hyperactivity for lead toxicity, although lead toxicity alone is generally not the only cause of ADHD.

• Thyroid Abnormalities

Any routine diagnostic workup should include routine measurements of thyroid and thyroid antibodies. The presence of thyroid antibodies may be caused by "autoimmune thyroiditis," a syndrome which may lead to hypothyroidism. Furthermore, as we have seen here, certain chemicals may take over thyroid hormone receptor sites and subsequently impair thyroid function. Abnormal thyroid tests should, of course, be evaluated by a qualified physician.

The First Step to Take: Rule Out Food Allergies

Eliminating the possibility of food allergies is key in establishing a healthy diet for individuals with attention disorders, as a number of food items may exacerbate symptoms in a small percentage of individuals. While food allergy tests can measure antibody levels and diagnose food allergies, most individuals can employ simple elimination diets without the risk of obtaining the false results common to some food allergy tests.

In simplest terms, you can begin an elimination diet by avoiding the most common allergenic foods for several days. These include milk, wheat, yeast, citrus, egg, chocolate, soy, corn, sugar, and the food additives and salicylates we listed above. Following this initial cleansing, your clinician can monitor behavioral and symptomatic responses as a single, potentially offending food is brought back into the diet at a time.

Although eliminating food allergies this way involves significant initial dietary modifications, this is the most cost-effective, efficient way to detect allergies. In one study conducted at the Institute of Child Health in London, for instance, using an elimination diet resulted in significantly improving the behavior of a group of hyperactive children. Their behavior worsened when they were challenged with allergy-provoking foods.

Similarly, in the prestigious medical journal *Lancet,* investigators reporting on a study with 185 hyperactive children on an elimination diet supported the concept that food allergies are associated with hyperactivity.

We recommend that all individuals considering this method of testing for food allergies do so under the guidance of a qualified nutritionist or physician.

The Second Step to Take: Explore the Role of Sugar in Causing Hyperactivity

As you already know, foods high in refined sugar are the major culprits responsible for poor eating habits leading to nutritional deficiencies. In addition, because of the potential relationship between refined sugar intake and abnormal cortisol rhythms among individuals with ADHD, and because of the impaired brain glucose metabolism found in many people with ADHD, we recommend assessing the patient with ADHD for both reactivity to sugar intake and potential glucose intolerance.

• *Don't Overlook the Possibility of High Lead Levels*

Given that so many studies have correlated the incidence of high lead levels with attention disorders, behavioral problems, and learning disabilities, your health care practitioner will no doubt question you about prenatal lead exposure and request the results of all lead tests. Most often, testing for lead is done through blood serum and urine; however, studies are currently underway to determine whether hair analysis is a viable alternative.

If testing confirms lead poisoning, your clinician may advise you to consider chelation therapy under a specialist's care. Chelation involves administering an agent that binds to the metal and promotes its excretion through the urine. However, although this type of therapy may possibly be valuable in treating lead poisoning in individuals with ADHD, it has potentially severe adverse effects and requires close monitoring, especially of kidney function.

In general, lead poisoning is promoted by zinc, calcium, and iron deficiencies. Therefore, a good route for parents concerned about lead toxicity may be to ensure that children are receiving adequate zinc, calcium, and iron (see below).

Nutritional Therapies You Should Consider Now

In addition to adopting the two-step healthy diet guidelines for healthy individuals we outline in *The Brain Wellness Plan*, individuals with ADHD should modify their diets according to the outcomes of food allergy elimination diets and assessment for both a reactivity to refined sugar and glucose intolerance.

• Add Chromium, Zinc, and the Complete B-Complex to Improve Glucose Metabolism

Individuals who demonstrate glucose intolerance should incorporate fully reacted chromium and zinc chelates and the complete B-complex vitamins into their diets. Chromium is essential for maintaining normal glucose control, while zinc and the B vitamins assist in the utilization of insulin and glucose.

RECOMMENDED DAILY DOSES WITH FOOD:

Chelated zinc	15 mg (children 6–12); 30 mg (adult)
Chelated chromium	100 mcg (children 6–12); 300 mcg (adult)
B-complex vitamins	As found in any children or adult multivitamin-mineral supplement

Look for fully reacted mineral chelates, as these are the best absorbed and utilized.

• Use Fatty Acids to Improve Brain Metabolism

Throughout this book, we have illustrated the importance of omega-3 and other essential fatty acids in building up cell membranes and improving their fluidity. In addition, essential fatty acids are necessary ingredients for the body to make prostaglandins and create myelin sheaths around nerve fibers, the white matter that facilitates cell-to-cell communication.

Independent investigators around the world have reached the conclusion that a deficiency in fatty acids may therefore adversely affect behavior, as a result of lowered prostaglandin production and poor communication between brain cells.

With respect to ADHD, a number of studies confirm the importance of fatty acids in improving the brain metabolism of children. For example, when Purdue University researchers studied the significance of fatty acids in metabolism among subjects with ADHD, they made a startling discovery: These people suffered from significantly lower plasma concentrations of the two most important fatty acids, EPA (eicosapentaenoic acid) and DHA (docosahexaenoic acid).

In another study, a subgroup of ADHD subjects with EFA deficiency symptoms demonstrated significantly lower DHA levels in plasma as compared to ADHD subjects who showed no deficiency in essential fatty acids. Investigators concluded that decreased cellular concentrations of DHA can adversely affect behavior by possibly decreasing the production of prostaglandins that act as modulators of nerve transmission, and believe that the cerebral cortex's proper function may be negatively affected since DHA is the predominant polyunsaturated fatty acid in that part of the brain.

Finally, animal studies have demonstrated that animals restricted to diets low in omega-3 fats have impaired behavioral and neurological functions.

We urge all individuals with attention disorders to consider being tested for fatty acid levels, and to boost fatty acid intake through a combination of DHA, fish oil omega-3 fats, and flaxseed oil. (Flaxseed oil contains linolenic acid, a precursor to the omega-3 fats.)

RECOMMENDED DAILY DOSES WITH FOOD:

DHA   100 mg (children 6–12), 300 mg (adult)
               (Look for the trademarked Neuromins™
                  from Martek Biosciences Corporation.)
Max EPA™   1–2 g (children), 3 g (adult)
Flaxseed oil   1 tbsp for children and adults
               (organic, cold pressed, keep refrigerated)
Vitamin E   100 IU (children 6–12), 400 IU (adult)

All these fatty acid boosters should be taken with meals.

• Keep Up Zinc Levels to Improve ADHD Symptoms

As we have seen in previous chapters, zinc plays a number of important roles in keeping you healthy—particularly when it comes to maintaining a vital immune system.

Now, as scientists continue to map out the various ways in which zinc is needed by your body, a number of studies are pointing to an association between zinc deficiency and ADHD. One such 1996 study, published in the *Journal of Child Psychology and Psychiatry,* revealed a statistically significant correlation between zinc and fatty acids, in that both were decreased in children with ADHD.

In another study, this one conducted at Ohio State University, investigators found a relationship between zinc deficiency and response to stimulant therapy among people with ADHD. (Stimulants such as Ritalin are commonly used to treat children with ADHD, as you will see in our section on medications.) Basically, this study showed that children diagnosed with ADHD may be zinc deficient, and that this deficiency may result in their poor response to stimulant therapy.

Investigators are now exploring the connection between associated deficiencies in zinc and fatty acid levels. The most likely explanation for the association is that zinc is necessary for the body to produce the enzyme which converts precursor ("parent") fat compounds into the essential fatty acid DHA.

Based on these results, we suggest that every individual diagnosed with ADHD be tested for a zinc deficiency. In the event that a zinc supplement proves necessary, we recommend a fully reacted zinc chelate.

RECOMMENDED DOSE: 15 mg for children (6–12) and 30 mg for adults, with a meal. Look for a fully reacted zinc chelate.

• *Amino Acids: Of Controversial Benefit*

Over the past ten years, a number of investigators have been examining the benefits of using the amino acids tyrosine and phenylalanine for treating ADHD. Interest in these amino acids stems from the association of ADHD with deficiencies in norepinephrine or dopamine. Researchers at Ohio State University, for example, have studied plasma amino acids in ADHD patients and found that these individuals had significantly lower levels of several, including tyrosine and tryptophan. These scientists concluded that a general deficit in amino acid transport, absorption, or both may lead to ADHD symptoms.

Since tyrosine and phenylalanine have been shown to increase catecholamine synthesis, scientists have reasoned that the therapeutic application of those amino acids might have positive effects. Unfortunately, several studies have reported no benefits in supplementing the diets of patients with ADHD with either amino acid. Further investigation into this area is ongoing.

Other Neuroimmunomodulating Substances to Discuss with Your Health Care Practitioner

• *SAMe: Improve the Brain's Housekeeping Ability*

The brain requires a continuous recycling of neurotransmitters. For a neurotransmitter to produce its desired effect, it can exist in its active form for only a very short time. It is then broken down by the brain, so that by-products can be recycled for future use in building fresh neurotransmitter messengers.

The brain recycles stale neurotransmitter by-products through two distinct detoxification mechanisms which we call "transulfation" and "transmethylation." As you can probably guess, "trans" means "transfer," and in this case the brain is transferring either a sulfur compound of a methyl compound out of the brain.

Why is it necessary for the brain to transfer these compounds anywhere? Because those forms are easier for the kidneys and liver to dispose of than the more complex compounds.

One key substance involved in transulfation is SAMe (s-adenosyl methionine). This hardy, high-energy compound helps break old neurotransmitters into compounds that can more easily be excreted from the body.

Researchers have discovered that increased levels of SAMe can significantly enhance the body's ability to detoxify itself of various substances, including old neurotransmitters. SAMe is currently under study as a potential therapeutic agent in ADHD as a result.

For instance, in a trial completed by researchers in Israel, adults diagnosed with ADHD took oral doses of SAMe and found that their symptoms improved significantly. Another study conducted by researchers at the University of California at Los Angeles revealed that 75 percent of adults diagnosed with ADHD reported feeling calmer, more in control, and slowed down enough to be more productive after taking SAMe.

Based on these and similar studies supporting the use of therapeutic SAMe in treating ADHD, investigators believe that SAMe may actually help mop up old neurotransmitter materials and improve the way fresh neurotransmitters bind to cell membranes.

While the mechanisms by which SAMe may benefit people with ADHD are still unclear, we suggest discussing the possibility of taking SAMe supplements with your health care practitioner.

RECOMMENDED DOSE: Consult with your health care practitioner about sources and dosages. We recommend that adults take 400 mg tablets, without exceeding 2400 mg per day. Children should be administered half that amount.

Medications Used to Treat ADHD

In most cases, medications are used as a last resort in treating the symptoms of ADHD, particularly in children. However, there are a number of medications on the market that are considered effective. We have listed those that are most commonly prescribed.

•Clonidine

If we prescribe any medication at all for a child diagnosed with ADHD, it is usually clonidine. Clonidine is actually a medication used for blood pressure, and acts on the receptors of the brain stem that receive dopamine and norepinephrine, the two neurotransmitters responsible for your ability to pay attention and monitor your own impulsive behavior. We typically do not prescribe Clonidine for children under five, as major side effects may include fatigue and hypotension.

•Ritalin

By far the most commonly prescribed medication of ADHD, Ritalin is a stimulant that treats only the symptoms of ADHD without addressing the underlying disease process. Furthermore, despite its wide use, Ritalin has become a subject of controversy in the past decade because of its potential side effects, including insomnia, diminished appetite, and the appearance of motor tics. We recommend Ritalin in only the most extreme cases of ADHD, and as a last resort.

•Effexor (venlafaxine)

A newly developed antidepressant, venlafaxine has been shown to be successful in treating some adults with ADHD. This medication appears to enhance neurotransmitter activity in the brain, and is a potent inhibitor of both norepinephrine and serotonin reuptake, which means more of these neurotransmitters are left around for the benefit of cell use.

•Piracetam

Originally introduced as a memory-enhancing medication, Piracetam improves the metabolism of brain cells through various mechanisms. Animal studies have shown that Piracetam has the potential to enhance learning and memory, and this medication is currently being investigated for its potential in treating neurological illnesses as wide-ranging as Alzheimer's and ADHD.

In adults with attention disorders, some clinicians are now

prescribing Piracetam to enhance attention. The drug has no appreciable effect on hyperactivity, and its effect on children has not been fully studied.

Putting It All Together

We were as determined as Clarissa to use medication as a last resort in treating her son Jon for ADHD. Instead, we began by referring the family to a nutritionist, who helped them eliminate allergies to certain foods and food additives and coached them in finding ways to improve Jon's eating habits. The elimination diet showed that Jon suffered from a significant milk allergy. Additional testing proved that Jon showed no evidence of abnormal glucose intolerance.

We immediately suggested that Jon discontinue drinking milk, and Clarissa began including juices and other nonmilk drinks in Jon's lunchbox for school. In addition, we added supplements of 400 mg of DHA, 3 g of fish oil, and 2 tablespoons of flaxseed oil to boost Jon's essential fatty acid intake and improve his brain metabolism, as Jon suffered from the excessive thirst and dry skin common to so many children with ADHD who are deficient in omega-3 fatty acids. We also recommended that Jon be given 15 mg daily of zinc, and assessed Jon for adequate calcium and iron intake as we offered suggestions for good dietary sources.

Clarissa and Ray began seeing a family counselor with Jon to learn how to better moderate their son's behavior, and worked closely with Jon's preschool and kindergarten teachers to assess his progress and adjust his learning environment where needed. Today, Jon is in the first grade, reads well, and is well liked by his classmates. Although he is still a highly energetic boy, he suffers none of the frustration in the classroom that he experienced in his early years, and is much more manageable at home.

Now that you have an overview of attention disorders and of how they may impact on brain metabolism, you are probably eager to begin investigating a complete ADHD treatment protocol for yourself or someone you love. We encourage all patients with ADHD to seek individual and family counseling to help resolve behavioral and emotional issues, and to investigate the educational support available through public and private schools.

Dietary Protocol

- Use elimination diets under the guidance of a professional to assess allergies to foods and food additives, and to evaluate the effect of sugar intake.
- Assess for adequate calcium and iron intake. If deficiencies exist, add 1000 mg of calcium, 400 mg of magnesium, and 15 mg of iron (use fully reacted mineral chelates).
- In the presence of glucose intolerance, add 200 mcg of fully reacted, chelated chromium taken twice daily.

Daily Nutritional Supplements

DHA (look for the preferred Neuromins™)	300 mg (adult), 100 mg (children)
Fish oil (look for MaxEPA™)	3 g (adult), 1–2 g (children)
Flaxseed oil (cold-pressed, organic, keep refrigerated)	1 tbsp
Chelated zinc	15 mg (children, 6–12); 30 mg (adult)
Vitamin E	400 IU (adult), 100 IU (children)

(For additional essential support, add 100 mg phosphatidyl-serine)
All supplements are to be taken with food.

Other Neuroimmunomodulating Substances to Discuss with Your Health Care Practitioner

SAMe (s-adenosyl methionine)

Medications

Clonidine
Ritalin
Effexor (venlafaxine)
Piracetam

CHRONIC FATIGUE SYNDROME

Alicia was thirty-seven when she came down with a particularly severe flu. She had always been able to kick that sort of thing within a few days, but this time was different. Although she stayed in bed for more than a week and her fever and headache did seem to ease a bit, she just couldn't seem to get enough rest to feel like herself again.

Admittedly, Alicia's job as a social worker left her feeling burned out—there were always too many clients and not enough time in the day to see them all—but something was definitely wrong with her. Even the simplest things, such as carrying the laundry downstairs, left her completely fatigued.

Weeks turned into months, and yet Alicia wasn't getting any better, despite the fact that her family physician had found nothing wrong. She was having trouble concentrating at work, she wasn't sleeping well, her lymph nodes felt swollen from time to time, and her headaches and fevers continued. Her husband was losing patience with her, and told her to "get a grip" on herself because he wasn't about to be married to someone who made him fetch and carry for her every day.

Finally, Alicia began seeing a round of specialists. A psychologist suggested depression, while an infectious disease specialist tested her for all sorts of illnesses she had never even heard of before. It was a full year, in fact, before a neurologist confirmed Alicia's diagnosis: She was suffering from chronic fatigue syndrome.

"Is this ever going to get better?" she pleaded. "I feel like I'm at death's door."

Chronic Fatigue Syndrome: An Overview

Chronic fatigue syndrome (CFS) began drawing the national spotlight in 1985, when Nevada physicians reported an unusually high number of unrelated patients suffering from disturbingly similar symptoms. Those symptoms included chronic fatigue, headaches, fevers, and aching muscles. The Centers for Disease Control recognized the condition and dubbed it "chronic fatigue syndrome" for its one common symptom—the debilitating exhaustion that affects everyone with CFS.

Today, interest in CFS has prompted investigators around the world to scrutinize its causes and pathways. What should be clearly stated at the outset of any discussion of CFS is this: Although up to a quarter of all U.S. adults attending primary care clinics report that fatigue is a major problem affecting their lives, the fatigue that serves as the hallmark symptom of CFS is much more persistent and severe.

Accompanying symptoms of CFS vary according to the individual, and may cover everything from joint pain to fevers, and decreased memory capability to depression. Because of this, a CFS diagnosis is usually made on the basis of symptoms lasting at least six months and only after eliminating other possible conditions that could be causing the fatigue and other symptoms described.

In fact, one of the biggest problems associated with the disease is lack of credibility—patients suffering from CFS have been accused by friends and coworkers of being hypochondriacs or of having "that yuppie flu." And despite the fact that an illness resembling CFS was described by an English physician, Sir Richard Manningham, as early as the mid-1700s, even some physicians refuse to be convinced that the condition is real. Patients often have to see several physicians, including specialists in neurology, immunology, and psychiatry before being successfully diagnosed—a process that is as frustrating as it is wearing.

To date, scientists have not yet uncovered the cause of CFS.

Most postulate that it is due to a combination of multiple factors acting together rather than the result of a single cause. The one common factor many patients report is the onset of a severe illness, such as bronchitis, gastrointestinal illness, sore throats, or hepatitis, just before developing CFS.

CFS is not a fatal disease, but at its most severe can be debilitating enough to impair an individual's ability to work, care for a household, or otherwise enjoy life. Although about 70 percent of the people diagnosed with CFS are young white women in the middle class, this disparate proportion may have to do with the fact that women are more apt to seek out medical care than men, or because the skepticism surrounding this diagnosis prevents individuals from other groups from seeking help.

Although neither cause nor cure has yet been discovered for this complex syndrome, our evolving biochemical knowledge about brain and immune system functions has brought us much closer to finding effective treatments for CFS.

In this chapter, we explore the most current theories developed to explain how CFS affects the brain and the immune system. We will then describe the disease in detail from onset to diagnosis, and present an aggressive treatment plan based on today's scientific findings in nutrition, neurology, and immunology.

What Goes Wrong in Chronic Fatigue Syndrome, and Why

Researchers at top medical centers around the world are conducting basic research and clinical studies to determine just what causes CFS.

To date, investigators have uncovered clues leading us to believe that (1) chronic fatigue syndrome may be an example of the hypothalamus failing to properly regulate the brain's influence on the immune system; (2) a clear relationship exists between CFS and one type of hypotension; (3) the symptoms of CFS may be produced, at least in part, by inadequate muscle metabolism of oxygen and nutrients; and (4) CFS may be due to an immune disorder.

• The Brain's Master Conductor Misses a Beat

From our earlier chapters on the brain-immune connection, you know that the hypothalamus is the key intersection for communication between your body's brain and immune system. Now, scientists believe that hypothalamic dysfunction may be at the root of CFS.

The tiny, pea-sized hypothalamus coordinates the activity of the brain and immune system by regulating the messenger molecules that travel between the two. In this way, the hypothalamus is the central control tower when it comes to coordinating the immune system; the endocrine system, which consists of the hormone-producing endocrine glands; and the autonomic nervous system, which regulates cardiac or smooth muscle cells and glands.

Among the most important glands to be under the control of your hypothalamus are the adrenal glands—small, triangular organs, one on top of each kidney. Although no more than a few centimeters in size, these glands are responsible for synthesizing some of your body's most essential hormones, including cortisol.

The hypothalamus produces a messenger hormone known as corticotropin-releasing hormone, or CRH, which is sent out by the brain as a chemical messenger to provoke the necessary responses among all three body systems mentioned above. CRH is especially critical for coordinating your body's response to stress because it provokes your adrenal glands to make cortisol.

Many people diagnosed with CFS suffer from low levels of CRH. Since that hormone is so essential in gearing up the adrenal glands to secrete cortisol, many people with CFS suffer from impaired adrenal gland function during times of infection or other types of stress. In other words, CFS is a state of relative adrenal insufficiency which occurs as a result of reduced CRH levels and, consequently, a reduced ability to manufacture cortisol. According to studies done at the National Institute of Mental Health and other research centers, cortisol is a necessary part of the body's defense against stressors such as toxins and infections. The low levels of CRH and, consequently, of cortisol could cause many of the common symptoms of CFS, such as fatigue, swollen lymph nodes, muscle and joint pain, insomnia, and depression.

As you will see later in this chapter, one of the revolutionary new treatments for people with CFS involves nutritionally supporting adrenal gland function as a way of restoring a healthy brain-immune connection.

• Hypotension and CFS: Why Do These Two So Often Go Together?

Recently, a landmark study performed at Johns Hopkins University proved that many people with CFS are also afflicted with a syndrome known as "neurally mediated hypotension" (NMH).

Just what is NMH? Under normal circumstances, your body is able to maintain a steady blood pressure and pulse while you change positions—from lying down to getting to your feet, for example. However, in NMH, the body has lost this ability to regulate the effects of heart rate and blood pressure during postural changes. This causes the blood pressure to decrease so much that, when the patient changes position, the result may be severe fatigue or headaches because of reduced blood flow to the brain.

NMH is typically diagnosed through a "tilt test," in which the patient lies on a table that the physician tilts in different directions, all the while monitoring the effects those position changes have on blood pressure and pulse. The Johns Hopkins study revealed that the majority of patients diagnosed with CFS also suffer precipitous falls in their blood pressure or heart rates during such tilt tests, indicating that they have NMH, too.

Why would CFS and hypotension go hand-in-hand so often?

Again, the answer boils down to having inadequate levels of CRH.

The autonomic nervous system is responsible for regulating the functions of cardiac and other smooth muscle cells in the body. One particular component of this system, the "sympathetic nervous system," specifically controls pulse and blood pressure.

As with the adrenal glands, the CRH hormone is the brain's lead messenger in regulating the sympathetic nervous system. If the brain is not producing enough of this hormone, it's like pressing the accelerator in a car that has run out of gas: there just isn't enough CRH to do the job. Consequently, the body is unable to maintain a steady blood pressure level or pulse rate.

The reasons for such a CRH deficiency are still under speculation. One possible explanation is that there has been a disruption in the normal feedback loop between the brain, the immune system, and the endocrine system, possibly owing to an infection or environmental toxin.

• Oxidative Muscle Metabolism: Not Enough Cellular Energy for Muscles

Many patients with CFS complain that they are so tired that they feel as if they are dragging about with their feet encased in heavy boots. Exercise may further aggravate their symptoms of fatigue and muscle pain.

Studies conducted with CFS patients performing heavy exercise have shown that these individuals exhibit higher heart rates than people without the disorder and are unable to fully activate skeletal muscles during intense fatigue. In addition, researchers have found abnormalities in the mitochondria of muscle cells—the tiny energy factory organelles responsible for cellular metabolism—among people with CFS.

At the Medical College of Pennsylvania, for example, investigators have studied people with CFS to see if the ability of their muscle cells to metabolize oxygen and other nutrients to produce energy in the form of ATP (adenosine phosphate) is affected by their condition.

They found that this ability was significantly reduced, and concluded that patients with CFS are affected by a functional abnormality in "oxidative muscle metabolism," or the way their muscle cells burn oxygen and other nutrients to produce energy. In our "Combined Medical and Nutritional Approach" section, you will discover that one particular nutritional supplement, coenzyme Q10, can help boost the ability of muscles to perform work among patients with CFS.

• What About Immune System Complications Owing to Epstein-Barr Virus and Other Viral Complications?

Early research indicated that some CFS patients had unusually high levels of antibodies to Epstein-Barr virus (EBV), the virus that causes infectious mononucleosis. Typically, acute illness eventually subsides in people infected with EBV, with the virus remaining dormant. However, in some CFS patients the antibody levels remained high, suggesting to some investigators that CFS might be a sort of chronic EBV.

Now, new evidence reveals that many other individuals without CFS also have high EBV antibody levels, leading most scientists to now conclude that EBV does not lead to CFS in most patients. However, recent studies do support the concept that EBV and a number of other viruses may be reactivated in patients with CFS, though whether this viral reactivation causes CFS or is a result of the syndrome remains to be seen.

Scientists are continuing to investigate the link between CFS and immune system complications that occur as a result of viral infections. Studies reveal that patients with CFS may have low levels of white blood cell activity, for example, or an abnormal distribution of white blood cells. Among those investigating the link between CFS and immune system breakdowns are researchers at the University of Miami School of Medicine. They have found that cytokines such as certain interleukins and tumor necrosis factor are elevated in patients with CFS, indicating that these patients suffer from the same sort of overzealous immune system activity prominent in so many other neurological illnesses.

Overall, then, in treating CFS, it is essential to ensure that patients receive the proper nutrition to build a healthy immune system.

A Combined Medical and Nutritional Approach to CFS

Although there is no cure for CFS, you can take aggressive steps now toward (1) adjusting your lifestyle to better manage the condition, (2) enhancing your brain's production of the

TABLE **8**

WHAT CAUSES CHRONIC FATIGUE SYNDROME?

- The hypothalamus produces inadequate levels of CRH (corticotropin-releasing hormone), which leads to a subsequent breakdown in adrenal gland production of cortisol.

- An association between neurally mediated hypotension and CFS.

- Insufficient energy metabolism by muscle cells.

- Immune system complications provoked by prior viral infections.

essential hormone CRH; (3) addressing the possible connection between hypotension and CFS; (4) boosting muscle metabolism; and (5) building back your immune system.

When Should You Suspect CFS?

CFS is often difficult to diagnose because individuals with the disorder vary widely in their symptoms, from being severely disabled and even bedridden to simply being unusually fatigued following stressful events. To add to the mysterious nature of this disorder, symptoms tend to come and go over time. CFS is often diagnosed only after many months and after other secondary causes of fatigue have been ruled out.

Generally, CFS is diagnosed according to these core criteria:

- Clinically evaluated, unexplained persistent or relapsing chronic fatigue that is not the result of ongoing exertion or alleviated by rest; this fatigue often results in an impaired ability to keep up with one's work, education, and social and personal life;
- The presence of four or more of the symptoms listed below, all of which must have lasted or recurred during at least six consecutive months since the fatigue first set in:
  - sleep disturbances

- tender lymph nodes
- sore throat
- short-term memory loss
- muscle pain
- joint swelling
- headaches

Secondary Causes of Fatigue to Be Ruled Out During Diagnosis

For a certain CFS diagnosis, it is first essential to rule out other possible causes of the pervasive fatigue experienced by patients, such as:

• Lyme Disease and Other Chronic Infections

A tick-borne illness characterized by rash and arthritis, Lyme disease is currently endemic to several areas of the United States. Two of the most frequent symptoms of Lyme disease are fatigue and malaise; in fact, estimates are that up to 80 percent of patients with Lyme disease experience significant and long-term fatigue.

Other infections that can cause fatigue include HIV, hepatitis, and chronic yeast infections. All these chronic infections can be ruled out through laboratory blood tests or spinal fluid analysis.

• Thyroid Disease

Hypothyroidism or low levels of circulating thyroid hormone characteristically produce fatigue and other associated symptoms, including constipation, slowed thinking, and excessively dry skin. Hypothyroidism can be ruled out through an analysis of thyroid-stimulating hormone (TSH) by ultrasensitive assay.

• Vitamin Deficiencies

A number of different vitamin deficiencies, especially low levels of B_{12}, are characterized by lassitude and fatigue. Again, the possibility of these deficiencies should be ruled out through laboratory tests in diagnosing CFS.

• Neurally Mediated Hypotension

Although NMH does not cause CFS, it may be useful for patients experiencing headaches and lightheadedness to have a "tilt test" to determine if NMH is causing those symptoms. As we discussed earlier, many patients with CFS also have NMH.

The First Step to Take in Treating CFS: Lifestyle Adjustments

Patients with CFS must take good care of themselves through adjusting their work or personal habits to minimize stress, improve sleep habits, and eat according to *The Brain Wellness Plan* guidelines for nutrition set out earlier in this book. The truth is, although this disease can be long-term and debilitating in some, many people do recover from CFS or manage the symptoms very well over time.

Dietary Suggestions You Can Incorporate Now

The nutritional therapy for CFS gives considerable attention to eliminating food allergies, enhancing immune and adrenal function, supporting the production of energy by muscle cells, addressing debilitating symptoms, and correcting nutritional deficiencies that might otherwise hamper rehabilitation.

Patients with CFS commonly experience gastrointestinal symptoms such as flatulence and poor digestive function. The "friendly bacteria" we describe in *The Brain Wellness Plan,* along with the other nutrients listed there that specifically support gastrointestinal functions, should help alleviate those symptoms.

• See a Qualified Nutritionist to Evaluate Individual Dietary Restrictions

Patients with CFS should seek the care of a qualified nutritionist to assess nutritional deficiencies and diagnose food allergies. In many cases, nutritionists treating CFS will advise an elimination diet, whereby all possible allergenic foods are avoided for a period of time and then reincorporated gradually to assess for food allergies.

The nutritionist will also evaluate whether the patient has a sugar intolerance, which would warrant a higher protein, moderate carbohydrate diet taken in small, frequent meals throughout the day.

Nutritional Supplements to Begin Taking Now

• NADH and Chronic Fatigue Syndrome

Rationale for Use of NADH in Chronic Fatigue Syndrome The etiology of chronic fatigue syndrome is currently unknown. As we mentioned earlier, a leading hypothesis suggests that defects in cellular energy production lead to decreased levels of ATP, as well as to the development of clinical symptoms like muscle cramps and fatigue. NADH increases energy production by stimulating mitochondria and, therefore, the manufacture of ATP.

Clinical Studies of NADH and Chronic Fatigue Syndrome A recent study at George Washington University Medical School involving 26 patients with chronic fatigue syndrome randomized the patients into two groups: the first received 10 mg of NADH over a one-month period and the second received a placebo. Approximately 30 percent of patients who received NADH reported relief of symptoms with no adverse effects.

RECOMMENDED DOSE: 10 mg daily, divided into two 5 mg doses.

• Transfer Factor and Chronic Fatigue Syndrome

What is transfer factor? Transfer factor is a large protein or peptide that assists in passive immunity. An example of passive immunity is when a mother breastfeeds her child and, in the process, passes on valuable antibodies that protect the child against infections. Transfer factor is found in human breast milk and in cow's milk. It is a natural stimulator of the immune system.

Rationale for Use of Transfer Factor in Chronic Fatigue Syndrome
Transfer factor has been found to be effective in various infectious diseases, such as herpes and other viral infections, including Epstein-Barr virus infection. CFS is often associated with these viruses.

Clinical Studies of Transfer Factor in Chronic Fatigue Syndrome
In a clinical trial performed at the viral epidemiology branch of the National Cancer Institute, researchers noted some dramatic improvements following the administration of transfer factor to patients with CFS. In the published report describing this study, follow-up studies were recommended, but have not been completed. However, many clinicians now employ transfer factor in treating immune disorders like CFS.

RECOMMENDED DOSE: Transfer factor is available in health food stores under the label "Cholostrum," but since it is unregulated, it is unclear how much transfer factor these preparations contain. Therefore, it's recommended that transfer factor be obtained from your health care practitioner. It is readily absorbed when taken orally. Precautions: Patients with autoimmune disease in which the immune system is already overactive should not take transfer factor.

• Boost Adrenal Function Through Nutrients and Herbs

The symptoms associated with low adrenal function include excessive fatigue, weakness, depression, insomnia, swollen lymph nodes, allergies, and headaches—a list of symptoms strikingly similar to the symptoms for CFS.

As we have noted earlier, people with CFS are often suffering from insufficient levels of adrenal hormones such as cortisol, owing to low levels of corticotropin-releasing hormone (CRH) and subsequently impaired adrenal gland function.

The adrenal glands contain the highest concentrations of

vitamin C in the body, and vitamin C is an essential cofactor in the enzyme precursor to making norepinephrine, the neurotransmitter which plays the largest role in regulating our sympathetic and parasympathetic nervous system. Therefore, it is essential that people with CFS limit adrenal gland stressors such as sugar and caffeine and incorporate the nutrients necessary for optimal adrenal support. These include vitamin C, zinc, vitamin B$_6$, pantothenic acid, and magnesium. These nutrients all play necessary roles in the manufacture of hormones by the adrenal glands.

For instance, a recent study published in *Lancet* revealed that patients with CFS have lower red cell magnesium and showed that magnesium supplements led to improved energy, better emotional states, and less pain among those patients.

Herbs have also proven beneficial in supporting the adrenal glands. For example, animal studies have shown that one of the best nutrients for supporting everything from enhancing adrenal gland hormone production to inhibiting adrenal atrophy is ginseng. The active ingredients in ginseng responsible for boosting adrenal function are "ginsenosides" in Panax ginseng extract and "eleutherosides" in Siberian ginseng; both have proven effective in promoting hormone production in the adrenal glands.

Another herb useful in managing CFS is standardized licorice extract (although this should be avoided if hypertension or depression is present). The ingredient in licorice that has proven active in affecting adrenal function is called "glycyrrhizin." Glycyrrhizin acts by stimulating the adrenal glands to produce cortisol and to prolong cortisol action. One 1995 article, published in the *New Zealand Medical Journal,* described the use of licorice in treating CFS and concluded that licorice upped cortisol production.

RECOMMENDED DAILY DOSES:

Vitamin C	4 g, in divided doses. The use of calcium ascorbate may help prevent GI tract upset.
Pantothenic acid	50 mg

Zinc	30 mg (Use a fully reacted mineral chelate for efficient absorption and utilization.)
Magnesium	600 mg in divided doses. (Use a fully reacted mineral chelate for efficient absorption and utilization.)
Ginseng	500 mg standardized Panax ginseng or Siberian ginseng
Licorice	150 mg standardized extract, as long as no hypertension or depression is present

All these nutritional supplements should be taken with meals.

• Enhance Muscle Metabolism

As we described earlier, many patients with CFS suffer from impaired energy metabolism in their muscle cells. In addition to the full B-complex vitamins we recommend in *The Brain Wellness Plan,* we suggest that all patients with CFS incorporate coenzyme Q10 and creatine to enhance muscle metabolism by assisting the production of ATP in muscle cells.

If you recall, ATP (adenosine triphosphate) is the energy currency of cells, serving as the chemical intermediate through which at least half of the energy of cells is released during the breakdown of carbohydrates, fats, and proteins. Half of the energy produced goes to the cell, while the other half is released as heat energy.

One of the most essential cellular ingredients for producing ATP is coenzyme Q10. And as an antioxidant, coenzyme Q10 helps protect the cell from free radical damage.

Creatine phosphate is just as essential to energy production in muscle cells, because ATP cannot be produced unless creatine phosphate is around to donate a phosphorus molecule. A nutrient naturally found in our bodies, creatine is made from the amino acids arginine, methionine, and glycine. It has been shown to increase muscle mass through promoting better protein synthesis within muscle fibers, and is essential for muscle contractions.

Researchers from the Queen's Medical Center in the United Kingdom established the important role of creatine in ATP muscle production. In addition, they have shown that supplemental creatine can significantly enhance muscle strength and reduce the amount of ATP lost during exercise.

We recommend that all patients with CFS incorporate a supplement of coenzyme Q10, and add creatine supplements if engaged in regular exercise.

RECOMMENDED DAILY DOSES:

Coenzyme Q10   200 mg, with food
Creatine monohydrate   5 g, on an empty stomach (Use
                           only if involved in a regular
                           exercise regime.)

• Rebuild Your Immune System Through General Multivitamin and Antioxidant Supplements

Because so many patients with CFS also have weakened immune systems, our "Combined Medical and Nutritional Approach" emphasizes supporting immune function through nutrients and herbs with proven roles as immune boosters.

Research in recent years has shown that a number of nutritional substances have the power to enhance the immune system. Studies have revealed the following:

- Reduced zinc levels are associated with decreased white blood cell activity.
- Vitamin A maintains the integrity of the immune system by stimulating and enhancing white blood cell activity and antibody response.
- Deficiencies in B vitamins can reduce antibodies and cell-mediated immune responses.
- Vitamin D can function as a steroid hormone, in that a number of white blood cells possess receptors for active vitamin D and are regulated by this vitamin.
- Selenium deficiency inhibits macrophage activity and the production of the tumor necrosis factor cytokine.

- Copper deficiency impairs macrophage function, the production of white blood cells, and healthy cytokine response.
- Vitamin C can modulate immune response by activating white blood cells and enhancing cytokine production.
- A deficiency in coenzyme Q10 is associated with viral infections.
- Vitamin E (tocopherols and tocotrienols) serve as antioxidants with immune-related functions, in that they can lower prostaglandin E2 levels and enhance immunity.

In general, all of the above nutrients are easy to come by, provided that patients with CFS follow our recommendations in Chapters 3 and 4 of *The Brain Wellness Plan*.

• *Enhance Glutathione Levels to Further Protect Cells from Free Radicals*

Free radical damage to DNA, proteins, and fats in cells is a major contributor to degenerative diseases such as CFS. In addition to the free radical damage done to cells during normal cellular metabolism, immune cell activity, and other processes, patients with CFS are also more vulnerable to damage by free radicals produced by external factors such as fatty foods, radiation, and cigarette smoke.

During any challenge to the immune system—as in CFS—additional antioxidants are required to help scavenge the free radicals produced as a result of immune system battles. The antioxidant complex described above will certainly help ameliorate any antioxidant deficiency. However, because patients with CFS are particularly vulnerable to fatigue, headaches, fevers, muscle pain, and other stresses on the immune system, we also recommend that these individuals boost their glutathione levels as extra insurance against free radical oxidation injury.

The ability of cells to maintain an adequate glutathione status is critical to our health. Additionally, through the activation of the enzyme glutathione transferase, glutathione inactivates toxic compounds that may hinder immune response.

The best strategy for boosting cellular glutathione levels is through supplements of NAC (n-acetyl-cysteine), lipoic acid, and selenium, which is an essential ingredient in making the glutathione transferase enzyme.

RECOMMENDED DAILY DOSES:

Lipoic acid   200 mg, with food
NAC   1 g, on an empty stomach
Selenium   200 mcg, with food (Do not exceed this amount.)

• Polyphenols: Strong Antioxidants to the Rescue

Polyphenols are strong antioxidants with a number of other important functions. For example, polyphenols can attach themselves to certain pro-oxidant metals, such as iron, thereby reducing the capacity of that metal to produce free radicals in the body. In addition, polyphenols can inhibit the effects of toxic arachidonic acid in the body by inhibiting lipoxygenase, the enzyme that converts arachidonic acid into leukotrienes (mediators of allergies and inflammation). Finally, polyphenols can gear up the immune system to combat viral infections.

One supplement of particular benefit in treating CFS is Pycnogenol®, a derivative extract from the bark of a French marine pine tree which contains a number of important polyphenolic components. As a dietary supplement, it acts as both an antioxidant and an immune system booster.

Animal studies conducted at the University of Arizona showed that Pycnogenol® has the power to maintain healthy immune system function by restoring cytokine imbalances and increasing white blood cell activity.

Our food supply is filled with polyphenols. Excellent sources include red wine, green tea, berries and other fruits, soybeans, and dark vegetables. The best supplement sources include Pycnogenol®, rhododendron extract, grape seed extract, pine bark extract, and herbs such as bilberry, ginkgo, and milk thistle.

RECOMMENDED DAILY DOSES: The best supplement sources include Pycnogenol®, fruit polyphenols, grape seed extract, pine bark extract, and herbs such as bilberry, ginkgo, and milk thistle. Choose one of the excellent sources of polyphenols listed below or look for a formula that combines several sources.

Pycnogenol® or pine bark extract	120 mg, with a meal
Grape seed extract	120 mg, with a meal
Fruit polyphenols	120 mg, with a meal

• Use Essential Fats to Strengthen Cells

Supplementing the diet of individuals suffering from immune-related disorders has proven that omega-3 fats such as EPA (eicosapentaenoic acid) and DHA (docosahexaenoic acid) can have a profound role in diminishing unwanted inflammation and building up immune function.

Omega-3 fatty acids from fish and algae sources can successfully compete with omega-6 fatty acids from corn and other vegetable oils, which can positively influence immune system function, as omega-6 fats have been shown to heighten inflammatory responses while suppressing the immune system.

In 1994, an article published in *Medical Hypotheses* demonstrated that offering supplements of omega-3 fats and gamma-linoleic acid (GLA) from primrose or borage oil significantly improved the immune systems of patients with CFS participating in the study. Scientists in other investigations have shown that omega-3 supplements can help reduce cytokine-mediated inflammation.

Food sources for omega-3 fats include fatty fish (salmon, mackerel, herring, and tuna). The omega-3 fatty acids can be easily obtained by using any of the following supplements: flaxseed oil, MaxEPA™ brand of fish oils, and the vegetarian source of DHA (look for the trademarked Neuromins™ brand). We also suggest adding primrose or borage oil.

RECOMMENDED DAILY DOSES:

MaxEPA™	2 g
DHA (Neuromins™)	300 mg
Primrose or borage oil	2 g

These supplements should all be taken with meals.

• Add These Herbs to Stimulate Your Immune System

Any immune nutritional protocol should include the following herbs for optimum support:

Astragalus membranaceous: 500 mg standardized extract daily. May be used long-term. Enhances antibody response, increases helper T-lymphocytes and natural killer cell activity, and promotes production of certain cytokines.

Echinacea: 250 mg standardized extract daily. Use for seven to ten days with three-week rest intervals. Stimulates macrophages, enhances white blood cells, and cytokine production.

Reishi mushroom: 4 g standardized extract daily. Increases production of cytokines and natural killer cells, boosts white blood cell activity. May be used long-term.

Shiitake mushroom: 4 g standardized extract daily. Stimulates white blood cell and natural killer cell activity, activates macrophages and promotes their recognition of antigens, and boosts white blood cell proliferation. May be used long-term.

Maitake mushroom: 4 g standardized extract daily. Activates macrophages, natural killer cells, and white blood cells. Also stimulates cytokine production. May be used long-term.

What Other Neuroimmunomodulators Should You Discuss with Your Health Care Practitioner?

• If the Tilt Test Reveals NMH, Consider Salt and Fludrocortisone

As so many patients with CFS also are diagnosed with NMH (neurally mediated hypotension), we advise our patients to have a tilt test. If the tilt test proves positive for NMH, we recommend increased salt intake or a mineral corticoid drug, Fludrocortisone, to reestablish your body's ability to maintain a steady blood pressure and pulse. Salt and Fludrocortisone do this by helping the kidneys to retain sodium and, therefore, to retain body fluids and maintain blood pressure.

• Address Sleep Disorders with Melatonin or Medication

Fatigue is the hallmark of CFS. Yet despite how tired they are, many patients with CFS report that they have difficulty getting to sleep and that their sleep is often disturbed. Whether CFS promotes sleep disturbances or sleep disturbances are simply a significant contributor to the overwhelming fatigue experienced by patients with the disorder, a health care practitioner should certainly thoroughly evaluate sleep patterns in treating patients with the disorder.

If sleep disturbances are reported, we recommend that patients try melatonin first to help restore normal sleep patterns. If that fails, there are a number of other herbs and medications that have proven beneficial in helping patients with CFS normalize sleep-wake cycles. Consult with your health care practitioner to find the proper type of sleeping aid and correct dosage.

• Improve Hypothalamus Function through SSRIs like Zoloft, Paxil, or Prozac

As we discussed at the outset of this chapter, one of the newest theories posed to explain CFS involves hypothalamic dysfunction. In treating patients, we often prescribe medications such as Zoloft, Paxil, or Prozac, as these SSRIs (selective serotonin reuptake inhibitors) have the ability to restore any abnormalities in serotonin receptors located in the hypothalamus.

As you may recall, the serotonin neurotransmitter plays a leading role in regulating sleep, appetite, sexual behavior, mood swings, the cardiovascular system, and immune system activity. Serotonin imbalances in the brain have been linked to a wide range of neurological disorders, including autism and depression.

Among its other features, serotonin is able to restore the activity of CRH, one of the body's most influential hormones. In a significant number of patients with CFS, SSRIs have demonstrated the ability to raise brain serotonin levels and reset CRH activity, therefore leading to healthier adrenal gland function.

Putting It All Together

In putting Alicia back on the road to good health, we encouraged her to take a close look at the long hours she was keeping in her position as a head social worker at a busy urban clinic. Alicia subsequently cut her hours in half and began taking a yoga class in the evenings.

Taking melatonin supplements restored Alicia's ability to get a good night's sleep, and she worked closely with a nutritionist to evaluate her eating habits and reduce her sugar intake. In addition, we referred Alicia to a medical center for a tilt test to rule out the possibility of NMH.

To support Alicia's flagging adrenal glands and immune system, we added all the nutritional supplements described in the protocol below. A month later, we estimated that Alicia had improved about 40 percent in most of her symptoms. She was less tired, experienced fewer headaches and fevers, and seemed to have a much higher energy level.

However, as Alicia still had relapses now and then, suffering occasional fevers and headaches during bouts of fatigue that caused her to cut back on her daily activities still further, we prescribed Zoloft. Now, more than two years later, Alicia has improved by more than 75 percent in all the symptoms she reported. She has been able to add a moderate exercise program and has returned to working full-time.

With this overview of chronic fatigue syndrome, you are probably anxious to begin—or to help someone you love get started—investigating the ways in which you can boost your immune function, muscle metabolism, and adrenal function through an aggressive protocol.

Here is our summary guideline for treatment.

| *Dietary Modifications* | Follow *The Brain Wellness Plan.* |

Daily Nutritional Supplements

Vitamin C	4 g in divided doses with food. The use of calcium ascorbate may help prevent GI tract upset.
Pantothenic acid	50 mg
Zinc*	30 mg of zinc glycinate or zinc histidinate with food
Magnesium*	600 mg of magnesium glycinate or magnesium citrate, taken in divided doses with food.
Licorice	150 mg of standardized extract, as long as no hypertension or depression is present
Coenzyme Q10	200 mg with a meal
Creatine monohydrate	5 g on an empty stomach (use only if involved in a regular exercise program)
Lipoic acid	200 mg with a meal
NAC (n-acetyl-cysteine)	1 g on an empty stomach
Selenium	200 mcg with a meal (Do not exceed this amount.)

Choose one:
Pycnogenol®	120 mg with a meal
Fruit polyphenols	120 mg with a meal
Grape seed extract	120 mg with a meal
MaxEPA™	2 g with a meal
DHA (Neuromins™)	300 mg with a meal
Primrose or borage oil	2 g with a meal
NADH	10 mg daily, divided into two 5 mg doses with or without food

* Look for fully reacted mineral chelates for efficient absorption and utilization.

To Stimulate Immune Function

Astragalus membranaceus	500 mg of standardized extract
Echinacea	250 mg of standardized extract (Use for seven to ten days with three-week stop intervals.)
Reishi mushroom	4 g of standardized extract
Shiitake mushroom	4 g of standardized extract
Maitake mushroom	4 g of standardized extract
Ginseng	500 mg of standardized Panax ginseng or Siberian ginseng

Additional Neuroimmunomodulators to Consider

Salt or Fludrocortisone
Melatonin

Medications

Medications to restore sleep patterns
Selective serotonin reuptake inhibitors (Prozac, Zoloft, Paxil, etc.)

CHAPTER 11

DEPRESSION

Despite her status as a star basketball player and senior class president, eighteen-year-old Doreen began suffering from mild episodes of depression. Generally, she worked her way through her infrequent "blue periods," as she called them, by forcing herself to continue to keep up with schoolwork even if she holed up at home and watched television for hours on end instead of socializing.

By the time Doreen was a junior in college, however, her episodes of depression had become frequent enough to interfere with her natural zest for life. She gradually lost interest in both sports and academics, and she dropped off the basketball team and began missing classes. Her appetite faltered and she began losing weight. Some mornings, she was too tired to drag herself out of bed, and when she did, she seldom bothered to dress. What was the point, when she didn't feel like going anywhere or seeing anyone?

Doreen tried using the college counseling service and was referred to a social worker, who attempted to address the source of her depression through therapy. However, Doreen could think of nothing to say that would shed any light on her mood.

"I feel so numb, I just can't enjoy things anymore," she confessed. "I feel hopeless all the time. And yet, someone looking at my life from the outside would say I have nothing to complain about."

The social worker recognized that Doreen was suffering from depression, and referred her to a psychiatrist, who suggested that Doreen continue her therapy once a week and try a prescription for antidepressants. While Doreen wanted to continue the therapy, she was resistant to the idea of medication. She sought help at our office because she was looking for an alternative solution.

"I just don't like the idea of medication," Doreen explained. "I'm the sort of person that doesn't even take aspirin for a headache. Isn't there something else I can try?"

Depression: An Overview

If you or someone you love is suffering from depression, rest assured that you are not alone. At present, one in twenty Americans suffers from clinical depression and requires medical treatment, and one person out of every five will suffer a depressive episode at some point. These statistics boost depression to the top of all public health problems in this country.

Abraham Lincoln suffered from depression most of his adult life. So did many famous musicians, writers, and artists including Peter Tchaikovsky, Robert Schumann, Gustav Mahler, Hans Christian Andersen, Ernest Hemingway, Charles Dickens, Isak Dinesen, Mary Shelley, Virginia Woolf, Michelangelo, and Paul Gauguin.

Yet, it is only in recent decades that depression has truly become understood for what it really is: a chronic disease of the brain that is completely different from the sort of mental anguish that follows loss, or the "down" cycles in life's ups and downs.

The risk for depression runs in families. However, many people are diagnosed with clinical depression who have no family history of the disease at all. Although people over sixty-five are four times more likely to suffer from depression than those in other age groups, children and teenagers can suffer from the disease, too. Currently, experts estimate that at least 5 percent of all adolescents suffer from depression. More than twice as many women are currently being treated for depression as men; however, this may be due to men denying that they need treatment. Almost two-thirds of the people who have one depressive episode will go on to have at least four more in their lifetime.

Where has research brought us so far in understanding this pervasive disease?

Scientists have at last succeeded in building a bridge between depression and brain mechanisms. Through two decades of research, we have come to understand that depression is closely linked to the dysfunction of two neurotransmitters in the brain, particularly serotonin. The diverse treatments that have emerged to treat depression as a result of this research—including mono-amine oxidase inhibitors, tricyclic antidepressants, and SSRIs—have been devloped on the basis of this research.

About two-thirds of all people diagnosed with clinical depression readily respond to treatment with short-term therapy combined with an antidepressant. People who do not respond to the first antidepressant prescribed will most likely respond to another, and symptoms of depression will ease within a few weeks' time as a result.

Tragically, however, many people with depression fail to find help in time. About fifteen percent of people with this disorder commit suicide as a result.

In this chapter, you will discover just what research has taught us about the ways in which depression alters brain function and metabolism, particularly in the relationship between the hypothalamus and the rest of the body.

More exciting still, you will learn how sophisticated studies in neurology and nutrition have contributed to our ability to prescribe a power-packed treatment plan to prevent and treat depression. This plan adds the latest breakthrough nutritional and hormonal therapies to our existing strategies of using therapy and antidepressants.

What Goes Wrong in Depression, and Why

In recent decades, a number of interesting scientific studies have begun to describe just what happens in the brain to affect the mood disorders characterizing clinical depression.

The most important of these findings include (1) the possibility that depression is an inherited disease, (2) the relationship between fatty acids and depression, (3) the breakdown in the hypothalamus's ability to regulate the production of an important hormone called CRH, and (4) the ways in which reduced brain levels of the norepinephrine and serotonin neurotransmitters alter brain chemistry and cause depression.

• For Some, Depression May Be in the Genes

Clinical studies conducted over the past decade have offered persuasive evidence that the risk for severe depression runs in families and is most likely genetic. Just as researchers have mined human chromosomes to determine how diseases such as Parkinson's and Alzheimer's are transmitted in families, so are a number of scientists at prestigious medical centers now racing to discover how gene mutations might account for depression.

However, clarifying just which genes are responsible for this debilitating illness is extremely complicated. For one thing, depression is so common in our population that scientists speculate the disorder must be due to several different gene mutations rather than just one.

And unlike the degenerative disorders we can describe according to the clear changes in brain structure they provoke, depression is variable in its pathways. This makes it much more difficult to track, both in individuals and in groups.

• A Deficiency in Omega-3 Fatty Acids: Weakened Cells Contribute to the Altered Brain Chemistry That Heralds Depression

Now, various studies have demonstrated that lowering plasma cholesterol through diet and medication may indeed be healthier for our hearts—but has the unwanted side effect of increasing episodes of depression and suicide.

For example, in the famous Framingham Study, the largest ever to examine the relationship between lowered cholesterol and decreased heart disease, researchers made this disconcerting discovery: People participating in the study who lowered their cholesterol did, in fact, suffer less from heart disease. However, more of the study's participants committed suicide compared to the rest of the population.

Yet other studies have shown that societies apt to consume large amounts of fish—which contain high amounts of omega-3 fatty acids—have lower cholesterol levels than other populations as well as a lower incidence of heart disease—*without* raising rates of depression.

Where does the discrepancy lie between our population and theirs? What are we doing wrong?

Researchers now believe that the answer lies in the types of fatty acids we consume. Over the past two decades, Americans have bought into the idea that eating margarine and corn oil can save our lives by lowering our cholesterol and preventing heart disease. Unfortunately, we have replaced saturated fat with too many omega-6 unsaturated fats, rather than the omega-3 unsaturated fats that are so essential to brain health.

Like all cells in your body, your brain cells are surrounded by membranes composed chiefly of fats (also called phospholipids). The basic function of those membranes is to regulate the way that biological substances travel in and out of cells.

A saturated fat when incorporated in a cell membrane differs considerably in structure and function from unsaturated fat in a cell membrane. Furthermore, as you learned from our general description of fatty acids in the general nutrition chapters of *The Brain Wellness Plan,* there are different types of polyunsaturated fats. The two broad groups are the omega-3 and omega-6 fatty acids.

Today, science supports the view that decreasing your intake of omega-3 fatty acids may impair brain function, increase your risk of heart disease, and raise your risk of suffering from depression. In other words, these essential fatty acids are vital to both your physical and psychological health.

Recently, as reported in the *American Journal of Clinical Nutrition,* scientists have shown that the omega-3 fatty acid phosphatidylserine (PS) increased dopamine, norepinephrine, and epinephrine concentrations in animals.

In another multicenter study conducted with 404 elderly patients, administering 300 mg of PS caused them to become less depressed. Studies like these have led many clinicians around the world to conclude that adequate omega-3 fatty acid intake may be essential in preventing and treating depression.

From all of this, we can conclude that omega-3 fatty acids are essential for all aspects of healthy brain cell metabolism. This is because the brain requires specific fatty acids to synthesize hormones, cell membranes, and components of the immune system.

If your diet is composed mostly of saturated fats (animal fats) and deficient in unsaturated fatty acids, the result is that your brain cell membranes will become less fluid—which can have a devastating effect on the way that neurotransmitters bind to their receptors.

But it's not enough simply to seek out unsaturated fatty acids; they have to be the right kind. The omega-3 unsaturated fatty acids are required to ensure healthy interactions between neurotransmitters and their receptors. A deficiency in omega-3 fatty acids results in the reduced ability of a neurotransmitter to bind to its receptor. Thus, omega-3 fatty acid deficiency is linked to depression, because the neurotransmitters we rely on to safeguard against depression—namely, norepinephrine and serotonin—cannot properly bind to their receptors and perform their function within the brain.

As part of our "Combined Medical and Nutritional Approach" in this chapter, we will show you just how you can help prevent and treat depression by raising your intake of essential omega-3 fatty acids.

• Inadequate Tryptophan May Lead to Low Brain Serotonin Levels . . . and Depression

The theory that low levels of serotonin in the brain may lead to clinical depression has been supported by numerous clinical studies examining the spinal fluid and brain tissue of people who died as a result of depression, usually by suicide. Those investigations have shown that these individuals did, indeed, have low levels of brain serotonin.

As we have already discussed, low levels of omega-3 fatty acids may impair the way serotonin binds to receptors on cell membranes. Now, new evidence has shown that reduced serotonin activity may also be the result of low levels of its essential chemical precursor, tryptophan. Individuals with depression have much lower tryptophan blood concentrations in relation to other amino acids than do people without the disorder.

Studies have shown that reducing the intake of dietary tryptophan can induce depression in some people, as there is simply not enough of this valuable ingredient to make the serotonin needed. In addition, tryptophan can be broken down by the liver before it's ever made into serotonin.

Interestingly, depressed patients often have an elevated cortisol level, as you will see in the discussion below, which in turn induces the activity of a certain liver enzyme capable of dismantling tryptophan. When the liver breaks down more tryptophan, less is around to act as a precursor to serotonin, and low levels of serotonin are clearly associated with depression. Because of the adverse effect of cortisol on the synthesis of serotonin from tryptophan, administering doses of tryptophan alone may prove to be an ineffectual treatment for depression.

In fact, using tryptophan as an antidepressant either by itself or with traditional antidepressant therapy has not demonstrated significant benefits; it may even have severe adverse effects if tryptophan is combined with any of the selective serotonin reuptake inhibitors (SSRIs) such as Prozac or Zoloft. That's because the combination of this nutrient with SSRIs may actually lead to the production of too much serotonin in the brain—a potentially life-threatening condition.

• A Faulty Hypothalamus Communication Loop May Lead to Depression

The hypothalamus is a tiny, pea-sized brain organ that serves as a sort of United Nations for important meetings between various body systems. The body systems that rely on the hypothalamus to orchestrate communication speak via chemical molecular messengers. They include the immune system; the endocrine system, which is made up of all hormone-producing glands; and the autonomic nervous system, which is responsible for monitoring cardiac and other smooth muscle functions.

As in so many neurological illnesses, depression can result when this miniature organ fails to orchestrate effective chemical communication. Over half of all patients diagnosed with severe depression exhibit striking abnormalities in brain metabolism that centers right in the hypothalamus. One of the most devastating consequences of this hypothalamic breakdown is that patients with depression experience a marked increase in the release of corticotropin-releasing hormone, or CRH.

What causes the hypothalamus to ratchet up CRH production when it shouldn't? And why should an abundance of this natural hormone lead to depression?

The mechanisms of the hypothalamic breakdown are still being explored. To date, we know only that the hypothalamus becomes overstimulated and sends too much CRH to your adrenal glands. These two small, triangular organs, which are just a few centimeters in size and located on top of your kidneys, respond to the frantic signaling by the hypothalamus in the only way they know how: they produce an overabundance of cortisol, your body's stress hormone.

As blood levels of cortisol rise in patients with depression, tryptophan production dips down and, consequently, leads to a reduced availability of that essential serotonin ingredient. The brain can then no longer make enough serotonin to go around. This leads to a Catch-22 situation, in that adequate brain serotonin is required to turn down the hypothalamus and slow down its production of CRH.

The different classes of antidepressants used to treat depression today all seem to work by increasing levels of serotonin, norepinephrine, and dopamine in the brain. Although we do not yet fully grasp just how increasing the concentrations of these neurotransmitters alleviates depression, most likely these medications change the way that the brain's cell membranes bind with these essential mood-altering neurotransmitters.

• What About the Relationship Between Vitamin Deficiencies and Depression?

In *The British Journal of Psychiatry* and other journals, scientists have reviewed the relationship between a number of vitamin

TABLE 9

WHAT CAUSES DEPRESSION?

- A genetic predisposition.

- Faulty neurotransmitter function owing to weakened brain cell membranes and impaired neuron receptor binding.

- Low levels of tryptophan, serotonin's key precursor.

- Overproduction of cortiocotropin-releasing hormone by the hypothalamus, causing the adrenal glands to produce too much cortisol.

- Vitamin deficiencies, which may cause depressive symptoms.

deficiencies and depressive states. Essentially, scientists have linked depression to deficiencies of riboflavin (B_2), pyridoxine (B_6), folic acid, and vitamin C.

This was not really a surprise, since the classic symptoms of these vitamin deficiencies mimic those of clinical depression. At Harvard Medical School's MacLean Geriatric Hospital, both geriatric and young adult depressive subjects were found to be deficient in B_2, B_6, and B_{12}. Their data support the hypothesis that poor nutritional status, especially in certain B vitamins, can contribute to depression.

In addition, several studies have demonstrated that impaired folic acid metabolism and folic acid deficiency are present in many patients diagnosed with depression. This may be because a folic acid deficiency impairs your body's ability to synthesize BH4, a cofactor essential for the body to make dopamine and serotonin. SAMe, which acts as an antidepressant, is also dependent on folic acid for its metabolism.

Glucose Metabolism and Depression

Glucose is required to fuel every organ in our bodies, including our brains. Researchers have recently correlated the brain's ability to utilize glucose with vulnerability to depression. Using a PET scan device, which measures how much glucose the brain uses, researchers compared elderly, depressed patients to a non-depressed control group. They found that depressed patients had a widespread decline in glucose metabolism throughout the brain. This inability to utilize glucose properly may be due to insulin resistance, which means that brain cells cannot mop up glucose for the purpose of utilizing it as fuel. This insight into the origins of depression may provide clues to the development of novel treatments that enhance the brain's ability to utilize glucose as a treatment for depression, along with new supplements like chiroinositol, and the natural hormone DHEA.

A Combined Medical and Nutritional Approach to Depression

As we have seen, the symptoms which doctors and therapists use to diagnose depression are linked to alterations in brain chemistry. Nobody knows exactly what event acts as a catalyst for the changes in brain metabolism in any one individual, as the disease varies so much in its pathways. Depression can be the result of hormonal changes, chemical effects owing to other chronic illnesses, spontaneous changes in chemistry, psychological triggers, or some combination of these factors.

Sometimes, this metabolic alteration returns to normal after a few years, even without medical treatment. Better still, up to 80 percent of all individuals diagnosed with clinical depression are readily treatable within a few weeks of diagnosis through a combination of therapy and antidepressant medications. In addition, revolutionary insights into the power of nutrients to boost brain health and mend faulty neurotransmitter synthesis and binding have led us to recommend aggressive nutritional therapies to restore healthy chemical balances in the brain.

When Should You Suspect Depression?

Everyone feels sad from time to time. So how do you determine if you're suffering from the "blues" or true, clinical depression?

Basically, in clinical depression, feelings are out of proportion to any external causes. In addition to feeling sad, depressed individuals may experience a numb or empty feeling and a noticeable loss in the ability to take pleasure in life. Depression is a disease of the brain, but it ends up as a "whole body" illness affecting they way you eat, sleep, and think. It is not a passing mood, and people with depression cannot simply pull themselves up by the bootstraps, keep their chin up, or put the best face on the situation. When it comes to depression, none of these clichés holds true.

The DSM-III-R, the official diagnostic and statistical manual for psychiatric illnesses, defines the most common types of depression according to these criteria:

•Major Depression

Major depression causes people who suffer from it to cease functioning normally. Treatments include medication and psychotherapy. Major depression is diagnosed if at least five of the following symptoms have been present during the same two-week period:

- Depression which lasts most of the day, nearly every day.
- Diminished interest or pleasure in most activities every day.
- Significant change in weight or appetite.
- Daily insomnia or feeling the need to sleep all of the time.
- Psychomotor agitation or retardation.
- Fatigue or loss of energy.
- Feelings of worthlessness or excessive guilt.
- Diminished ability to think or concentrate.
- Recurrent thoughts of death or suicide.

•Dysthymia

While this form of depression is milder, it is chronic, lasting for two years or more. Although most people with this disorder continue to function at work or school, they are often going through the motions and not taking any pleasure in life's activities. Dysthymia is treated with both antidepressants and psychotherapy. It is diagnosed if at least two of the following symptoms are present for a minimum of two years:

- Poor appetite or overeating.
- Insomnia or sleeping all the time.
- Low energy or fatigue.
- Low self-esteem.
- Poor concentration or an inability to make decisions.
- Feelings of hopelessness.

•Adjustment Disorder with Depressed Mood

Generally, people suffering from this type of depression have a precipitating event that begins the depression, such as losing a job or ending an intimate relationship. Many people are able to recover from adjustment disorders on their own. The condition is diagnosed if most of the following are present:

- A reaction to an identifiable stressor that occurred within three months of the depression.
- Impairment in functioning at school, at work, or in social relationships.
- Symptoms in excess of a normal reaction to the stressor.
- The disturbance is not merely one instance of a pattern of overreaction to stress.
- The maladaptive reaction persists no longer than six months.
- The disturbance does not meet the criteria for any specific mental disorder.

Diagnosing Depression: Rule Out Associated Conditions

In addition to using the criteria listed above to diagnose depression, a health care practitioner must rule out other conditions that may be linked to depressive states. These include:

•Hypothyroidism

Hypothyroidism develops slowly in most individuals, taking many months or even years to become full-blown. It is characterized by lethargy and decreased sexual interest, among other things, in addition to an inability to regulate body temperature, dry skin, and constipation. Because some of these symptoms are common in patients with depression, too, it is necessary to conduct laboratory tests to rule out the possibility of hypothyroidism in a person who seems to be suffering from depression. The best way to do this is through laboratory tests that can analyze the different forms of the thyroid hormone and thyroid-stimulating hormone as well as antibodies in the blood.

•Hypercalcemia

This condition, which is diagnosed by laboratory tests and characterized by raised serum calcium, may be caused by a malignancy that has spread to the bones. Hypercalcemia can also be a result of hyperparathyroidism, a condition in which one or more of the parathyroid glands produces an overabundance of their hormone, causing calcium concentrations in the blood to rise. Hypercalcemia may be confused with depression because both cause symptoms of indefinite fatigue and general listlessness.

•Pancreatic Cancer

The possibility of pancreatic cancer should be ruled out in diagnosing depression, particularly among elderly patients who report a new onset of depression, decreased appetite, and weight loss. They may also exhibit jaundice, an abnormal yellow appearance to the skin. Diagnosis of pancreatic cancer should be made only by an experienced physician.

•Vitamin Deficiencies

A number of vitamin deficiencies, especially in B_{12} and folic acid, result in many of the same mood changes and behaviors associated with depression. It is important to rule these out, as vitamin deficiencies are readily treated with supplements, alleviating the patient's depressive symptoms.

• Parkinson's Disease

Nearly half of all patients diagnosed with Parkinson's disease also suffer from depression. Symptoms of depression may occur early in the course of Parkinson's, even prior to the onset of classic motor symptoms.

The First Step to Take in Treating Depression: Ensure a Healthy Diet and Incorporate an Exercise Regimen

Dietary intake may be severely compromised in depression, as individuals with depression are likely to experience significant changes in appetite. From anorexia to poor eating habits, depression sets the stage for a malnourished state. One study, published in 1994 in the *Journal of the American College of Nutrition*, reported that individuals diagnosed with moderate to severe depression had such poor dietary intake that they suffered from demonstrated deficiencies in a number of important nutrients.

Therefore, one of the first steps anyone diagnosed with depression can take toward health is to follow the guidelines we set forth earlier, in the complete *Brain Wellness Plan* nutrition guidelines. This plan includes a number of important supplements with proven benefits in treating depression, particularly the B vitamins.

In addition, we recommend that people diagnosed with depression work with a health care professional in adding a regular exercise routine, as exercise has been shown to raise serotonin levels in the brain. Patients should also consider the role sugar and hypoglycemia plays in contributing to depressive symptoms (see below).

The Three R's of Depression: Reduce Excessive Inflammation, Raise Mitochondrial Activity, and Rebalance Neurotransmitter Levels

Depression is multifactorial, which means that several variables contribute to the disease. *Depression is a disease.* The biological influence on depression is no different from the biological influence on the development of diabetes, cancer, or heart disease.

The diverse biological factors involved in depression include the role of the immune system, the role of signals sent from one cell to another that influence the activity of mitochondria, and neurotransmitter effects.

A compelling body of evidence suggests that the immune system is disturbed in depressed patients. For example, certain types of immune cells, natural killer cells, are markedly lower in depressed patients as compared to nondepressed patients. Furthermore, with antidepressant therapy, natural killer cell levels are restored to normal. This observation clearly supports the brain-immune connection in depression. Various other aspects of the immune system also affect our mood, including an immunotransmitter referred to as substance P and the hormone corticotropin-releasing factor (CRF). Each of these immune messengers plays a vital role in the development of depression and chronic stress.

Substance P is markedly elevated in inflamed tissue, and it's possible that depression is actually a state of low-grade inflammation caused by elevated substance P levels. Lowering substance P levels, then, is an important anti-inflammatory strategy in treating depression.

The second neurotransmitter related to depression is cortisol. As we've discussed, elevated cortisol levels are clearly associated with depression and chronic anxiety. Release of cortisol from our adrenal glands is stimulated by the hormone CRF, which directly raises cortisol levels. This is a necessary physiological process that helps us deal with short-term situations which require a "fight or flight" response. It is eventually terminated by an elaborate feedback system in which cortisol tells the brain to stop producing CRF. Under normal circumstances, when CRF release is inhibited, cortisol levels return to normal. In depressed patients, however, cortisol fails to repress the release of CRF. With the continual release of CRF by the brain, cortisol levels remain elevated. The long-term consequences of this effect are alterations in mood and memory.

Strategies to Reduce Inflammation

Since we can now view depression as a state of low-grade inflammation of the brain, various anti-inflammatory strategies can be devised to "put the fire out" or dampen the negative effects of the immune system on the brain. This strategy would include methods to reduce both substance P and cortisol.

• Substance P Blockers and Depression

Rationale for Use of N-acetyltryptophan in Depression An important new development in the treatment of depression is the identification of specific receptors, called substance P receptors, that are abnormally active in depressed patients. Substance P coordinates the perception of pain in the brain. We may conclude from this new research, in fact, that psychic and physical pain are identical in their effects on our brains, since both psychic and physical pain are processed by substance P receptors. Substance P receptor blockers are aggressively being explored as effective agents against depression.

Stress is also mediated in the brain by substance P. Blocking the receptors in the brain that bind substance P has been shown to block the effects of stress on the brain. Identification of substance P receptor blockers, like N-acetyltryptophan, has opened the door to an exciting new way of controlling depression.

While N-acetyltryptophan is currently unavailable for use, it is the opinion of this author (Dr. Lombard) that substance P receptor–blocking compounds will become a major new therapeutic advance in the treatment of depression.

Clinical Studies of N-Acetyltryptophan in Depression It has recently been demonstrated that blocking the substance P receptor causes an antidepressant effect. Researchers have identified numerous substance P blockers, including a derivative of the amino acid L-tryptophan named N-acetyltryptophan. N-acetyltryptophan and derivatives are currently under intensive study.

• DHEA and Depression

Rationale for Use of DHEA in Depression DHEA is a neuroactive steroid produced by the adrenal glands. One of its functions is to regulate the level of cortisol, a hormone produced in response to stress, in our bodies. As we've discussed, cortisol levels are elevated in many patients with depression, which suggests that they are in a chronic state of stress. DHEA, by neutralizing the inflammatory effects of cortisol, allows the brain to utilize it more effectively.

Clinical Studies Supporting the Use of DHEA in Depression Researchers at the University of California Department of Psychiatry examined 22 patients with major depression and administered either DHEA or placebo over a six-week period. DHEA was associated with a significant decrease in depression rating scores (compared to the patients who took the placebo), with approximately 50 percent of patients who used DHEA reporting an overall 50 percent reduction of symptoms of depression.

RECOMMENDED DOSE: 10–100 mg daily. Discuss the use of DHEA with your health care practitioner. Men with prostate problems should use DHEA with caution.

• Phosphatidylserine and Depression

Rationale for Use of Phosphatidylserine in Depression One of the possible benefits of PS in depression may have to do with its anti-inflammatory effects. Phosphatidylserine acts as an anti-TNF factor. As you may recall, tumor necrosis factor is a pro-inflammatory immunotransmitter that directs the immune system in some kind of antagonistic way against the brain. By reducing TNF, phosphatidylserine may help to put out the inflammation of depression.

As we have seen throughout this book, our brain health

depends on PS more than on any other single fatty acid. Besides maintaining and improving brain cell membranes, PS is essential for cells to efficiently metabolize glucose for energy and successfully release and bind with neurotransmitters. PS also serves as an added barrier against free radicals pummeling our brain cell membranes. Patients diagnosed with clinical depression have shown marked improvement as a result of taking PS daily.

PS is also an anti-inflammatory compound that reduces destructive cytokines like tumor necrosis factors. TNF and other cytokines may be elevated in depression, again suggesting that this disorder is related to alterations in the immune system.

Clinical Studies of PS in Depression Administration of phosphatidylserine was assessed in ten elderly, depressed patients for 15 days and compared with patients who received a placebo. The dose of phosphatidylserine was 300 mg daily. The Hamilton Rating Scale, a widely regarded, standardized score to assess the degree of depression, was performed before and after PS therapy in each group. In the group that received phosphatidylserine, clinical improvement in depressive symptoms was demonstrated on the scale. The researchers also noted that the patients treated with PS had improved memory.

RECOMMENDED DOSE: 300 mg daily. Precautions: None.

• Omega-3 Fatty Acids and Depression

Rationale for Use of Omega-3 Fatty Acids in Depression Omega-3 fatty acids are essential fatty acids derived from either cold water fish or plant sources. Cold water fish (like fatty tuna, mackerel, and salmon) contain the essential fatty acids EPA (eicosapentaenoic acid) and DHA (docosahexanoic acid). Flaxseed oil, derived from the flax plant, contains another omega-3 fatty acid called linoleic acid.

Omega-3 fatty acids are also natural anti-inflammatories because of their ability to reduce the potentially harmful effects of arachidonic acid and to decrease our pro-inflammatory prostaglandins.

Omega-3 fatty acids have been best studied in bipolar or

"manic" depression. In this disorder, patients experience extreme mood swings characterized by either intensely depressed moods or mania (overexcitement). Omega-3 fatty acids may benefit these patients by dampening the second messenger system, described earlier. They accomplish this by stabilizing brain cell membranes, as well as preventing excessive stimulation or excitement of these cells.

Clinical Studies of Omega-3 Fatty Acids and Bipolar Depression In a recent study performed at the Psychopharmacology Unit of Brigham and Women's Hospital in Boston, Massachusetts, 30 patients with bipolar disorder received either 9 grams of omega-3 fatty acids or a placebo over a four-month period. In the omega-3 fatty acid group, there was a significantly longer period of remission from bipolar disorder, and treated patients improved in every outcome, compared to the placebo group.

RECOMMENDED DOSE: 5 grams of fish oil or flaxseed oil once or twice daily. Precautions: Consult your health care practitioner prior to using omega-3 fatty acids if you are currently taking blood thinners. Fish oils may increase the likelihood of bleeding and, therefore, should be used with care in this population of patients.

Strategies to Raise Mitochondrial Activity

• *Mitrochondria, Depression, and Signal Transduction*

Mitochondria are either activated or inhibited by signals they receive from the internal chamber of a cell. For instance, increased calcium within a cell will initially activate the mitochondria but will ultimately fatigue them, a process known as excitotoxicity. Other factors, referred to as second messengers, also influence the activity of the mitochondria via a process known as signal transduction. There exists a family of second messengers found on all cell membranes including brain cells. Each member of the second messenger molecule family can either activate or inhibit the mitochondria.

In fact, neurotransmitters like serotonin and dopamine exert their effects on a cell by these second messenger systems. Ultimately the message delivered to the cell by the neurotransmitter is intended to influence the activity of the mitochondria.

In depression specific second messengers known as G-proteins play an inhibitory role on mitochondrial activity. These proteins blunt the message of a neurotransmitter, inhibiting its intended mood-lifting effects. Interestingly, a specific protein known as G alpha 12 is increased in depressed patients and is lowered after antidepressent therapy. The relationship between mitochondria, depression, and signal transduction offers an exciting insight into the basic mechanisms of depression, and may help us develop a specific marker which can be measured in blood cells to monitor the clinical effects of antidepressant therapy.

To explain it another way: Cells are either activated or inactivated by neurotransmitters. When a cell is activated by a neurotransmitter, that is due to increased interactions between calcium and the mitochondria. Conversely, certain neurotransmitters can down-regulate receptors, which results in *decreased* interactions between calcium and mitochondria. It's like an on/off switch: The light is "turned on" by calcium, and "turned off" by mitochondria not releasing calcium. Therefore, the mitochondria play a crucial role in the activation of cells.

Two natural compounds, inositol and lithium, increase the effectiveness of antidepressive therapy by influencing the activity of calcium and mitochondria in brain cells. Each has demonstrated an antidepressent effect. With regard to inositol, this vitamin B–based compound binds to receptors found on the mitochondria, which regulates and enhances calcium release within the cell. This, in turn, results in the activation of the cell. We can envision depression as a condition in which brain cells have dead batteries. Inositol may help "jump-start" cells by recharging our biological battery, the mitochondria.

• Inositol and Depression

Rationale for Use of Inositol in Depression Inositol serves as the substrate of a compound known as phosphatidylinositol. Phosphatidylinositol is involved in a process in the brain called the "second messenger system," which works like this: When an antidepressant substance meets a receptor in the brain, it induces changes within this receptor that modify the brain cell's function. This neurotransmitter-receptor interaction is known as the second messenger system. All antidepressants ultimately carry out their functions through changes in the phosphatidylinositol second messenger system. Therefore, it has been speculated that enhancing the second messenger system would be a useful strategy for treating depression.

Clinical Studies of Inositol in Depression In animal studies, high doses of inositol result in decreased behavioral markers of depression. In human studies, a recent double-blind, controlled study of 28 patients administered 12 grams of inositol daily to the treatment group, and a placebo substance to the control group. In the treated group, inositol exhibited a significant antidepressant effect (as measured on the Hamilton Rating Scale of Depression).

Inositol has also been shown to enhance the antidepressant effect of prescription antidepressent medications in a manner similar to the effects of lithium.

RECOMMENDED DOSE: 6–12 g daily. Precautions: None.

• Lithium and Depression

Rationale for Use of Lithium in Depression Lithium has long been one of the cornerstones of therapy for manic depression, but its use in augmenting the effects of antidepressant therapy, especially in patients who are treatment resistant, is less appreciated. Approximately 10 percent of depressed patients are nonresponders—that is, they remain depressed, despite any antidepressant medication given to them. Using lithium in addition to an antidepressant medication is the most substantiated, effective treatment strategy in treatment-resistant depression.

Lithium, like inositol, acts on the second messenger system. Furthermore, lithium increases brain ATP production, the by-product of mitochondria and the energy currency of the cell. Lithium has also been suggested to act as a neuroprotective factor by favorably influencing mitochondrial activity.

Lithium helps to break down the phosphatidylinositol molecules contained in the cell membranes of brain neurons. The breakdown of phosphatidylinositol releases calcium into the cells, amplifying the second messenger antidepressant-signaling effect.

Clinical Studies of Lithium in Treatment-Resistant Depression Two randomized, double-blind, placebo-controlled studies have demonstrated that the addition of lithium to standard antidepressant therapy is an effective strategy. A response rate of 50–60 percent of patients has been reported when using lithium in treatment-resistant depression patients. Lithium is available only by prescription.

> **RECOMMENDED DOSE:** Lithium, a prescription medication, should only be used under the direct supervision of a physician. Potentially serious side effects of lithium include kidney damage, and levels need to be monitored frequently.

Strategies to Rebalance Neurotransmitter Levels

As you now know, the neurotransmitter serotonin is severely depleted in people with depression. Numerous compounds, both natural substances and prescription drugs, raise serotonin levels in depressed patients and alleviate many of their symptoms involving mood, sleep, anxiety, appetite, and energy levels.

• Antidepressant Medications and Depression

As we mentioned earlier, about two-thirds of all individuals diagnosed with depression are likely to respond well to one of the antidepressant medications. People taking antidepressants generally feel the depressive symptoms gradually lift; they are still able to feel sadness or joy at appropriate times. In other words, antidepressants are not ''happy'' pills. At best, these medications simply relieve depression and allow individuals to return to their normal activities and enjoy life again.

There are many classes of antidepressants. Two of them, the tricyclic antidepressants and the monoamine oxidase inhibitors, have been used successfully for decades. The most popular new class of antidepressants are the selective serotonin reuptake inhibitors (SSRIs). Most recently, venlafaxine (Effexor) was added to the roster of available antidepressants.

We have listed the most commonly prescribed antidepressants below. Naturally, you should discuss proper administration, drug interactions, and the potential benefits and side effects of each with your health care practitioner.

The important thing to remember here is that, even if the first antidepressant you try does not relieve symptoms after several weeks, there is another that will most likely work.

- *Tricyclic Antidepressants*
  imipramine (Tofranil)
  amitriptyline (Elavil)
  nortriptyline (Aventyl and Pamelor)
  desipramine (Norpramin)

- *Monoamine Oxidase Inhibitors*
  tranylcypromine (Parnate)
  phenelzine (Nardil)

- *Selective Serotonin Reuptake Inhibitors*
  fluoxetine (Prozac)
  sertraline (Zoloft)
  paroxetine (Paxil)
  fluvoxamine (Luvox)

- *Others*
  bupropion (Wellbutrin)
  traxodone (Desyrel)
  venlafaxine (Effexor)

• S-Adenosyl Methionine (SAMe) and Depression

Rationale for Use of SAMe in Depression SAMe is a naturally occurring physiological substance that is involved in a multitude of biochemical processes within our bodies. SAMe is also a major source of methyl groups in the brain. The process of methylation in the brain in which SAMe participates so intimately is essential to the synthesis, activation, and metabolism of various neurotransmitters.

The antidepressant effects of SAMe are unique and distinctive from prescription medications. Both serotonin and dopamine levels are increased by SAMe administration. These neurotransmitters are linked to mood, sleep, anxiety, appetite, and energy levels, all of which are commonly disturbed in depression.

Clinical Studies of SAMe in Depression In a study completed at the Massachusetts General Hospital, researchers gave 195 patients 450 mg of SAMe over a two-week period. This open, multicenter study demonstrated that SAMe is effective for depression, and has no serious side effects.

In a small study, also conducted at Massachusetts General Hospital, 20 patients with major depression were given oral SAMe. The compound was found to be effective in approximately 50 percent of depressed patients. In fact, two patients who had been previously unresponsive to all other conventional therapies also responded favorably to SAMe administration.

SAMe was also found to be effective in depressed post-menopausal women in a thirty-day double-blind, placebo-controlled study. Eighty women who met criteria for major depression or dysthymia received either 1600 mg of SAMe or placebo. In the treated group, there was a statistically significant improvement in depressive symptoms, compared to the control group.

RECOMMENDED DOSE: 400–800 mg daily. A person should not take higher doses unless under a health care practitioner's supervision. Precautions: People who want to take SAMe for depression should consult with their health care practitioners, especially if they are taking SAMe in conjunction with other antidepressant medications.

• St. John's Wort and Depression

Rationale for Use of St. John's Wort in Depression Extracts of St. John's wort are now widely used for the treatment of depression and have been used in European folk medicine for centuries. In Germany, St. John's wort is one of the most widely prescribed antidepressants. The mechanism of St. John's wort in depression is not entirely clear, but may be similar to different classes of antidepressants.

Some researchers have suggested that St. John's wort acts as a monoamine oxidase inhibitor. This enzyme is responsible for the breakdown of certain neurotransmitters, including serotonin, norepinephrine, and dopamine. Other researchers speculate that St. John's wort may act similarly to the antidepressants known as selective serotonin reuptake inhibitors (SSRIs). Reuptake inhibitors, which include medications like Prozac and Zoloft, block the inactivation of serotonin, causing the neurotransmitter to have a prolonged effect on the receptors in the brain.

Within St. John's wort are several active constituents that may be responsible for its pharmacological effects. Among them are the hypericum and the hyperforin portions of the plant. Until recently, the antidepressant action of St. John's wort has been attributed to the hypericum extract. In fact, the most commonly available St. John's wort preparations are standardized for hypericum. Recently, however, it has been proposed that it is the hyperforin, not the hypericum, content of St. John's wort that is responsible for its antidepressant effects. This is not an insignificant distinction, because the amount of hyperforin in St. John's wort can vary widely, and may determine whether you get relief from depression or not.

Hyperforin has several biochemical effects in the brain, supporting the theory that it may be the active ingredient producing the antidepressant effect of St. John's wort. Hyperforin raises brain concentrations of serotonin, norepinephrine, and dopamine, and leads to changes in brain wave activity that are similar to those produced by prescription medications for depression.

In a randomized, double-blind, placebo-controlled study, the hypericum extract of St. John's wort was compared to the hyperforin extract. At the end of the treatment period, patients with major depression who received hyperforin exhibited a significant reduction of symptoms, while patients taking the hypericum extract had results similar to those taking the placebo substance.

Clinical Studies of St. John's Wort in Depression In a meta analysis of controlled, double-blind studies using St. John's wort for depression, it was found to be approximately 1.5 times as effective as placebo, and had fewer side effects than typical tricyclic antidepressant therapies.

> RECOMMENDED DOSE: 300 mg, standardized for hyperforann extract. Precautions: Patients should not use St. John's wort in conjunction with other antidepressant prescription medications unless they are doing so under the direct supervision of a health care practitioner, to avoid potentially serious side effects.

A Cocktail Approach to Treating Depression

I. Reduce inflammation.

1. Substance P blockers: These include the compound N-acetyltryptophan, which is currently under study for depression. No dosage has been established for this compound in treating depression.

2. DHEA: This neuroactive steroid is produced by the adrenal glands. It regulates the level of the stress hormone cortisol. Dosages range from 10–100 mg daily. Be sure to discuss the use of DHEA with your health care practitioner. Men with prostate problems should use DHEA with caution.

3. Phosphatidylserine: PS is essential for cells to metabolize glucose efficiently, so it can bind to neurotransmitters. It also acts as an antioxidant. Recommended dose is 300 mg daily.

4. Omega-3 fatty acids: These essential fatty acids stabilize brain cell membranes and prevent excessive stimulation of brain cells. Recommended dose is 5–9 g daily.

II. Raise mitochondrial activity.

1. Inositol enhances the interaction of calcium and mitochondria. Recommended dose: 6–12 grams daily.

2. Lithium: Lithium positively influences mitochondrial activity. It should be used only in patients with treatment-resistant

depression and under the care of a health care practitioner. It is a prescription medication.

III. Rebalance neurotransmitter levels.

1. Antidepressant medications: The most commonly prescribed antidepressant medications are the selective serotonin reuptake inhibitors, also called SSRIs. These include Prozac, Zoloft, and Paxil. Prozac has the longest half-life of all the SSRI medications, and therefore, side effects are more likely. Paxil may have some effects on blocking acetylcholine activity and, therefore, may not be as useful in patients who are elderly and exhibit concurrent memory symptoms. Zoloft has the shortest half-life of the currently available SSRIs, and is generally well tolerated. All of these are prescription medications.

2. S-adenosyl methionine (SAMe): This supplement acts to enhance the production of neurotransmitters like serotonin and dopamine. Recommended dose: 400–800 mg daily.

3. St. John's wort: As mentioned earlier in this chapter, the active extract of St. John's wort may be hyperforin, so consult with your health care practitioner with regard to finding a St. John's wort that contains a significant amount of this extract.

CHAPTER 12

AUTISM

Robert and Sharon's first child, Adam, was born right on schedule without any prenatal or postdelivery complications. Although healthy in many ways, Adam had frequent ear infections that required numerous visits to the pediatrician. Otherwise, he was an affectionate, active child who began to say his first words and take his first steps during his first year of life.

When he was eighteen months old, however, Adam received his immunizations, and shortly thereafter, he developed a high fever and cried inconsolably for three days. Eventually these symptoms resolved, but afterward, Adam appeared withdrawn. He seemed to be "in his own world," uninterested in his surroundings. Adam stopped making eye contact or pointing to things, as he'd done previously. He began to line up objects and play incessantly with a single one for hours on end.

Alarmed, Robert and Sharon took Adam to their pediatrician, who was not exactly sure what to make of this bizarre cluster of symptoms. A pediatric neurologist at the local university was consulted. Adam underwent a series of tests, including an MRI scan of his brain, an EEG (a brain wave test), blood tests, and genetic testing, all of which failed to reveal a specific cause for his developmental regression. The pediatric neurologist sat Adam's parents down, and gave them the bad news: The doctor suspected Adam was autistic. Robert and Sharon were devastated. A behavioral program was recommended but Robert and Sharon, not satisfied, sought other recommendations for Adam's treatment. By the time Adam was three years old, he'd undergone countless examinations by doctors, numerous blood tests, and various therapies that failed to influence the bizarre cluster of behavioral symptoms that is characteristic of autism.

An Overview of Autism

Very few conditions are as confusing to families and physicians alike as the autistic syndrome. Many physicians do not recognize the symptoms of autism unless the presentation is so characteristic and stereotypical that it is hard to miss. Often, the symptoms of autism are not so clear-cut. Children can manifest autistic symptoms in a variety of ways, including disturbances in language, socialization, and behavior.

Autism is most often exhibited in boys, usually when they're eighteen to twenty-four months old. Parents are often the first to recognize the symptoms of autism, which include absent or delayed speech, loss of previously acquired speech, and delay in achieving social milestones. One of the behavioral symptoms associated with autism can be a lack of interest in other children, but this is not always the case. Children with autism also display excessive anxiety, tactile defensiveness, sleep disturbances, poor focusing, hand-flapping behavior, and labile mood.

Prevalence of Autism

It is difficult to make valid prevalence estimates of autism because of disagreement on the exact criteria for its diagnosis. Furthermore, counting children with autism spectrum disorder, who exhibit some mild to moderate symptoms of autism without developing the full-blown syndrome, would raise any calculated incidence of the disorder. Based upon current estimates, 1 in 500 children is affected by this disease, which accounts for approximately 1 million children in the United States alone.

What Causes Autism?

The etiology of autism is currently unknown. Many theories have been proposed, including genetic factors, insults during brain development, immune factors, and environmental factors.

Genetics clearly plays a role in a percentage of autism cases. Studies of identical twins reveal that both are more likely to develop autism than are fraternal twins. In most children, a defective gene or genes would result only in an increased vulnerability to autism; however, this genetic vulnerability may interfere with normal brain development when it is triggered by specific environmental factors.

• Environmental Factors and Autism

During pregnancy, the fetal brain is growing rapidly. The process of brain growth in the prenatal period is complex; it involves brain cells growing in specific directions and forming connections with other brain cells, a process known as "synaptic connectivity." This process within the developing brain is very elaborate and intricate. Any disturbance in it can result in defects in a child's language, social, and mental functioning.

Recently, some researchers have reported a correlation between environmental toxins and autism. These toxins include certain forms of benzenes, which are in commonly used chemical solvents. These chemicals have also been linked to neural tube defects (like spina bifida and anencephaly), supporting the claim that they can interfere with normal brain development. Studies of clusters of autistic individuals who live near hazardous waste sites, with a high exposure to these toxins, will help to confirm the association between environmental chemicals and autism.

• The Immune System and Autism

Many children have abnormalities in immune system functioning. This can manifest as frequent ear infections, but immune problems have also been found in children with recurrent ear infections by sophisticated analyses of immune parameters. The role of the immune system in brain development is critical. An overactive or underactive immune system can result in misguided direction of neurons, an abnormal growth pattern of neurons, or changes in the brain's biochemistry. For instance, certain cytokines, the messenger chemicals of the immune system, can alter the way tryptophan (an amino acid) is processed. While tryptophan is a precursor of the neurotransmitter serotonin, it can also be converted into a compound known as kynurenine, which is an antiserotonin compound. Increases in brain kynurenitic levels produce aggression and stereotypical behaviors that resemble autism.

The immune system is critical in determining the fate of tryptophan. When the immune system is excessively activated, the cytokine gamma interferon is turned on. Gamma interferon, in turn, stimulates the enzyme that converts tryptophan to kynurenine, in essence shuttling away available tryptophan and making it inaccessible for the synthesis of serotonin. This results in lowered levels of serotonin.

• Immunizations and Autism

Some clinicians believe there is a connection between autism and immunizations. This belief comes from the observation that, in some children, regression is closely associated with administration of the MMR (mumps, measles, and rubella) vaccine. Some recent studies have found the presence of active measles virus in the intestinal lining of autistic children, but other researchers dispute these findings. Clearly this issue needs more study before any definite recommendations about the relationship of immunizations to autism can be made.

• Epilepsy and Autism

In a small percentage of autistic children, behavioral regression is associated with abnormal brain wave activity, which can be seen on an EEG. However, it is difficult to document these brain wave abnormalities because they may be intermittent, not continuous. If this epileptic activity occurs in areas of the brain responsible for speech, it can result in a language disorder. In fact, an epileptic condition known as Landau-Kleffner syndrome is characterized by speech regression. There are many similarities

262   THE BRAIN WELLNESS PLAN

between this regression and autism, which has led researchers to suggest that autism may also be due to abnormal electrical activity in the brain. Treatment of these children involves antiepileptic medication or steroids.

• Porphyria and Autism

Porphyria is a rare neurological disorder that affects the liver, blood, and brain. It is characterized by severe anxiety, restlessness, nausea, and psychotic episodes. In patients routinely screened for porphyria in psychiatric hospitals a significant percentage of patients were found to be affected by this disorder, compared to the general population.

Porphyria is caused by disturbances in the production of heme. Heme has several vital functions in the body including carrying oxygen to every tissue including the brain, binding toxic metals and disarming them, and increasing the synthesis of tryptophan so that it is available to manufacture serotonin. In porphyria the enzymes that are heme-dependent are adversely affected, resulting in decreased concentrations of tryptophan and subsequently neurotoxicity.

A possible relationship between autism and porphyria has been speculated by the author Dr. Jay Lombard. Autistic children, when deemed appropriate by the clinician, can be screened for porphyria by specific blood and urine tests.

• Biochemistry of Autism

Neurotransmitter abnormalities have frequently been associated with autism and represent the "final common pathway" of altered behavior, cognition, and language in this disorder. Virtually every neurotransmitter has been proposed as contributing to the etiology of autism, but it is not likely that a single biochemical defect could produce the wide array of symptoms that is seen in autism. Rather, a complex combination of abnormalities probably exists in the brains of autistic children, including disturbances of serotonin, dopamine, and glutamate.

Serotonin and Autism Decreased blood serotonin is found in approximately 30 percent of autistic patients. You will recall that

serotonin acts as a neurotransmitter, and its depletion is implicated in other neurological disorders, including depression. Serotonin can also act as a nerve growth factor, which could be
particularly important in the development of autism, since it
typically appears in 18- to 24-month-olds, in whom the brain is
still developing. Depletion of serotonin's precursor tryptophan,
which leads to decreases in serotonin neurotransmission, exacer-
bates symptoms of autism. Furthermore, medications that increase brain serotonin levels, such as the selective serotonin reuptake inhibitors (SSRIs), improve symptoms of autism in some
children.

Dopamine and Autism Dopamine is intimately involved in attention, motivation, and perception. Several researchers have found
elevated metabolites of dopamine in autistic patients, suggesting
that autistic children are experiencing a hyperdopaminc condition. In some ways, this condition may resemble schizophrenia
with its characteristic disturbances in perception, anxiety, and
cognition, all of which are linked to excessive dopamine activity.

Glutamate and Autism Glutamate in an excitatory neurotransmitter. It is involved in a memory-forming process called "long-
term potentiation," which governs the likelihood that a thought
will be placed into long-term memory. If there is increased potentiation, there is a decrease in the amount of time needed to form
a memory—that is, increased potentiation results in increased
memory formation. Glutamate assists in the brain's capacity to
form new memories. Recently, it has been speculated that autism
may be due to low glutamate levels in the brain. This observation
has been supported by the fact that certain drugs that block
glutamate receptors also produce symptoms identical to autism
and schizophrenia.

Diagnosis of Autism

There is no biochemical or brain imaging study that confirms
the diagnosis of autism. Its diagnosis is made by specific diagnostic
criteria as defined in the *Diagnostic Statistical Manual* used by
psychiatrists. When testing is done for an autistic child, it is most

often used to exclude other diseases that mimic autism. These include a genetic disorder known as Fragile X syndrome, an epileptic condition called Landau-Kleffner syndrome, and certain inborn errors of metabolism. Usually a pediatric neurologist is required to determine if an MRI, brain wave test, or blood and urine tests are required in this scenario.

The Three R's of Managing Autism: Reduce Inflammation, Raise Mitochondrial Action, and Rebalance Neurotransmitter Levels

Various nutritional and pharmacological recommendations have been suggested for use in autism. A whole book could be written on this topic alone; therefore, we will address the more common treatment recommendations.

These include drugs and supplements that reduce inflammation, including antifungal medications (if candida is diagnosed or suspected), drugs like secretin and supplements like Serenaid that help break down proteins (and so combat excessive inflammation), the drug Naltrexone (which controls pain by reducing immune system overactivity), and the supplement CDP choline (which helps slow overactive immune systems); supplements that support mitochondrial functioning, like creatine, d-ribose, and CDP choline; vitamins or drugs that raise brain glutamate levels, including DMG; drugs that block dopamine, including the atypical neuroleptic medications; and drugs that raise brain serotonin levels, such as SSRIs.

Strategies Based on Reducing Inflammation

Excessive inflammation is produced, in part, by an overactive immune system. Since children with autism are known to have overactive immune systems: decreasing inflammation may help to control the symptoms of autism. Numerous substances may help to ameliorate the effects of inflammation in autistic children.

An overgrowth of fungus (due to a weakened immune system or excessive antibiotic use) may be producing inflammation in children who have autism, so medications that treat fungal infections may also affect the symptoms of the disorder. Compounds like secretin, which increases the pancreatic enzymes necessary to break down proteins during digestion, may help to regulate the inflammation that poorly digested proteins can generate. Also available as an oral alternative to secretin is the dietary supplement Serenaid. Naltrexone, a medication that lowers the levels of circulating endorphins, may correct the insensitivity to pain that some children with autism exhibit, which may also be linked to an inflammatory response. And CDP choline, a form of choline that stimulates the production of phosphatidylcholine, is thought to slow overactive immune responses.

•Nystatin and Other Antifungal Therapies and Autism

Rationale for Use of Antifungal Therapies in Autism Yeast are fungi that are normally found in our bodies, but which can cause disease when the immune system is weak. Symptoms of yeast infection can include rash, bloating, and other gastrointestinal disturbances. It is speculated that yeast can cause behavioral problems like those seen in autism because of their ability to ferment sugar into alcohol. Although blood alcohol levels have never been measured in autism, metabolites of yeast activity have been detected through specific biochemical tests (including analysis of urine organic acids). Furthermore, maternal alcohol use during pregnancy has been associated with both autism and attention deficit disorder. Increased levels of blood alcohol have adverse effects in the brain stem. The brain stem controls the production and release of several neurotransmitters including serotonin, and we know that serotonin levels are abnormal in autism.

Clinical Studies of Antifungal Therapies in Autism There are no clinical studies exploring the effects of Nystatin in autism; however, many researchers, including this author (Dr. Lombard), have reported beneficial effects of antifungal therapy in children with autism, including decreased hyperactivity, better eye contact, and better bowel habits.

> RECOMMENDED DOSE: Nystatin is very safe, because it does not enter the bloodstream. Dosages are between 100,000 and 500,000 units three times daily. It is only available by prescription. Many clinicians recommend the concurrent use of nutritional compounds known as probiotics, which are microorganisms found in the intestinal tract that control the overgrowth of yeast. Probiotics also help the gut assimilate vitamins. The most commonly utilized probiotics are *Lactobacillus acidophilus* and *Bifido bifidum.*

• Secretin and Autism

Rationale for Use of Secretin in Autism Secretin is a physiological stimulant that increases pancreatic enzymes necessary to break down proteins properly during digestion. These digestive enzymes, known as peptidases, may be underactive in autism.

The inability to break down protein, which results from pancreatic dysfunction (i.e., when the pancreas doesn't produce the necessary pancreatic enzymes mentioned above), may lead to absorption of large proteins. These absorbed large proteins may activate the immune system in harmful ways. For example, incompletely digested proteins from casein (called caseomorphins) and gluten (called gluteomorphins) may have morphine-like effects on the brain, since they appear to bind to and stimulate brain opiate receptors. Pancreatic dysfunction contributes to an inability to break down these morphine-like proteins, and possibly result in the behavioral disturbances found in autism.

Dr. Horvath, at the University of Maryland School of Medicine, first noted a dramatic benefit of secretin in autistic children who were undergoing testing for pancreatic function. During this testing, secretin was administered intravenously to monitor the pancreatic response. Within several weeks of this infusion, it was noted by parents that the children exhibited increased eye contact and improved language.

Despite suggestions that secretin affects protein digestion in autistic children, it's not precisely understood how secretin may be helpful. One recent theory suggests that an ingredient in the secretin preparation, cysteine, is responsible for the changes observed during secretin therapy. Cysteine is a sulfur amino acid that detoxifies cells. While secretin does not cross the blood-brain barrier, cysteine does; therefore, it's possible that the cysteine in secretin crosses into the brain and affects behavior.

Cysteine also stimulates glutamate receptors. As mentioned earlier, patients with autism may have a relative deficiency of glutamate. This is suspected because blocking glutamate receptors with drugs (thereby artificially creating a glutamate deficiency) can produce symptoms that are identical to autism and even psychosis. Conversely, by enhancing the effects of glutamate, cysteine may ameliorate some of the symptoms of autism that are characterized by glutamate deficiency.

Clinical Studies of Secretin in Autism Currently, there are no data available regarding the use of secretin in autism; the only reports are anecdotal. Double-blind studies are currently under way to determine the efficacy of secretin in autism.

RECOMMENDED DOSE: Speak to your health care practitioner about availability and use of secretin therapy for autism.

• Serenaid and Autism

Rationale for Use of Serenaid in Autism Serenaid, an enzymatic dietary supplement, helps the pancreas break down harmful proteins that have been incompletely digested. Because of this effect, Serenaid may be an oral alternative to Secretin therapy in children with autism who have pancreatic dysfunction. Serenaid consists of a unique enzyme, peptidase, that helps to break down large proteins.

Clinical Studies of Serenaid in Autism A Phase II pilot study involving 62 autistic children will evaluate the effect of Serenaid on autistic symptoms. Preliminary data suggest that a substantial percentage of patients experience improvement after two weeks of treatment.

RECOMMENDED DOSE: It is recommended that children with autism ingest 1–2 capsules per meal. Dosage may be increased until the desired result is achieved. Precautions: None.

•Naltrexone and Autism

Rationale for Use of Naltrexone in Autism Various researchers and clinicians have observed that some autistic children are insensitive to pain, which may be because they possess higher levels of naturally occurring opioids (or "endorphins") than healthy children. This hypothesis is supported by recent findings of elevated endorphin levels in autistic children (compared to age-matched, controlled groups of healthy children). One theory about these elevated levels of endorphins suggests that they are derived from the diet. Recently, it has been demonstrated by researchers at the University of Liverpool in England that endorphins affect the immune system in several ways. While endorphins stimulate the activity of white blood cells, very high levels of endorphins can reduce immune system activity. In particular, endorphins reduce natural killer cell activity. These vital immune system cells help fight off yeast and other infections, so this effect of endorphins is deleterious and may explain why autistic children have more yeast infections. Clearly, high circulating endorphins disturb both the immune system and the brain.

Drugs that block this excessive opiate activity may help autistic children by restoring the immune system and reducing the adverse effects of opiates on the brain. Naltrexone, an opiate-blocking drug that lowers the levels of circulating endorphins, does precisely that, and so may help autistic children. It is only available by prescription.

Clinical Studies of Naltrexone in Autism Eleven children, ages 3 to 8, were treated wtih Naltrexone daily in a double-blind, placebo-controlled study at Children's Hospital of Pittsburgh in 1997. Objective measurement studies were conducted, evaluating behavior, hyperactivity, and language. Three of the eleven children improved on one or more of the measurements in the study group, compared to those in the placebo group. However, in a follow-up study by the same researchers, no improvement was seen in language disturbance, which is a core symptom of autism.

In a study conducted by researchers at the University of Milan, Italy, another group of eleven autistic children were examined in a study of Naltrexone. These investigators found a direct correlation between reduced endorphin levels and decreased autistic symptoms, including improvement in speech and stereotypical motor behavior. This second study, therefore, suggests that Naltrexone may be helpful to some children with autism.

RECOMMENDED DOSE: Naltrexone should only be used under the guidance of a physician. Treatment doses in the above studies were 1 mg per kg of body weight.

Strategies Based on Increasing Mitochondrial Function

It has recently been proposed by the author (Dr. Lombard) that autism may be related to dysfunction of the mitochondria, the energy-producing units of our cells. One of the clinical manifestations of mitochondrial disorder is the reduction of motor tone, also known as hypotonia, which many children with autism have. Furthermore, ongoing clinical research suggests that a significant percentage of autistic children have defects in mitochondrial DNA.

Creatine and CDP choline both help to stimulate mitochondrial function, and so may be helpful to autistic children. Both creatine and CDP choline contribute to the production of ATP, our cells' main source of energy, which is produced by the mitochondria.

• Creatine and Autism

Rationale for Use of Creatine in Autism Creatine is a dietary supplement that protects the brain. It has been shown that taking creatine orally increases brain creatine concentrations as well as brain ATP concentrations. Creatine also protects the mitochondria from free radical injury.

Clinical Studies of Creatine in Autism There are no controlled clinical studies examining the effects of creatine in autism. However, creatine has important functions in the brain, and the observation that levels of creatine are diminished in autistic patients makes this compound worthy of future study.

> RECOMMENDED DOSE: Creatine should be administered under the guidance of a health care practitioner. Recommended doses are between 500 mg and 1 g daily; however, much lower doses are required in children, and kidney functions should be monitored.

• CDP Choline and Autism

Rationale for Use of CDP Choline in Autism CDP choline is a natural supplement that is essential for the synthesis of key phospholipids in the brain. It also improves mitochondrial activity and brain energy metabolism. In an elaborate study performed by Dr. Nancy Minschew (at the Department of Psychology, University of Pittsburgh), levels of brain phospholipids and creatine were measured in autistic patients and compared to normal control groups. In autistic children, there was a significant decline of phosphocreatine, resulting in alterations in brain energy and phospholipid metabolism. These findings suggest that either the undersynthesis of brain phospholipids or their increased degradation is associated with decreased mitochondrial function. This may be the underlying defect in autism.

Dr. Richard Wertmann at the Massachusetts Institute of Technology has suggested that CDP choline acts as an anti-inflammatory compound in the brain, because of its ability to remove certain pro-inflammatory fatty acids, like arachidonic acid. CDP choline helps to sequester arachidonic acid in cell membranes, preventing its activation of the immune system. Therefore, CDP choline could be useful because it reduces inflammation, or because it enhances mitochondrial function, which is why we suggest using it in both of those strategies of treating autism.

Clinical Studies of CDP Choline in Autism While there are currently no studies of choline in autism, because of its important physiological effects on brain mitochondria and brain phospholipid metabolism, it is strongly suggested by the authors that CDP choline be considered for future study. Furthermore, in Dr. Lombard's practice, he has noted moderate improvements in autistic symptoms with the use of CDP choline.

> RECOMMENDED DOSE: Consult with your health care practitioner about using CDP choline to treat autism. Precautions: None.

Strategies Based on Rebalancing Neurotransmitter Levels

The neurotransmitter abnormalities in autism include low glutamate levels, increased dopamine levels, and serotonin imbalances. Let's look at some strategies to rebalance the levels of these crucial neurotransmitters in the brains of autistic children.

• Strategies Based on Raising Brain Glutamate Levels: Dimethylglycine (DMG) and Autism

Rationale for Use of DMG in Autism DMG is a modification of the amino acid glycine. Glycine acts similarily to glutamate in the brain, stimulating excitatory receptors. Schizophrenic patients with negative symptoms (i.e., withdrawn behavior and decreased socialization) have been shown to improve when given high doses of glycine. DMG, which increases glycine levels in the brain, may help normalize the low level of glutamate in the brains of autistic patients.

Clinical Studies of DMG in Autism Although DMG has been widely recommended for use in autism, there is only one double-blind, placebo-controlled study, which was recently reported in the *Journal of Autism and Developmental Disorders* (1999). In a small sample of patients ranging from four to thirty years of age, low-dose DMG was administered over a three-and-a-half-month period. There were no changes in any behavioral measurements when the treatment and placebo groups were compared. The problem with interpreting this study is that the sample size is too small—only eight patients—and a low dose of DMG was used. In clinical experience, many clinicians and parents report that DMG has a beneficial effect.

> RECOMMENDED DOSE: 125 mg daily. Precautions: None. However, DMG can sometimes produce a state of excitation and hyperactivity that requires lowering the dose.

• Strategies Based on Decreasing Dopamine Levels: Atypical Neuroleptics (Risperidone) and Autism

Rationale for Use of Risperidone and Other Atypical Neuroleptics in Autism As mentioned earlier, dopamine levels may be excessive in certain children with autism, leading to abnormal cognitive and behavorial symptoms. Risperidone is a selective dopamine-blocking drug that specifically acts in the regions of the brain that control these higher functions.

Clinical Studies of Risperidone in Autism In a double-blind, placebo-controlled study performed at the Indiana University School of Medicine in 1998, 31 adults with autistic disorder received Risperidone or a placebo over a twelve-week period. Fifty-seven percent of the patients who received Risperidone were characterized as "responders," compared to none of those in the placebo group. Risperidone reduced repetitive behavior, aggression, and anxiety.

In an open-label study of ten autistic children, ranging from four to ten years of age, researchers at the University of Toronto gave Risperidone in doses of 1 to 2.5 mg a day over a three-month period. These researchers noted that eight out of the ten children responded favorably in all behavioral indices.

> RECOMMENDED DOSE: Risperidone is available only by prescription and should be taken only under the care and supervision of a health care practitioner. Precautions in Risperidone use include weight gain and sedation, which are common side effects. Infrequently, a paradoxical increase in irritability and crying spells is seen with Risperidone therapy. Side effects like adventitious (jerky and irregular) movements are rare.

Strategies Based on Increasing Brain Serotonin Levels

It's suspected that the symptoms of autism may result, in part, from nerve cells failing to make the proper synaptic connections during a child's early development. One factor that might contribute to this failure to form proper synapses is a lack of serotonin which, in addition to being a neurotransmitter, also acts as a nerve growth factor. Since autism typically appears in toddlers whose brains are still developing neuronal synaptic pathways, a lack of serotonin might cause their synaptic pathways to form inappropriately, resulting in the symptoms of autism. Increasing brain serotonin levels, using serotonin selective reuptake inhibitors (SSRIs), appears to be helpful in treating children with autism, possibly lending support to this theory. Natural substances that increase brain serotonin levels, including St. John's wort and SAMe, may also ameliorate autistic behaviors.

• Sertraline and Autism

Rationale for Use of Setraline and Other SSRIs in Autism Sertraline and other SSRIs are prescription medications that raise brain serotonin levels. Many children with autism display behavioral problems including excessive anxiety, sleep disturbances, and irritability. These symptoms may be linked to a serotonin deficiency. By raising brain serotonin levels through the use of SSRIs, some of these symptoms may be ameloriated.

Clinical Studies of Sertraline in Autism Researchers at the Massachusetts General Hospital administered Sertraline to nine patients averaging 6–12 years of age over a 2–8-week period. Eight of nine patients showed a clinically significant improvement with minimal side effects during therapy.

RECOMMENDED DOSE: Sertraline and other SSRIs are available only by prescription. In my clinical experience (Dr. Lombard), much lower doses are used than those reported in clinical studies. Starting dose is usually 5–10 mg with a maximum of 25 mg daily, but this drug is given only by prescription under the care of a supervising physician.

• S-Adenosyl Methionine (SAMe)

Rationale for Use of S-Adenosyl Methionine in Autism SAMe is a naturally occurring compound that affects neurotransmitters. SAMe participates intimately in the process of methylation in the brain; methylation is essential to the synthesis, activation, and metabolism of various neurotransmitters. Levels of the neurotransmitter serotonin are increased by SAMe administration. Serotonin is linked to mood, sleep, anxiety, appetite, and energy levels, all of which are disturbed in autistic children.

Clinical Studies of SAMe and Autism Currently there are no clinical studies on SAMe and autism. However, Dr. Lombard has observed in many of his patients that autistic symptoms are reduced with the administration of SAMe.

RECOMMENDED DOSE: Consult with your health care practitioner regarding correct dosage. Precautions: A paradoxical increase in irritability, hyperactivity, and crying spells is sometimes seen.

• St. John's Wort and Autism

Rationale for Use of St. John's Wort in Autism As mentioned in Chapter 11, "Depression," St. John's wort is a natural herbal substance that acts in a similar way to the SSRI antidepressants. The active constituents of St. John's wort may include hyperforin and hypericum. Hyperforin, in particular, raises brain concentrations of serotonin, norepinephrine, and dopamine.

Clinical Studies of St. John's Wort in Autism There are currently no controlled studies measuring the effects of St. John's wort in autism. Nevertheless, this compound is of theoretical interest, because it can increase neurotransmitter levels. However, one must *never* take both St. John's wort and a prescription SSRI drug simultaneously.

RECOMMENDED DOSE: Dosage: Consult with your health care practitioner regarding correct dosage. Precaution: Never take St. John's wort and an SSRI drug simultaneously.

A Cocktail Approach to Treating Autism

I. Strageties based on reducing excessive inflammation.

1. Antifungal therapy: It is speculated that yeast can cause behavioral problems like those seen in autism because of their ability to ferment sugar into alcohol. Recommended dosage of the antifungal prescription drug Nystatin is 100,000–500,000 units three times daily.

2. Secretin: This prescription drug increases the pancreatic enzymes necessary to break down proteins during digestion. Speak to your health care provider about the availability of secretin.

3. Serenaid: This natural substance increases the pancreatic enzymes necessary to break down proteins during digestion. Recommended dosage for children is 1–2 capsules at mealtime; dosage can be increased until the desired result is achieved.

4. Naltrexone: This prescription drug decreases the level of circulating endorphins found in autistic children. Naltrexone should be used only under the guidance of a physician. Treatment doses in studies are 1 mg per kg of body weight.

II. Strategies based on increasing mitochondrial function.

1. Creatine is a building block of ATP, our cells' energy source. Recommended doses are between 500 mg and 1 g daily; however, much lower doses are required in children, and kidney functions should be monitored.

2. CDP choline is a building block of ATP, our cells' energy source. Consult your health care provider about using CDP choline for autism.

III. Strategies based on rebalancing neurotransmitter levels.

1. Raising brain glutamate levels: The amino acid dimethylglycine, or DMG, increases glycine levels in the brain, and may

help normalize the low level of glutamate in the brains of autistic patients. Dosage: 125 mg a day. Precaution: May sometimes produce hyperactivity, and require a lower dose.

2. Decreasing dopamine levels: Risperdal, a typical narcoleptic, decreased dopamine, which is thought to be elevated in autistic children. Dosage of this prescription medication is determined individually by treating physicians.

3. Increasing brain serotonin levels.

a. Serotonin reuptake inhibitor medications (SSRIs) increase brain levels of serotonin. Dosages of these prescription medications are determined individually by treating physicians.

i. Sertraline is a prescription SSRI that raises brain serotonin levels. Starting dose is usually 5–10 mg, with a maximum of 25 mg daily, but this prescription drug is administered only under the supervision of a physician.

b. S-adenosyl methionine (SAMe) increases levels of the neurotransmitters serotonin and dopamine. Dosage to be determined by your health care practitioner.

c. St. John's wort increases brain levels of serotonin. Dosage to be determined by your health care practitioner.

RESOURCES

The following organizations offer additional information and support to patients and their families.

Alzheimer's
Alzheimer's Association
70 East Lake Street
Suite 600
Chicago, IL 60601
(312) 853-3060
(800) 621-0379

Parkinson's
National Parkinson's
   Foundation
1501 Northwest Ninth Avenue
Bob Hope Road
Miami, FL 33136
(305) 547-6666
(800) 327-4545

Parkinson's Disease
   Foundation
Columbia-Presbyterian
   Medical Center
650 West 168th Street
New York, NY 10032
(800) 457-6676

Multiple Sclerosis
National Multiple Sclerosis
   Society
733 Third Avenue
New York, NY 10017
(212) 986-3240
(800) 624-8232

Amyotrophic Lateral Sclerosis
The ALS Association
21021 Ventura Boulevard
Suite 321
Woodland Hills, CA 91364
(818) 340-7500
(800) 782-4747

Attention Deficit Hyperactivity Disorder
CHADD
1859 North Pine Island Road
Suite 185
Plantation, FL 33322
(954) 587-3700

Chronic Fatigue Syndrome
CFIDS of America
P.O. Box 220398
Charlotte, NC 28222
(800) 442-3437

Depression
National Foundation for
   Depressive Illnesses
P.O. Box 2257
New York, NY 10116
(800) 248-4344

NUTRITION ASSOCIATIONS

The following is a list of professional organizations that will serve as useful resources of information on herbs, nutrition, and preventive medical care.

American Botanical Council
P.O. Box 201660
Austin, TX 78720-1660
(512) 331-8868;
fax (512) 331-1924

American College of
   Alternative Medicine
(800) 532-3688

American Holistic Medical
   Association
4101 Lake Boone Trail
Suite 201
Raleigh, NC 27607
(919) 787-5146

American Preventive Medical
   Association
P.O. Box 2111
Tacoma, WA 98401
(206) 926-0551;
fax (206) 922-7583

Citizens for Health
P.O. Box 2260
Boulder, CO 80306-1195
(303) 417-0772;
fax (303) 417-9378

Council for Responsible
  Nutrition (CRN)
1300 Nineteenth Street NW
Suite 310
Washington, DC 20036-1609
(202) 872-1488

Herb Research Foundation
1007 Pearl Street, Suite 200
Boulder, CO 80302-5124
(303) 449-2265;
fax (303) 449-7849

NUTRITIONAL SUPPLEMENT RESOURCES

The following companies have products described in this book
which are available in health food stores everywhere.

Retail Health Food Store Brands

Source Naturals®
23 Janis Way
Scotts Valley, CA 95066
1-800-815-2333
http://www.sourcenaturals.com

Acetyl-L-Carnitine
250 mg and 500 mg tablets

GABA—Gamma Amino Butyric
  Acid
(Chief inhibitory neuro-
  transmitter in the brain)
750 mg tablets

GABA Calm™
Sublingual Delivery System
GABA Complex tablets

Phosphatidyl Serine
(Important constituent of nerve
  cell membranes)
100 mg, 150 mg, 500 mg tablets

J.R. Carlson® Laboratories
15 College Drive
Arlington Heights, IL 60004-
  1985
1-800-323-4141
http://www.carlsonlabs.com

Alpha Lipoic Acid
100 mg, 300 mg tablets

Phosphatidyl Serine
100 mg soft gels

E·Gems® Plus
Vitamin E
200 IU, 400 IU, 800 IU soft gels

Raw Material Suppliers of Brain Nutrients

General Nutrition Center (GNC)
300 Sixth Ave
Pittsburgh, PA 15222

For a store nearest you call:
(800) 477-4462
http://www.gnc.com

For all your nutritional supplement needs visit GNC or buy online at Drugstore.com.

Nutratech, Inc.
208 Passaic Avenue
Fairfield, NJ 07004
Phone (973) 882-7773
Fax (973) 882-9666

Nutratech is a leading supplier, manufacturer, research and development and marketing resource. They carry many of the brain wellness nutrients covered in this book.

Martek
Supplier of Neuromins® DHA
(a special micro-algae, non-fish DHA product in softgel form)

For information and a list of companies carrying Neuromins®, call 1-800-662-6339.

Marco HI-Tech JV Ltd.
1 Penn Plaza, Suite 2514
New York, NY 10119
Phone (212) 798-8109
Fax (212) 631-0971
E-mail: Richard.Sequeira@juno.com

Marco HI-Tech JV Ltd. discovers, develops and commercializes, through its network of marketing relationships, nutraceuticals that address important unmet medical needs, with a concentration on compounds that support healthy neurological function.

Contact Marco HI-Tech for all of your raw material needs.

FOOD SOURCES FOR THE BRAIN WELLNESS NUTRIENTS RECOMMENDED THROUGHOUT THE BOOK

None of the foods listed can be eaten in sufficient amounts to elicit a nutritional therapeutic effect, and therefore, we do recommend supplements. However, these foods do provide the basis for a healthy diet and optimum brain wellness.

Nutrient	*Food Sources*
Phosphatidylserine (PS)	Lecithin
Docosahexaenoic Acid (DHA)	Fatty fish, fish oil
Genistein	Soy foods, soy protein
NAC (N-acetyl-cysteine)	Protein foods, such as fish and poultry
ALC (acetyl-L-carnitine)	Protein foods, such as fish
Glutamine	Protein foods, such as fish
Threonine	Protein foods, such as fish and poultry
Lipoic acid	Liver, yeast
Polyphenols, proanthocyanidins	Red wine; green tea; fruit, grapes; grape seed and pine bark extracts; and herbs such as bilberry, ginkgo, and milk thistle.

Vitamin E	
Tocopherols	Polyunsaturated vegetable oils, seeds, nuts
Tocotrienols	Barley and rice oils
Coenzyme Q10	Every plant and animal cell
Vitamin C	Citrus fruits, broccoli, peppers, and other dark-colored vegetables and fruits
B vitamins	
Thiamine	Brown rice, soybeans, seeds, yeast
Riboflavin	Yeast, organ meats, almonds, wheat germ
Niacin	Eggs, organ meats, fish, brown rice, seeds
B_6	Seeds, whole grains, beans, bananas, nuts
Biotin	Cheese, soybeans, organ meats, brown rice
Pantothenic acid	Fish, poultry, milk, nuts, soybeans, brown rice
Folic acid	Green leafy vegetables, beans, wheat germ, nuts
B_{12}	Organ meats, milk, fish, cheese, meat
Choline	Grains, beans, cauliflower, whole grains, lettuce
Inositol	Whole grains, citrus fruits, nuts, seeds, beans
Minerals	
Calcium	Dairy products, tofu, kale, green leafy vegetables, seaweed
Magnesium	Tofu, beans, seeds, nuts, whole grains, green leafy vegetables

Zinc	Shellfish, fish, meats, whole grains, beans, seeds
Manganese	Nuts, whole grains, dried fruits, green leafy vegetables
Selenium	Wheat germ, nuts, whole grains, Swiss chard, garlic
Vanadium	Parsley, mushrooms, shellfish, soybeans, corn
Carotenoids: alpha and beta	Carrots, tomatoes, squash, kale
Carotene, lutein, lycopene	Collards, broccoli, yams, other dark-colored fruits and vegetables

REFERENCES

Part I

• Chapter 1: Brain-Immune Connection Basics

Bindoni M., et al. Interleukin-2 modifies the bioelectrical activity of some neurosecretory nuclei in the rat hypothalamus. Brain Res 1988; 462: 10–14.

Black P. Psychoneuroimmunology. Brain and immunity. Sci. American 1995 Nov–Dec: 16–25.

Blum F. and Kupfer D., eds. Psychopharmacology, the Fourth Generation of Progress. Raven Press, 1995.

Carpenter M., ed. Core Text of Neuroanatomy, 4th ed. Williams and Wilkins, 1991.

Fabris N., Markovic B.M., Spector N.H., Jankovic B.D., eds. Neuroimmunomodulations: the state of the art. Ann NY Acad Sci 1994; Vol. 741.

Ganong W.F., Dallman M.F., Roberts J.L., eds. The hypothalamic pituitary adrenal revisited. Ann NY Acad Sci 1987; Vol. 512.

Jankovic B.D., Markovic B.M., Spector N.H., eds. Neuroimmune interactions. Ann NY Acad Sci 1987; Vol. 496.

Netter F. Ciba Collection of Medical Illustrations. Nervous System Anatomy and Physiology, Vol. 1. Ciba-Geigy, 1991.

Scriver C.R., Beaudet A.L., Sly W.S., Valle D.S., eds. Metabolic and Molecular Bases of Inherited Disease, 7th ed. McGraw-Hill Inc., 1995.

Shatz, C. The developing brain. Sci American 1992 Sept; 267(3): 60–7.

Snyder S. Nitric oxide: first in a new class of neurotransmitter. Science 1992 Jul; Vol. 253.

Streight W.J. and Kincaid-Colton C.A. The brain's immune system. Sci American 1995 Nov; 273 (5): 54–61.

• Chapter 2: Communication Breakdown

Barinaga M. Cell suicide: by ICE, not FIRE. Science 1994 Feb. 11; 263: 754–6.

Beal M.F. Aging, energy and oxidative stress in neurodegenerative diseases. Ann Neurol 1995 Sept; 38(3): 357–68.

Chan T.H. and Fishman R.A. Free fatty acids, oxygen free radicals and membrane alterations and brain ischemia and injury. In Cerebrovascular Disease, Plum F. and Pulsinell W., eds. Raven Press, 1985: 161–71.

Heyes M.P. Relationship between interferon gamma, indoleamine, #2-3 dioxygenase and tryptophans. FASEB J 1991; 5: 3003–4.

Murphy T., et al. Arachidonic acid metabolism in glutamate neurotoxicity in arachidonic metabolism in the nervous system. Ann NY Acad Sci 1989; 559.

Olanow C.W. A radical hypothesis for neurodegeneration. Trends in Neuroscience 1993; 16: 439–44.

Oldstone M.B. Molecular mimicry and autoimmune disease. Zell 1987 Sept; 50(6): 819–20.

Opp M.R., et al. Cytokine involvement in the regulation of sleep. Proc Soc Exp Biol Med 1992; 201: 16–27.

Palmer A.M., Burns M. Selective increase in lipid peroxidation in the inferior temporal cortex in Alzheimer's disease. Brain Res 1994; 645: 338–47.

Rothstein J., et al. Chronic inhibition of the superoxide dismutase produces apoptotic death of spinal neurons. Proc Nat Acad of Sci 1994 May; 91: 4155–9.

Rubbo H., et al. Nitric oxide regulation of superoxide and peroxynitrate dependent lipid peroxidation. J of Biol Chem 1994; 269(42): 26066–75.

Sapolsky R.M., et al. Inhibition of glucocorticoid secretion by the hippocampal formation in the primate. J of Neuroscience 1991; 11: 3695–704.

Steinman L. Autoimmune disease. Sci American 1993 Sept; 107–14.

Vandenabelle P., et al. Is amyloidogenesis during Alzheimer's disease due to IL-1/Il-6 mediated acute phase response in the brain? Immunol Today 1991; 12: 217–9.

• Chapter 3: Food for Thought

Ahnert-Hilger G. and Bigalke H. Molecular aspects of tetanus and botulinum neurotoxin poisoning. Progress in Neurobiology 1995; 46: 83–96.

Bland J. New perspectives in nutritional therapies. Health Com. Inc., 1996.

Dawks D. Disorders of copper transport. In Metabolic and Molecular Bases of Inherited Diseases, 7th ed., Vol 2. Scriver C., Beaudet A., Sly W. and Valle D., eds. McGraw-Hill Inc., 1995.

Eastwood S.L. and Harrison P.J. Decreased synaptophysin in the medial temporal lobe in schizophrenia demonstrated using immunoautoradiography. Letters to Neuroscience 1995; 69: 339–343.

Frederickson C.J. Neurobiology of zinc and zinc-containing neurons. Rev Neurobiol 1989; 31: 146–238.

Gibson R.S., et al. A growth-limiting, mild zinc deficiency syndrome in some South Ontario boys with low height percentiles. Am J of Clin Nutrition 1991; 49: 1266–73.

Huan Y., et al. Further study on the magnesium-mediated change in physical state of phospholipid modulates mitochondrial ATP ASE activity. Magnesium Res 1993; 6: 321–7.

Krieger D., Bronstein M., Martin J., eds. Brain Peptides. John Wiley and Sons Inc., 1983.

Lindenbaum J., et al. Neuropsychiatric disorders caused by cobalamin deficiency in the absence of anemia or macrocytosis. N Engl J Med 1988 Jun 30; 318(26): 1720–8.

Lockwood A.H. Hepatic encephalopathy and other neurological diseases associated with gastrointestinal disease. In Neurology and General Medicine, Aminoff M. ed. Churchill Livingston Publishing, 1989.

Magistretti P.J., Pellerin L., Martin J.L. Brain energy metabolism: an integrative cellular perspective. In Psychopharmacology: The Fourth Generation of Progress. Bloom F. and Kupfer D., eds. Raven Press, 1995.

Ramadan N. and Welch K. Migraine and cluster headaches. In Current Therapy in Neurological Diseases, 4th ed., Johnson R. and Griffin J., eds. Mosby Yearbook, 1990.

Rowland L. Nutritional deficiency in gastrointestinal disease. In Merrits Textbook of Neurology, 8th ed., Rowland L. ed. Lea & Febiger Publishing, 1989.

Shaw W., et al. Increased urinary excretion of analogs of krebs cycle metabolites and arabinose in two brothers with autistic features. Clin Chem 1995; 1094–104.

• Chapter 4: The Brain Wellness Plan

Agostoni C., et al. Neurodevelopmental quotients of healthy term infants at 4 months and feeding practice: the role of long-chain polyunsaturated fatty acids. Ped Res 1994 Aug; 38: 262–6.

Asahi M., Fujii J., Suzuki K., Seo H.G., et al. Inactivation of glutathione peroxidase by nitric oxide. Implication for cytotoxicity. J Biol Chem 1995 Sept 8; 270(36): 21035-9.

Baldessarini R.J. The neuropharmacology of S-adenosyl methionine. Am J of Med 1987; 83: 95–103.

Barbiroli B., Medori R., Tritschler H.J., et al. Lipoic (thioctic) acid increases brain energy availability and skeletal muscle performance as shown by in vivo 31P-MRS in a patient with mitochondrial cytopathy. J Neurol 1995 Jul; 242(7): 472–7.

Barbour B. Arachidonic acid induces a prolonged inhibition of glutamate uptake into glial cells. Nature 1989; 342: 918–20.

Bottigleri T. Cerebrospinal fluid S-adenosyl methionine in depression and dementia: effects of treatment with parenteral and oral S-adenosyl methionine. J of Neurol, Neurosurg and Psych 1990; 53: 1056–98.

Boutard V., Fouqueray B., Philippe C., et al. Fish oil supplementation and essential fatty acid deficiency reduce nitric oxide synthesis by rat macrophages. Kidney Int 1994 Nov; 46(5): 1280–6.

Duval D.L., Sieg D.J., Billings R.E. Regulation of hepatic nitric oxide synthase by reactive oxygen intermediates and glutathione. Arch Biochim Biophys 1995 Feb 1; 316(2): 699–706.

Fridel H.A., et al. S-adenosyl methionine. A review of its pharmacological properties and therapeutic potential in liver dysfunction and affective disorders in relation to its physiological role in cell metabolism. Drugs 1989; 38: 389–416.

Gaiti, A. The Aging Brain. Arachidonic Acid Metabolism in the Nervous System. Barkai A. and Bazan N.G., eds. Ann NY Acad Sci, Vol. 559: 1989.

Hall E. Free radicals and CNS injury. Crit Care Clinics 1989 Oct; 5(4): 793–805.

Han D., Tritschler H.J., Packer L. Alpha-lipoic acid increases intracellular glutathione in a human T-lymphocyte Jurkat cell line. Biochim Biophys Res Commun 1995 Feb 6; 207(1): 258–64.

Hellerstein M.K., Wu K., McGrath M., et al. Effects of dietary n-3 fatty acid supplementation in men with weight loss associated with the acquired immune deficiency syndrome: relation to indices of cytokine production. J Acquir Immune Defic Syndr Hum Retrovirol 1996 Mar 1; 11(3): 258–70.

Hogg N., Singh R.J., Kalyanaraman B. The role of glutathione in the transport and catabolism of nitric oxide. FEBS Lett 1996 Mar 18; 382(3): 223–8.

Justaffson L.E. Mechanisms involved in the action of prostaglandins as modulators of neurotransmission. Ann NY Acad Sci 1989; 559: 178–91.

Kiens B., Rasmussen L.B., Pedersen B.K., Richter E.A. Significance of fatty acid composition in plasma and in food for cellular immune function in elderly men. Ugeskr Laeger 1994 Oct 24; 156(43): 6388–91.

Kuo P.C. and Abe K.Y. Nitric oxide-associated regulation of hepatocyte glutathione synthesis is a guanylyl cyclase-independent event. Surgery 1996 Aug; 120(2): 309–14.

Lizasoain I., Moro M.A., Knowles R.G., et al. Nitric oxide and peroxynitrite exert distinct effects on mitochondrial respiration which are differentially blocked by glutathione or glucose. Biochem J 1996 Mar 15; 314(Pt 3): 877–80.

Majewska M., et al. Neuronal action of DHEA: possible role in brain development, aging and memory. Ann NYAcad Sci 1994; 774: 11–12.

Mayer M. and Noble M. N-acetyl-L-cysteine is a pluripotent protector against cell death and enhancer of trophic factor-mediated cell survival in vitro. Proc Natl Acad Sci 1994 Aug 2; 91(16): 7496–500.

Miller B., et al. Potentiation of NMDA receptor currents by arachidonic acid. Nature 1992; 355: 722–5.

Moore S.A., et al. Role of the blood-brain barrier in the formation of long chain omega-3 and omega-6 fatty acids from essential fatty acid precursors. J of Neurochem 1990; 55: 391–402.

Muller U. and Krieglstein J. Prolonged pretreatment with alpha-lipoic acid protects cultured neurons against hypoxic-glutamate-, or iron-induced injury. J Cereb Blood Flow Metab 1995 Jul; 15(4): 624–30.

Ordway R.W., et al. Direct regulation of ion channels by fatty acids. Trends in Neuroscience 1001; 14: 96–100.

Orentreich N., et al. Long-term measurement of plasma DHEA sulfate in normal men. J of Clin Endocrin and Metabolism 1992; 75: 1002–5.

Packer L., Witt E.H., Tritschler H.J. Alpha-lipoic acid as a biological antioxidant. Free Rad Biol Med 1995 Aug; 19(2): 227–50.

Pani A., Marongiu M.E., La Colla P. Modulatory effect of N-acetyl-L-cysteine on the HIV-1 multiplication in chronically and acutely infected cell lines. Antiviral Res 1993 Sept; 22(1): 31–43.

Petit J.F., Nicaise M., Lepoivre M., et al. Protection by glutathione against the antiproliferative effects of nitric oxide. Biochem Pharmacol 1996 Jul 26; 52(2): 205–12.

Pettegrew J.W., et al. Clinical and neurochemical effects of acetyl-

L-carnitine in Alzheimer's disease. Neurobiol of Aging 1995 Jan-Feb; 16(1-4).

Rasmussen L.B., Kiens B., Pedersen B.K., Richter E.A. Effect of diet and plasma fatty acid composition on immune status in elderly men. Am J Clin Nutr 1994 Mar; 59(3): 572-9.

Regelson W. Dehydroepiandrostone (DHEA), the multi-functional steroid: effects on the central nervous system, cell proliferation, metabolic and vascular clinical and other effects. Ann NY Acad Sci 1994; 564: 564-75.

Scarlett J.L., Packer M.A., Porteous C.M., Murphy M.P. Alterations to glutathione and nicotinamide nucleotides during the mitochondrial permeability transition induced by peroxynitrite. Biochem Pharmacol 1996 Oct 11; 52(7): 1047-55.

Scott B.C., Aruoma O.I., Evans P.J., et al. Lipoic and dihydrolipoic acids as antioxidants. A critical evaluation. Free Radic Res 1994 Feb; 20(2): 119-33.

Shibanuma M., Kuroki T., Nose K. Inhibition by N-acetyl-L-cysteine of interleukin-6 mRNA induction and activation of NF kappa B by tumor necrosis factor alpha in a mouse fibroblastic cell line, Balb/3T3. FEBS Lett 1994 Oct 10; 353(1): 62-6.

Van der Vliet A., Smith D., O'Neill C.A., et al. Interactions of peroxynitrite with human plasma and its constituents: oxidative damage and antioxidant depletion. Biochem J 1994 Oct 1; 303 (Pt. 1): 295-301.

Vatassery G.T. Oxidation of vitamin E, vitamin C, and thiols in rat brain synaptosomes by peroxynitrite. Biochem Pharmacol 1996 Aug 23; 52(4): 579-86.

Walker M.W., Kinter M.T., Roberts R.J., Spitz D.R. Nitric oxide–induced cytotoxicity: involvement of cellular resistance to oxidative stress and the role of glutathione in protection. Ped Res 1995 Jan; 37(1): 41-9.

Weber P.C. Membrane phospholipid modification by dietary N-3 fatty acids: effects on eicosanoid formation and cell function in biological membranes. In Aberrations in Membrane Structure and Function, Liss A., ed., 1988: 263-74.

White A.C., Maloney E.K., Boustani M.R., et al. Nitric oxide increases cellular glutathione levels in rat lung fibroblasts. Am J Respir Cell Mol Biol 1995 Oct; 13(4): 442-8.

Whiteman M., Tritschler H., Halliwell B. Protection against peroxynitrite-dependent tyrosine nitration and alpha 1-antiproteinase inactivation by oxidized and reduced lipoic acid. FEBS Lett 1996 Jan 22; 379(1): 74–6.

Part II

• Chapter 5: Alzheimer's Disease

Adams J.D., et al. Alzheimer's and Parkinson's disease brain levels of glutathione, glutathione disulfide, and vitamin E. Mol and Chem Neuropathol 1991; 14: 213–23.

Aisen P.S. and Davis K.L. Inflammatory mechanisms in Alzheimer's disease: implications for therapy. Am J Psychiatry 1994 Aug; 151(8): 1105–13.

Amaducci L. Phosphatidylserine in the treatment of Alzheimer's disease: results of a multicenter study. Psychopharmacol Bull 1988; 24(1): 130–4.

Amaducci L., Crook T.H., Lippi A., et al. Use of phosphatidylserine in Alzheimer's disease. Ann NY Acad Sci 1991; 640: 245–9.

Aureli T., Miccheli A., Ricciolini R., et al. Aging brain: effect of acetyl-L-carnitine treatment on rat brain energy and phospholipid metabolism. Brain Res 1990; 526: 108–12.

Bastianetto S., et al. Dehydroepiandrosterone (DHEA) protects hippocampal cells from oxidative stress-induced damage. Brain Res Mol Brain Res 1999 Mar 20; 66:35.

Behl C. Vitamin E and other antioxidants in neuroprotection. Int J Vitam Nutr Res 1999 May; 69:213.

Birkmayer J.G. Coenzyme nicotinamide adenine dinucleotide. Ann Clin Lab Sci 1996 Jan–Feb; 26:1.

Bissette G., Seidler F.J., Nemeroff C.B., Slotkin T. High affinity choline transporter status in Alzheimer's disease tissue from rapid autopsy. Ann NY Acad Sci 1996 Jan 17; 777: 197–204.

Breitner J.C., Gau B.A., Welsh K.A., Plassman B.L., et al. Inverse association of anti-inflammatory treatments and Alzheimer's disease: initial results of a co-twin control study. Neurology 1994 Feb; 44(2): 227–32.

Brenner D.E., et al. Postmenopausal estrogen replacement therapy and the risk of Alzheimer's disease: population-based case-controlled study. Am J of Epidemiology 1994; 140; 262–7.

Bruno G., Scaccianoce S., Bonamini M., et al. Acetyl-L-carnitine in Alzheimer's disease: a short-term study on CSF neurotransmitters and neuropeptides. Alzheimer Dis Assoc Disord 1995 Fall; 9(3): 128–31.

Caamano J., Gomez J.J., Franco A., Cacabelos R. Effects of CDP-choline on cognition and cerebral hemodynamics in patients with Alzheimer's disease. Methods Find Exp Clin Pharmacol 1994 Apr; 16(3): 211–18.

Cacabelos R., Alvarez X.A., Franco-Maside A., Fernandez-Novoa L., Caamano J. Effect of CDP-choline on cognition and immune function in Alzheimer's disease and multi-infarct dementia. Ann NY Acad Sci 1993 Sept. 24; 695: 321–3.

Cacabelos R., Caamano J., Gomez M.J., Fernandez-Novoa L., et al. Therapeutic effects of CDP-choline in Alzheimer's disease. Cognition, brain mapping, cerebrovascular hemodynamics, and immune factors. Ann NY Acad Sci 1996 Jan 17; 777: 399–403.

Carta A., Calvani M., Bravi D., Bhuachalla S.N. Acetyl-L-carnitine and Alzheimer's disease: pharmacological considerations beyond the cholinergic sphere. Ann NY Acad Sci 1993 Sept. 24; 695: 324–6.

Castano E.M., Prelli F., Wisniewski T., Golabek A., et al. Fibrillogenesis in Alzheimer's disease of amyloid beta peptides and apolipoprotein E. Biochem J 1995 Mar 1; 306 (Pt. 2): 599–604.

Castorina M. and Ferraris L. Acetyl-L-carnitine affects aged brain receptorial system in rodents. Life Sci 1994; 54(17): 1205–14.

Cenacchi T., Bertoldin T., Farina C., et al. Cognitive decline in the elderly: a double-blind, placebo-controlled multicenter study on efficacy of phosphatidylserine administration. Aging 1993; 5: 123–33.

Cheney D.L., exec. ed. Pathology of Alzheimer's disease. Neuroscience Facts 1991 Mar; 2(5): 1.

Crook T., Petrie W., Wells C., Casadei M.D. Effects of phosphatidylserine in Alzheimer's disease. Pharmacology Bull 1992; 28(1): 61–5.

Crook T.H., Tinklenberg J., et al. Effects of phosphatidylserine in age-associated memory impairment. Neurology 1991; 41: 644–9.

Davenport A. and Goodall R. Aluminum and dementia. Lancet 1992 May 16; 39: 1236.

Davis S., Markowska A.L., Wenk G.L., Barnes C.A. Acetyl-L-carnitine: behavioral, electrophysiological, and neurochemical effects. Neurobiol Aging 1993 Jan-Feb; 14(1): 107–15.

Dedman D., et al. Iron and aluminum in relation to brain ferritin in normal individuals and Alzheimer's disease and chronic renal dialysis patients. Biochem Journal 1992; 509–14.

De Feudis F.V. Ginkgo biloba extract (EGb 761): pharmacological activities and clinical applications. Elsevier, 1991.

Doraiswamy P.M.J. and Steffens D.C. Combination therapy for early Alzheimer's disease. J Am Geriatr Soc 1998 Oct; 46:1322.

Dumont E., D'Arbigny P., Nouvelot A. Protection of polyunsaturated fatty acids against iron-dependent lipid peroxidation by a ginkgo biloba extract (EGb 761). Methods Find Exp Clin Pharmacol 1995 Mar; 17(2): 83–8.

Eisinger J., et al. Erythrocyte transketolase in Alzheimer's disease: the thiamine hypothesis. J of the Advancement of Med 1994 Summer; 7(2): 69–75.

Engel R.R., Satzger W., Gunther W., et al. Double-blind cross-over study of phosphatidylserine vs. placebo in patients with early dementia of the Alzheimer type. Eur Neuropsychopharmacol 1992 Jun; 2(2): 149–55.

Engel R.R., et al. Double-blind cross-over study phosphatidylserine vs. placebo in patients with early dementia of the Alzheimer type. Eur Neuropsychopharmacol 1992 Jun; 2:149.

Ershler W.B. Interleukin-6: a cytokine for gerontologists. JAGS 1993 Feb; 41(2): 176–81.

Farooqui A.A., Wells K., Horrorocks L.A. Breakdown of membrane phospholipids in Alzheimer's disease. Mol Chem Neuropathol 1995 Jun-Aug; 25(2–3): 155–73.

Fillit H. Estrogens in the pathogenesis and treatment of Alzheimer's disease in postmenopausal women. Ann NY Acad Sci 1994 Nov 14; 743: 223–8.

Forbes, et al. Aluminum and Alzheimer's disease. Can Med Assoc Journal 1992; 146(9): 1534.

Forloni G., Angeretti N., Smiroldo S. Neuroprotective activity of acetyl-L-carnitine: studies in vitro. J Neurosci Res 1994 Jan; 37(1): 92–6.

Franco-Maside A., Caamano J., Gomez M.J., Cacabelos R. Brain mapping activity and mental performance after chronic treatment with CDP-choline in Alzheimer's disease. Methods Find Exp Clin Pharmacol 1994 Oct; 16(8): 597–607.

Frolich L. and Riederer P. Free radical mechanisms in dementia of the Alzheimer's type and the potential for antioxidative treatment. Drug Res 1995; 45(1): 3A: 443–6.

Funfgeld E.W., Baggen M., Nedwidek P., et al. Double-blind study with phosphatidylserine (PS) in parkinsonian patients with senile dementia of Alzheimer's type (SDAT). Prog Clin Biol Res 1989; 317: 1235–46.

Gandy S.E., Bhasin R., Ramabhadran V., et al.: Alzheimer B/A4 amyloid precursor protein: evidence for putative amyloidogenic fragment. J Neurochem 1992; 58: 383–6.

Glick J. Dementias: the role of magnesium deficiency and hypothesis concerning the pathogenesis of Alzheimer's disease. Med Hypothesis 1990; 31: 211–25.

Gold M., et al. Plasma and red blood cell thiamine deficiency in patients with dementia of the Alzheimer's type. Arch Neurol 1995 Nov; 52: 1081–5.

Good P.F., Perl D.P., Bierer L.M., Schmeidler J. Selective accumulation of aluminum and iron in the neurofibrillary tangles of Alzheimer's disease: a laser microphobe (LAMMA) study. Ann of Neurol 1992 Mar; 31(3): 286–92.

Hardy J.A. and Higgins G.A. Alzheimer's disease: the amyloid cascade hypothesis. Science 1992 Apr 10; 256: 184–5.

Heiss W.D., Kessler J., Mielke R., et al. Long-term effects of phosphatidylserine, pyritinol, and cognitive training in Alzheimer's disease. A neuropsychological, EEG, and PET investigation. Dementia 1994 Mar-Apr; 5(2): 88–98.

Henderson V.W., Paganinin-Hill A., Emanuel C.K., Dun M.E., Buckwalter J.G. Estrogen replacement therapy in older women. Arch Neurol 1994 Sept; 51(9): 896–900.

Ho L., et al. Regional distribution of cyclooxygenase-2 in the hippocampal formation in Alzheimer's disease. J Neurosci Res 1999 Aug 1; 57:295.

Ikeda T., et al. Vitamin B12 levels in serum and cerebrospinal fluid of people with Alzheimer's disease. ACTA Psychiatr Scand 1990; 82: 327–9.

Imagawa M. Iron, B6 and coenzyme Q10 in Alzheimer's. The Nutrition Report 1994 Oct; 12(10): 75.

Imagawa M. Therapy with a combination of iron, vitamin B_6 and coenzyme Q10 in the long term for sporadic Alzheimer's disease. Neurobiol 1994; A15: S101.

Imagawa M., et al. Coenzyme Q10, iron and vitamin B_6 in genetically-confirmed Alzheimer's disease; Lancet 1992 Sept 12; 40: 671.

Inestrosa N.C., et al. Cellular and molecular basis of estrogen's protection. Mol Neurobiol 1998 Winter; 17:73.

Jacobs, R.W., et al. Alzheimer dementia and reduced nicotinamide adenine dinucleotide (NADH)-diaphorase activity in senile plaques and the basal forebrain. Neurosci Lett 1981 Jan 7; 53:39.

Jeandel C., et al. Lipid peroxidation and free radical scavengers in Alzheimer's disease. Gerontology 1989; 35: 275–82.

Johnson R. Estrogen/Alzheimer's link found. Medical Tribune 1993 Dec 9; 34(23): 1–8.

Kanowski S., et al. Proof of efficacy of the ginkgo biloba special extract EGb 761 in outpatients suffering from mild to moderate primary degenerative dementia of the Alzheimer type or multiinfarct dementia. Pharmacopsychiat 1996; 29: 47–56.

Klegeris A., Walker D.G., McGeer P.L. Activation of macrophages by Alzheimer beta amyloid peptide. Biochem Biophys Res Commun 1994 Mar 15; 199(2): 984–91.

Kose K. and Dogan P. Lipoperoxidation induced by hydrogen peroxide in human erythrocyte membrane. J Int Med Res 1995 Jan-Feb; 23(1): 1–8.

Kraus A.S. and Forbes W. Aluminum, fluoride and prevention of

Alzheimer's disease. Can Journal of Public Health 1992 Mar-Apr; 83:(2): 97–100.

Kunkel H. EEG profile of three different extractions of ginkgo biloba. Neuropsychobiol 1993; 27(1): 40–5.

Laganiere S., et al. Acute and chronic studies with the anticholinesterase Huperzine A. Neuropharmacology 30:763.

LeBars P.L., et al. A placebo-controlled, double-blind, randomized trial of an extract of Ginkgo biloba for dementia. JAMA 1997 Oct. 22/29; 278: 1327.

Levitt A.J., et al. Folate, vitamin B_{12} and cognitive impairment in patients with Alzheimer's disease. Acta Psychiatr Scand 1992; 86: 301–5.

Lipsky P.E. The clinical potential of cyclooxygenase-2-specific inhibitors. Am J Med 1999 May 31; 106:51S.

Liu R.Y., et al. Decreased melatonin levels in postmortem cerebrospinal fluid in relation to aging, Alzheimer's disease, and apoliproprotein E-epsilon4/4 genotype. J Clin Endocrinol Metab 1999 Jan; 84:323.

Lukiw, W.J., and Bazan N.G. Strong nuclear factor-kappaB-DNA binding parallels cyclooxygenase-2 gene transcription in aging and in sporadic Alzheimer's disease superior temporal lobe neocortex. J Neurosci Res 1998 Sep 1; 53:583.

Maitra I., Marcocci L., Droy-Lefaix M.T., Packer L. Peroxyl radical scavenging activity of ginkgo biloba extract EGb 761. Biochem Pharmacol 1995 May 26; 49(11): 1649–55.

Marcocci L., Maguire J.J., Droy-Lefaix M.T., Packer L. The nitric oxide–scavenging properties of ginkgo biloba extract EGb 761. Biochem Biophys Res Commun 1994 Jun 15; 201(2): 748–55.

Markesbery W.R. and Carney J.M. Oxidative alterations in Alzheimer's disease. Brain Pathol 1999 Jan; 9:133.

Mason R.P., Trumbore M.W., Pettegrew J.W. Molecular membrane interactions of a phospholipid metabolite. Ann NY Acad Sci 1996 Jan 17; 777: 368–73.

Mastrogiacomo F., et al. Brain thiamine, its phosphate esters, and its metabolizing enzymes in Alzheimer's disease. Ann Neurol 1996; 39: 585–91.

McCaddon A. and Kelly C. Familial Alzheimer's disease and vitamin B_{12} deficiency. Age and Aging 1994 Jul; 23: 334–7.

McCaddon A. and Kelly C. Vitamin B_{12} and Alzheimer's disease. The Nutrition Report 1994 Oct; 12(10): 75.

McGeer P.L., McGeer E.G, Rogers J., Sibley J., Anti-inflammatory drugs and Alzheimer's disease. Lancet 1990; 335: 1037.

McGeer P.L. and Rogers J. Anti-inflammatory agents as a therapeutic approach to Alzheimer's disease. Neurology 1992; 42: 447–8.

Nilsson L., et al. The essential role of inflammation and induced gene expression in the pathogenic pathway of Alzheimer's disease. Front Biosci 1998 Apr 16; 3:d436.

Nolan K.A., et al. A trial of thiamine in Alzheimer's disease. Arch Neurol 1991 Jan; 48: 81–3.

Oyama Y., Hayashi A., Ueha T. Ca(2+)-induced increase in oxidative metabolism of dissociated mammalian brain neurons: effect of extract of ginkgo biloba leaves. Jpn J Pharmacol 1993 Apr; 61(4): 367–70.

Paganinin-Hill A; Henderson V.W. Estrogen deficiency and risk of Alzheimer's disease in women. Am J Epidemiol 1994 Aug 1; 140(3): 256–61.

Palmer A.M. and Burns M.A. Selective increase in lipid peroxidation in the inferior temporal cortex in Alzheimer's disease. Brain Res 1994 Feb; 645: 338–42.

Palmert M.R., Usiak B.S., Mayeux R., et al. Soluble derivatives of the B amyloid protein precursor in cerebrospinal fluid. Neurology 1990 Jul; 40: 1028–34.

Pan Y., et al. Evidence for up-regulation of brain-derived neuro-trophic factor mRNA by soy phytoestrogens in the frontal cortex of retired breeder female rats. Neurosci Lett 1999 Feb 12; 261:17.

Parnetti L., Gaiti A., Mecocci P., Senin U. Pharmacokinetics of IV and oral acetyl-L-carnitine in a multiple dose regimen in patients with senile dementia of Alzheimer type. Eur J Clin Pharmacol 1992; 42: 89–93.

Pasinetti G.M. Cyclooxygenase and inflammation in Alzheimer's disease. J Neurosci Res 1998 Oct 1; 54:1.

Pereira, C., et al. Involvement of oxidative stress on the impairment of energy metabolism induced by A beta peptides on PC12 cells. Neurobiol Dis 1999 Jun; 6:209.

Pettegrew J.W., Klunk W.E., Kanal E., et al. Changes in brain membrane phospholipid and high-energy phosphate metabolism precede dementia. Neurobiol Aging 1995 Nov-Dec; 16(6): 973–5.

Pettegrew J.W., Klunk W.E., Panchalingam K., Kanfer J.N., McClure R.J. Clinical and neurochemical effects of acetyl-L-carnitine in Alzheimer's disease. Neurobiol Aging 1995 Jan-Feb; 16(1): 1–4.

Pike C.J. Estrogen modulates neuronal Bcl-xL expression and beta-amyloid induced apoptosis. J Neurochem 1999 Apr; 72:1552.

Pincemail J., Dupuis M., Nasr C., Hans P., et al. Superoxide anion scavenging effect and superoxide dismutase activity of ginkgo biloba extract. Experientia 1989 Aug 15; 45(8): 708–12.

Ramassamy C., et al. Oxidative damage and protection by antioxidants in the frontal cortex of Alzheimers's disease is related to the apolipoprotein E genotype. Free Radic Biol Med 1999 Sep; 27:544.

Reiter R.J. Oxidative damage in the central nervous system. Prog Neurobiol 1998 Oct; 56:359.

Ren Z., Ding W., Su Z., Gu X., et al. Mechanisms of brain injury with deep hypothermic circulatory arrest and protective effects of coenzyme Q10. J Thorac Cardiovasc Surg 1994 Jul; 108(1): 126–33.

Rich J.B., Rasmusson D.X., Folstein M.F., Carson K.A. et al. Nonsteroidal anti-inflammatory drugs in Alzheimer's disease. Neurology 1995 Jan; 45(1): 51–5.

Robb-Nicholson C. and Merz B., eds. Estrogen and Alzheimer's Disease. Women's Health Watch 1996 Nov; Vol. IV (3): p. 1–3.

Rogers J. Inflammation as a pathogenic mechanism in Alzheimer's disease. Arzneimittel-Forschung/Drug Res 1995; 45(I), 3a, 439–42.

Rogers J., Kirby L.C., Hempelman S.R., et al. Clinical trial of indomethacin in Alzheimer's disease. Neurology 1993 Aug; 43: 1609–10.

Rogers S.L., Friedhoff L.T. and the Donepezil Study Group. Dementia 1996; 7: 293–303.

Rosler M., et al. Free radicals in Alzheimer's dementia. J Neural Trans Suppl 1998; 54:211.

Sano M., et al. A controlled trial of selegiline, alpha-tocopherol, or both as treatment for Alzheimer's disease. N Engl J Med 1997 Apr 24; 336:1216.

Sano M., Bell K., Cote L., et al. Double-blind parallel design pilot study of acetyl levocarnitine in patients with Alzheimer's disease. Arch Neurol 1992 Nov; 49: 1137–41.

Sano M. et al. A controlled trial of selegiline, alpha-tocopherol or both as treatment for Alzheimer's disease. N Engl J Med 1997 Apr: 1216–1222.

Saunders A.M., Hulette C., Welsh-Bohmer K.A., Schmechel D.E., et al. Specificity, sensitivity and predictive value of apolipoprotein-E genotyping for sporadic Alzheimer's disease. Lancet 1993 Jul; 348: 90.

Shin R.W., Lee V.M., Trojanowski J.Q. Neurofibrillary pathology and aluminum in Alzheimer's disease. Histol Histopathol 1995 Oct; 10(4): 969–78.

Simpkins J.W., et al. Role of estrogen replacement therapy in memory enhancement and the prevention of neuronal loss associated with Alzheimer's disease. Am J Med 1997 Sep 22; 103:19S.

Singh V.K. Studies of neuroimmune markers in Alzheimer's disease. Mol Neurobiol 1994 Aug-Dec; 9(1–3): 73–81.

Sisodia S.S., Koo E.H., Beyreuther K., Unterbeck A., Price D.L. Evidence that B-amyloid protein in Alzheimer's disease is not derived by normal processing. Science 1990; 248: 492–5.

Soderberg M., Edlund C., Kristensson K., Dallner G. The fatty acid composition of brain phospholipids in aging and in Alzheimer's disease. Lipids 1991 Jun; 26(6): 421–5.

Spagnoli A., et al. Long-term acetyl-L-carnitine treatment in Alzheimer's disease. Neurology 1991 Nov; 41: 1726–32.

Steventon G.B., et al. Xenobiotic metabolism in Alzheimer's disease. Neurology 1990 Jul; 40: 1095–8.

Stoll S., Scheuer K., Pohl O., Muller W.E. Ginkgo biloba extract (EGb 761) independently improves changes in passive avoidance learning and brain membrane fluidity in the aging mouse. Pharmacopsychiat 1996 Jul; 29(4): 144–9.

Subbaramaiah K., et al. Resveratrol inhibits cyclooxygenase-2 transcription and activity in phorbol ester-treated human mammary epithelial cells. J Biol Chem 1998 Aug 21; 273:21875.

Svec F. and Lopez A. Antiglucocorticoid actions of dehydroepiandrosterone and low concentrations in Alzheimer's disease. Lancet 1989 Dec 2: 1335–6.

Taylor G.A., et al. Gastrointestinal absorption of aluminum in Alzheimer's disease: response to aluminum citrate. Age and Aging 1992; 21: 81–90.

Thal L.J., et al. A one-year, multicenter placebo controlled study of ALC in patients with Alzheimer's. Neurology 1996; 477: 705–11.

Volicer L., Crino P.B., et al. Involvement of free radicals in dementia of the Alzheimer type: a hypothesis. Neurobiol of Aging 1990; 11: 567–71.

Wang T. and Tang X.C. Reversal of scopolamine-induced deficits in radial maze performance by huperzine A. European Journal of Pharmacology 1998; 349:137.

Williams A. Alzheimer's disease and nutrition. British J of Hospital Med 1991 Jan; 45: 12.

Winograd C.H., et al. Nutritional intake in patients with senile dementia of the Alzheimer's type. Alzheimer's Disease and Associated Disorders 1991; 5(3): 173–80.

Xu, H., et al. Estrogen reduces neuronal generation of Alzheimer beta-amyloid peptides. Nature Medicine 1998 Apr; 4:447.

Yankner B.A. and Mesulam M. B-amyloid and the pathogenesis of Alzheimer's disease. N Engl J Med 1991 Dec. 26; 325(26): 1849–57.

Yatin S.M., et al. The antioxidant vitamin E modulates amyloid beta-peptide-induced creatine kinase activity inhibition and increased protein oxidation. Neurochem Res 1999 Mar; 24:427.

Yokel R.A. Aluminum exposure produces learning and memory deficits: a model of Alzheimer's disease. In Toxin-Induced Models of Neurologic Disorders, Woodruff, M.I. and Nonneman A., eds. Plenum Press 1994, Chap. 11; 301–18.

Yokoyama H., Lingle D.M., Crestranello J.A., et al. Coenzyme Q10 protects coronary endothelial function from ischemia reperfusion injury via an antioxidant effect. Surgery 1996 Aug; 120(2): 189–96.

Zhou Y., Richardson J.S., Mombourquette M.J., Weil J.A. Free radical formation in autopsy samples of Alzheimer and control cortex. Neurotoxic Lett 1995 Aug 4; 195(2): 89–92.

Zubenko G.S., Wusylko M., Cohen B.M., Boller F., Telpy I. Family study of platelet membrane fluidity in Alzheimer's disease. Science 1987; 238: 539–42.

• Chapter 6: Parkinson's Disease

Abbott R.A., Cox M., Markus H., Tomkins A. Diet, body size and micronutrient status in Parkinson's disease. Eur J Clin Nutr 1992 Dec; 46(12): 879–84.

Adams J.D., Klaidman L.K., Odunze I.N., et al. Alzheimer's and Parkinson's diseases. Brain levels of glutathione, glutathione disulfide, and vitamin E. Biol Chem Neuropathol 1991 Jun; 14(3): 213–2.

Astarloa R., Mena M.A., Sanchez V., et al. Clinical and pharmacokinetic effects of a diet rich in insoluble fiber on Parkinson's disease. Clin Neuropharmacol 1992 Oct; 15(5): 375–80.

Bast A., et al. The pharmacology of the antioxidant lipoic acid. Gen Pharmacol 1997 Sep; 29:315.

Bast A., et al. Mechanism of the reaction of ebselen with endogenous thiols. Mol Pharmacol 1990 Mar; 37:412–22.

Beal M.F. Aging, energy, and oxidative stress in neurodegenerative diseases. Ann Neurol 1995; 38: 357–66.

Beal M.F. Does impairment of energy metabolism result in excitotoxic neuronal death in neurodegenerative illnesses? Ann Neurol 1992; 31: 119–30.

Beuter A., Mergler D., de Geoffroy A., et al. Diadochokinesimetry: a study of patients with Parkinson's disease and manganese exposed workers. NeuroToxicology 1994 Fall; 15(3): 655–64.

Birkmayer G.J., Vrecko C., Volc D., Birkmayer W. Nicotinamide adenine dinucleotide (NADH)—a new therapeutic approach to Parkinson's disease. Acta Neurol Scand 1993; 87: Suppl 146: 32–5.

Birkmayer W. and Birkmayer G.J.D. Strategic and tactic of modern Parkinson therapy. Acta Neurol Scand 1989; 126: 63–6.

Blandini F., et al. Quantitative study of mitochondrial complex I in platelets of parkinsonian patients. Mov Disord 1998 Jan; 13:11.

Burkhardt C.R. and Weber H.K. Parkinson's disease: a chronic, low-grade antioxidant deficiency? Med Hypotheses 1994 Aug; 43(2): 111–4.

Cabrera-Valdivia F., Jimenez-Jimenez F.J., Molina J.A., et al. Peripheral iron metabolism in patients with Parkinson's disease. J Neurol Sci 1994 Aug; 125(1): 82–6.

Carter J.H., Nutt J.G., Woodward W.F., et al. Amount and distribution of dietary protein affects clinical response to levodopa in Parkinson's disease. Neurology 1989 Apr; 39(4): 552–6.

Carvey P.M., et al. The potent use of a dopamine neuron antibody and a striatal neurotrophic factor as diagnostic markers in Parkinson's. Neurology 1995; 41: S3–8.

Cheng W., et al. Selenium-dependent cellular glutathione peroxidase protects mice against a pro-oxidant-induced oxidation of NADPH, NADH, lipids, and protein. FASEB J 1999 Aug; 13(11):1467.

Croxson S., et al. Dietary modification of Parkinson's disease. Eur J of Clin Nut 1991; 45: 263–6.

Dexter D.T., Carayon A., Javoy-Agid F., et al. Alterations in the levels of iron, ferritin and other trace metals in Parkinson's disease and other neurodegenerative diseases affecting the basal ganglia. Brain 1991; 114: 1953–75.

Dizdar N., Kagedal B., Lindvall B. Treatment of Parkinson's disease with NADH. Acta Neurol Scand 1994 Nov; 90(5): 345–7.

Fahn S. An open trial of high-dose antioxidants in early Parkinson's disease. Am J of Clin Nut 1991; 53: 380S–382S.

Faucheu B.A., et al. Expression of lactoferrin receptors is increased in the mesencephalon of patients with Parkinson disease. Proc Natl Acad Sci USA 1995 Oct 10;92:9603.

Gil A., et al. Neonatal dietary gangliosides. Early Human Dev 1998 Dec; 53:S135.

Gimenez-Roldan S. and Mateo D. Predicting beneficial response to a protein-redistribution diet in fluctuating in Parkinson's disease. Acta Neurol Bel 1991; 91(4): 189–200.

Gimenez-Roldan S., Mateo D., Garcia A.A., Garcia P.P. Proposal for a protein redistribution diet in the control of motor fluctuations in Parkinson's disease: acceptance and efficacy. Neurologia 1991 Jan; 6(1): 3–9.

Gorell J.M., et al. Increased iron-related MRI contrast in the substantia nigra in Parkinson's disease. Neurol 1995 Jun; 45(6): 1138–43.

Griffiths P.D. and Crossman A.R. Distribution of iron in the basal ganglia and neocortex in postmortem tissue in Parkinson's disease and Alzheimer's disease. Dementia 1993 Mar-Apr; 4(2): 61–5.

Grimes J.D., Hassan M.N., Thakar J. Antioxidant therapy in Parkinson's disease. Can J Neurol Sci 1987 Aug; 14(3 Suppl): 483–7.

Hagen, T.M., et al. (R)-alpha-lipoic acid-supplemented old rats have improved mitochondrial function, decreased oxidative damage, and increased metabolic rate. FASEB J 1999 Feb; 13:411.

Halliwell B., et al. Conjugates of catecholamines with cysteine and GSH in Parkinson's disease. J Neurochem 1998 Nov; 71:2112.

Hantraye P., Brouillet E., Ferrante R., Palfi S., et al. Inhibition of neuronal nitric oxide synthase prevents MPTP-induced parkinsonism in baboons. Nature Medicine 1996 Sept; 2(9): 1017.

Harley Al, Cooper J.M., Schapira A.H. Iron induced oxidative stress and mitochondrial dysfunction: relevance to Parkinson's disease. Brain Res 1993 Nov 12; 627(2): 349–53.

Iida M., et al. Dopamine D2 receptor-mediated antioxidant and neuroprotective effects of ropinirole, a dopamine agonist. Brain Res 1999 Aug 14; 838:51.

Jellinger K.A., et al. The role of iron in neurodegeneration. Drugs Aging 1999 Feb; 14:115.

Jellinger K.A., Kienzl E., Rumpelmaier G., et al. Iron and ferritin in substantia nigra in Parkinson's disease. Adv Neurol 1993; 60: 267–72.

Jener P. Altered mitochondrial function, iron metabolism and glutathione levels in Parkinson's disease. Acta Neurol Scand Suppl 1993; 146: 6–13.

Jimenez-Jimenez F.J., Molina J.A., Aguilar M.V., et al. Serum and urinary manganese levels in patients with Parkinson's disease. Acta Neurol Scand 1995 May; 91(5): 317–20.

Kalra J., Rajput A.H., Mantha S.V., Prasad K. Serum antioxidant enzyme activity in Parkinson's disease. Mol Cell Biochem 1992 Mar 25; 110(2): 165–8.

Karstaedt P.J. and Pincus J.H. Protein redistribution diet remains effective in patients with fluctuating parkinsonism. Arch Neurol 1992 Feb; 49: 149–51.

Karstaedt P.J., Pincus J.H., Coughlin S.S. Standard and controlled-release levodopa/carbidopa in patients with fluctuating Parkinson's disease on a protein redistribution diet. A preliminary report. Arch Neurol 1991 Apr; 48(4): 402–5.

Koller W., Vetere-Overfield B., Gray C., et al. Environmental risk factors in Parkinson's disease. Neurology 1990 Aug; 40: 1218–21.

Kolm R.H., et al. Isothiocyanates as substrates for human glutathione transferases. Biochem J 1995 Oct 15; 311:453.

Kuhn W. Parenteral application of NADH in Parkinson's disease. J Neural Transm 1996; 103:1187.

Leveugle B., et al. Cellular distribution of the iron-binding protein lactotransferrin in the mesencephalon of Parkinson's disease cases. Acta Neuropathol (Berl) 1996; 91:566.

Lichter D., Kurlan R., Miller C., Shoulson I. Does pergolide slow the progression of Parkinson's disease? A 7-year follow-up study. Neurology 1988 Mar; 38(Suppl 1): 122.

Loeffler D.A., Connor J.R., Juneau P.L., et al. Transferrin and iron in normal, Alzheimer's disease, and Parkinson's disease brain regions. J Neurochem 1995 Aug; 65(2): 710–24.

Mann V.M., Cooper J.M., Daniel S.E., et al. Complex I, iron, and ferritin in Parkinson's disease substantia nigra. Ann Neurol 1994 Dec; 36(6): 876–81.

McClain D.E., et al. Ebselen inhibition of apoptosis by reduction of peroxides. Biochem Pharmacol 1996 Jun 14;51:1443.

Mayeux R., et al. Altered systemic iron metabolism in Parkinson's disease. Neurology 1997 Sep; 49:714.

Meister A. Mitochondrial changes associated with glutathione deficiency. Biochim et Biophys Acta 1995; 1271: 35–42.

Menegon A., et al. Parkinson's disease, pesticides, and glutathione transferase polypmorphisms. Lancet 1998 Oct 24; 352:1344.

Mizuno Y., Ikebe S., Hattori N., et al. Role of mitochondria in the etiology and pathogenesis of Parkinson's disease. Biochim Biophys Acta 1995 May 24; 1271(1): 265–74.

Mizuno Y., Shin-ichirou I., Nobutaka H., et al. Role of mitochondria in the etiology and pathogenesis of Parkinson's disease. Biochim et Biophys Acta 1995; 1271: 265–74.

Mohr E., et al. Neuropsychological and glucose metabolic profiles in asymmetric Parkinson's disease. Can J of Neurol Sci 1992; 19: 163–9.

Monte D., et al. Glutathione in Parkinson's disease: a link between oxidative stress and mitochondrial damage. Ann Neurol 1992; 32: S111–S15.

Montgomery E.B. Heavy metals and the etiology of Parkinson's disease and other movement disorders. Toxicology 1995 Mar 31; 97(1–3): 3–9.

Morris C.M. and Edwardson J.A. Iron histochemistry of the substantia nigra in Parkinson's disease. Neurodegeneration 1994 Dec; 3(4): 277–82.

Moutet M., et al. Glutathione peroxidase mimics prevent TNF-alpha- and neutrophil-induced endothelial alterations. Free Radic Biol Med 1998 Aug; 25:270.

Nutt J.G. and Carter J.H. Therapy of Parkinson's disease and diet issues in the treatment of Parkinson's disease. In Therapy of Parkinson's Disease, Elsevier Science Inc. 1990, Chapter 28.

Offen D., et al. Prevention of dopamine-induced cell death by thiol antioxidants. Exp Neurol 1996 Sep; 141:32.

Olanow C.W., et al. Dopamine agonists and neuroprotection in Parkinson's disease. Ann Neurol 1998; Suppl 1:5167.

Olanow C.W., et al. The causes of Parkinson's disease are being unraveled and rational neuroprotective therapy is close to reality. Ann Neurol 1998; 44 (Suppl 1): 5196.

Olanow C.W. An introduction to the free radical hypothesis in Parkinson's disease. Ann Neurol 1992; 32: S2–S9.

Olanow C.W., et al. The effect of deprenyl and levodopa on the progression of Parkinson's. Ann Neurol 95; 38: 71–8.

Packer L., et al. Antioxidant activity and biologic properties of procyanidin-rich extract from pine (Pinus maritima) bark, pycnogenol. Free Radic Biol Med 1999 Sep; 27:704.

Packer L., et al. Hydroxyl and superoxide anion radical scavenging activities of natural source antioxidants using the computerized JES-FR30 ESR spectrometer system. Biochem Mol Biol Int 1997 Jun; 42:35.

The Parkinson Study Group. Effect of deprenyl on the progression of disability in early Parkinson's disease. N Engl J Med 1989 Nov 16; 321(20): 1364–71.

The Parkinson Study Group. Effects of tocopherol and deprenyl on the progression of disability in early Parkinson's disease. N Engl J Med 1993 Jan 21; 328(3): 176–83.

Peppard R.F., et al. Cerebral glucose metabolism in Parkinson's disease with and without dementia. Arch Neurol 1992 Dec; 49: 1262–8.

Riley D. and Lang A.E. Practical application of a low-protein diet for Parkinson's disease. Neurol 1988 Jul; 38(7); 1026–31.

Rothblat D.S. and Schneider J.S. Effects of GM1 ganglioside treatment on dopamine innervation of the striatum of MPTP-treated mice. Ann NY Acad Sci 1998 Jun 19; 845:274.

Ryu B.R., et al. Attenuation of corticol neuronal apoptosis by gangliosides. J Pharmacol Exp Ther 1999 Aug; 290:811.

Sanchis G., Mena M.A., Martin del Rio R., et al. Effect of a controlled low-protein diet on the pharmacological response to levodopa and on the plasma levels of L-dopa and amino acids in patients with Parkinson's disease. Arch Neurobiol 1991 Nov-Dec; 54(6): 296–302.

Schapira A.H. Evidence for mitochondrial dysfunction in Parkinson's disease—a critical appraisal. Mov Disord 1994 Mar; 9(2): 125–38.

Schapira A.H., Cooper J.M., Dexter D., Clark J.B., Jenner P., Marsden

C.D. Mitochondrial complex I deficiency in Parkinson's disease. J of Neurochem 1990; 54(3): 823–7.

Schapira A.H., Hartley A., Cleeter M.W., Cooper J.M. Free radicals and mitochondrial dysfunction in Parkinson's disease. Biochem Soc Trans 1993 May; 21(2): 367–70.

Schneider J.S., et al. Parkinson's disease. Neurology 1998 Jun; 50:1630.

Schulz J.B., Henshaw D.R., Matthews R.T., Beal M.F. Coenzyme Q10 and nicotinamide: a free radical spin trap protect against MPTP neurotoxicity. Experimental Neurol 1995; 135(2): 279–83.

Sechi G., et al. Reduced intravenous glutathione in the treatment of early Parkinson's disease. Prog Neuropsychopharmacol Biol Psychiatry 1996 Oct; 20:1159.

Shultz C.W., et al. Absorption, tolerability, and effects on mitochondrial activity of oral coenzyme Q10 in parkinsonian patients. Neurology 1998 Mar; 50:793.

Shultz C.W., et al. A possible role of coenzyme Q10 in the etiology and treatment of Parkinson's disease. Biofactors 1999; 9:267.

Sian J., Dexter D.T., Lees A.J., et al. Alterations in glutathione levels in Parkinson's disease and other neurodegenerative disorders affecting basal ganglia. Ann Neurol 1994; 36: 348–55.

Singer T.P., Ramsay R.R., Ackresll B.A. Efficiencies of NADH and succinate dehydrogenases in degenerative diseases and myopathies. Biochim Biophys Acta (Netherlands) 1995 May 24; 1271 (1): 211–9.

Snyder S.H. No NO prevents parkinsonism. Nature Medicine 1996 Sept; 2(9): 965–6.

Stevenson G.B., et. al. Xenobiotic metabolism in Parkinson's disease. Neurology 1989; 883–7.

Swerdlow R.H. Is NADH effective in the treatment of Parkinson's disease? Drugs Aging 1998 Oct; 13:263.

Tanner, C.M. Liver enzyme abnormalities in Parkinson's disease. Geriatrics 1991 Aug; 46 (Suppl 1): 60–3.

Tanner C.M. and Langston J.W. Do environmental toxins cause Parkinson's disease? A critical review. Neurology 1990; 40 (Suppl 3): 17–30.

Taylor D.J., Drige D., Barnes P.R., Kemp G.J., et al. A 31P magnetic resonance spectroscopy study of mitochondrial function in skeletal muscle of patients with Parkinson's disease. J Neurol Sci 1994 Aug; 125(1): 77–81.

Tetrud J.W. and Langston J.W. The effect of deprenyl (selegiline) on the natural history of Parkinson's disease. Science 1989 Aug; 4: 519–22.

Vatassery G.T. Vitamin E neurochemistry and implications for neuro-degeneration in Parkinson's disease. Ann NY Acad Sci 1992 Sept 30; 669: 97–109.

Vieregge P., et al. Lifestyle and dietary factors early and late in Parkinson's disease. Can J of Neurol Sci 1992; 19 (2): 170–3.

Yasui M., et al. Calcium, magnesium and aluminum concentrations in Parkinson's disease. NeuroToxicology 1992; 13: 593–6.

Youdim M. New perspectives in nutritional therapies. Ann NY Acad Sci 1994; 738: 64–7.

Youdim M.B., Ben-Shachar D., Eshel G., et al. The neurotoxicity of iron and nitric oxide. Relevance to the etiology of Parkinson's disease. Adv Neurol 1993; 60: 259–66.

Youdim M.B., Ben-Shachar D., Riederer P. The possible role of iron in the etiopathology of Parkinson's disease. Mov Disord 1993; 8(1): 1–12.

Youdim M.B. and Riederer P. The role of iron in senescence of dopaminergic neurons in Parkinson's disease. J Neural Transm 1993; 40 (Suppl): 57–67.

• Chapter 7: Multiple Sclerosis

Aberg J.A., et al. Prostaglandin production in chronic progressive mutiple sclerosis. J of Clin Lab Analysis 1990; 4: 246–50.

Ansari K.A. and Shoeman D.W. Arachidonic and docosahexanoic acid content of bovine brain myelin: implications for the pathogenesis of multiple sclerosis. Neurochem Res 1990 Jan; 15(1): 7–11.

Bates D., Cartlidge N.E.F., French J.M., et al. A double-blind controlled trial of long chain n–3 polyunsaturated fatty acids in the treatment of multiple sclerosis. Journal of Neurology, Neurosurgery, and Psychiatry 1989; 52: 18–22.

Beck W. Megaloblastic anemias. Cecil Textbook of Medicine. Wyngarden and Smith, eds. 17th ed., W.B. Saunders, 1985.

Ben-Shlomo Y., Davey S.G., Marmot M.G. Dietary fat in the epidemiology of multiple sclerosis; has the situation been adequately assessed? Neuroepidemiology 1992; 11 (4–6): 214–25.

Bolanos, J.P., et al. Evaluation of the efficacy of potential therapeutic agents at protecting against nitric oxide synthetase mediated mitochondrial damage in activated astrocytes. Brain Res Protoc 1997 Aug; 1:258.

Boullerne A.I., Petry K.G., Geffard M. Circulating antibodies directed against conjugated fatty acids in sera of patients with multiple sclerosis. J Neuroimmunol 1996; 65: 75–81.

Bray P.F., Luka J., Bray P.F., Culp K.W., Schlight J.P. Antibodies against Epstein-Barr nuclear antigen (EBNA) in multiple sclerosis CSF, and two pentapeptide sequence identities between EBNA any myelin basic protein. Neurology 1992; 42: 1798–1804.

Cantorna M.T., et al. 1-25-dihydroxyvitamin D3 reversibly blocks the progression of relapsing encephalomyelitis, a model of multiple sclerosis.

Chelmicka-Schorr E. and Aranson B.G. Nervous system–immune system interactions and their role in multiple sclerosis. Ann Neurol 1994; 36: S29–S32.

Demerens C., et al. Eliprodil stimulates CNS myelination. Neurology 1999 Jan 15; 52:346.

Fitzgerald G., Harbige L.S., Forti A., Crawford M.A. The effect of nutritional counselling on diet and plasma EFA status in multiple sclerosis patients over 3 years. Hum Nutr Appl Nutr 1987 Oct; 41(5): 297–310.

Frequin S.T., Wevers R.A., Braam M., et al. Decreased vitamin B_{12} and folate levels in cerebrospinal fluid and serum of multiple sclerosis patients after high-dose intravenous methylprednisolone. J Neurol 1993 May; 240(5): 305–8.

Goldberg P., Fleming M.C., Picard E.H. Multiple sclerosis: decreased relapse rate through dietary supplementation with calcium, magnesium and vitamin D. Med Hypotheses 1986 Oct; 21 (2): 193–200.

Goodkin D.E., Jacobsen D.W., Green R. Biologically significant serum vitamin B_{12} deficiency in multiple sclerosis inadequately documented. Arch Neurol 1992 Jul; 49 (7): 683–4.

Grasso G. and Muscettola M. Possible role of gamma interferon in ovarian function. Ontogenetic and Phylogenetic Mechanisms of Neuroimmunomodulation. Fabris N., Jankovic B., Markovic B. and Spector N., eds. Ann NY Acad Sci 1992; Vol. 650.

Gruener D.M., Kunkel E.J., Snyderman D.A., et al. Dietary vitamin B_{12} deficiency in a patient with multiple sclerosis. Gen Hosp Psychiatry 1994 May; 16 (3): 224–8.

Hauser S., et al. Antispasticity effect of threonine in MS. Arch Neurol 1992 Sept; 49: 923–6.

Heales S.J., et al. Nitric oxide, mitochondria, and neurological disease. Biochim Biophy Acta 1999 Feb 9; 1410:215.

Holman R.T., Johnson S.B., Kokmen E. Deficiencies of polyunsaturated fatty acids and replacement by nonessential fatty acids in plasma lipids in multiple sclerosis. Proc Natl Acad Sci 1989 Jun; 86: 4720–4.

Hutter C.D. and Laing P. Multiple sclerosis: sunlight, diet, immunology and aetiology. Med Hypotheses 1996 Feb; 46 (2): 67–74.

Jacobs L.D., et al. Intramuscular interferon beta 1-A for disease progression in relapsing multiple sclerosis. Ann Neurol 1996; 39: 285–94.

Johnson K.P. Experimental therapy of relapsing-remitting multiple sclerosis with copolymer-1. Ann Neurol 1994; 36: S115–17.

Johnson K.P., Brooks B.R., Cohen J.A., et al. Copolymer 1 reduces relapse rate and improves disability in relapsing-remitting multiple sclerosis: results of a phase III multicenter, double-blind, placebo-controlled trial. Neurology 1995 Jul; 45: 1268–75.

Karp C. Editorial: Interleukin-12: Amiss in MS. Ann Neurol 1999 June; 45:690.

Kim S., et al. Estriol ameliorates autoimmune demyelinating disease. Neurology 1999 Apr 12; 52:1230.

Kira J., Tobimatsu S., Goto I. Vitamin B_{12} metabolism and massive-dose methyl vitamin B_{12} in Japanese patients with multiple sclerosis. Intern Med 1994 Feb; 33 (2): 82–6.

Kruger P.G. and Nyland H.I. The role of mast cells and diet in the onset and maintenance of multiple sclerosis: a hypothesis. Med Hypotheses 1995 Jan; 44 (1): 66–9.

Lehmann D., Karussis D., Misrachi-Koll R., et al. Oral adminstration of the oxidant-scavenger N-acetyl-L-cysteine inhibits acute experimental autoimmune encephalomyelitis. J Neuroimmunol 1994; 50: 35–42.

Lemire J.M., et al. Immunosuppressive actions of 1,25-dihydroxy-vitamin D_3. J Nutr 1995 Jun; 125:1704S.

Logigian E.L., Kaplan R.F., Steere A.C. Chronic neurologic manifestations of Lyme disease. N Engl J Med 1990 Nov 22; 323 (21): 1438–44.

Mai J., et al. High dose antioxidant supplementation to MS patients: effects on glutathione peroxidase, clinical safety, and absorption of selenium. Biol Trace Element Res 1990; 24: 109–17.

Manley P. Diet in multiple sclerosis. Practitioner 1994 May; 238 (1538): 358–63.

Miller A., et al. Treatment of multiple sclerosis with copolymer-1 (Copaxone). J Neuroimmunol 1998 Dec 1; 92:113.

Monastra G., Cross A.H., Bruni A., Raine C.S. Phosphatidylserine, a putative inhibitor of tumor necrosis factor, prevents autoimmune demyelination. Neurology 1993 Jan; 43: 153–62.

Neu I., et al. Leukotrienes in the cerebrospinal fluid of multiple sclerosis patients. Acta Neurol Scand 1992; 86: 586–7.

Nieves J., Cosman F., Herbert J., et al. High prevalence of vitamin D deficiency and reduced bone mass in multiple sclerosis. Neurology 1994 Sept; 44 (9): 1687–92.

Nightingale S., Woo E., Smith A.D., et al. Red blood cell and adipose tissue fatty acids in mild inactive multiple sclerosis. Acta Neurol Scand 1990; 82: 43–50.

Nijst T.Q., Wevers R.A., Schoonderwaldt H.C., et al. Vitamin B_{12} and folate concentrations in serum and cerebrospinal fluid of neurological patients with special reference to multiple sclerosis and dementia. J Neurol Neurosurg Psychiatry 1990 Nov; 53 (11): 951–4.

Ozenci V., et al. Multiple sclerosis. Scand J Immunol 1999 May; 49:554.

Packer L., et al. Antioxidant activity and biologic properties of a procyanidin-rich extract from pine bark, pycnogenol. Free Radic Biol Med 1999 Sep; 27:704.

Reynolds E.H. Multiple sclerosis and vitamin B₁₂ metabolism. J Neuroimmunol 1992 Oct; 40 (2–3): 225–30.

Reynolds E.H. Multiple sclerosis and vitamin B₁₂ metabolism. J Neurol Neurosurg Psychiatry 1992 May; 55 (5): 339–40.

Reynolds E.H., Bottigliere T., Laundy M., et al. Vitamin B₁₂ metabolism in multiple sclerosis. Arch Neurol 1992 Jun; 49 (6): 649–52.

Reynolds E.H., Linnell J.C., Faludy J.E. Multiple sclerosis associated with vitamin B₁₂ deficiency. Arch Neurol 1991 Aug; 48 (8): 808–11.

Rieckmann P., Albrecht M., Kitze B., Weber T., et al. Tumor necrosis factor-alpha messenger RNA expression in patients with relapsing-remitting multiple sclerosis is associated with disease activity. Ann Neurol 1995 Jan; 37 (1): 82–88.

Robinson M.K. Glutathione deficiency and HIV infection. Lancet 1992 Jun 27; 339: 1603–4.

Sandyk R. and Awerbuch G.I. Vitamin B₁₂ and its relationship to age of onset of multiple sclerosis. Int J Neurosci 1993 Jul-Aug; 71 (1–4): 93–9.

Schwartz G.G. Hypothesis: calcitriol mediates pregnancy's protective effect on multiple sclerosis. Arch Neurol May 1993; 50: 455.

Sharief M.K. and Hentges R. Association between tumor necrosis factor-alpha and disease progression in patients with multiple sclerosis. N Engl J Med 1991 Aug 15; 325 (7): 467–71.

Sharief M.K., Noori M.A., Ciardi M., Cirelli A., Thompson E.J. Increased levels of circulating ICAM-1 in serum and cerebrospinal fluid of patients with active multiple sclerosis. Correlation with TNF-alpha and blood-brain barrier damage. J Neuroimmunol 1993 Mar; 43 (1–2): 15–21.

Soldan S.S., et al. Association of human herpes virus 6 (HHV-6) with multiple sclerosis. Nat Med 1997 Dec; 3:1394.

Sommer N., et al. Therapeutic potential of phosphodiesterase type 4 inhibition in chronic autoimmune demyelinating disease. J Neuroimmunol 1997 Oct; 79:54.

Stanislaus R., et al. Amelioration of experimental allergic encephalomyelitis in Lewis rats by lovastatin. Neurosci Lett 1999 Jul 9; 269:71.

Steinman L. Autoimmune disease: misguided assaults on the self produce multiple sclerosis, juvenile diabetes and other chronic illnesses. Promising therapies are emerging. Scientific American 1993 Sept: 107–14.

Stewart V.C., et al. Pretreatment of astrocytes with interferon-alpha/ beta prevents neuronal mitochondrial respiratory chain damage. J Neurochem 1998 Jan; 70:432.

Sumaya C.V., Myers L.W., Ellison G.W., Ench Y. Increased prevalence and titer of Epstein-Barr virus antibodies in patients with multiple sclerosis. Ann Neurol 1985; 17: 371–77.

Swank R.L. Multiple sclerosis; fat-oil relationship. Nutrition 1991 Sept-Oct; 7 (5): 368–76.

Swank R.L. and Dugan B.B. Effect of low saturated fat diet in early and late causes of multiple sclerosis. Lancet 1990 Jul 7; 336 (8706): 37–9.

Teitelbaum D., et al. Immunomodulation of experimental autoimmune encephalomyelitis by oral administration of copolymer 1. Proc Natl Acad Sci USA 1999 Mar 30; 96:3842.

Toshniwal P. and Zarling E. Increased free radicals in multiple sclerosis. Neurochem Res 1992; 17: 207–7.

Wong E.K., Enomoto H., Leopold I.H., et al. Intestinal absorption of dietary fat in patients with multiple sclerosis. Metab Pediatr Syst Ophthalmol 1993; 16 (3–4): 39–42.

Yasui M., et al. Magnesium concentration in brains from multiple sclerosis patients. Acta Neurol Scand 1990; 81: 197–200.

Yoon C.K. MS study yields mixed results. Science 1993 Feb; 259: 1263.

• Chapter 8: Amyotrophic Lateral Sclerosis

Aschner M. Methylmercury in astrocytes—what possible significance? NeuroToxicology 1996; 17 (1): 93–106.

Ashmead, H.D. Increased superoxide dismutase activity resulting from ingested amino acid chelated minerals. Paper presented at

Albion Laboratories International Conference on Human Nutrition, Salt Lake City, Utah, Jan 21–22, 1995.

Barrett-Connor E., Khaw K.T., Yen S.S.C. Prospective study of dehydroepiandrosterone sulfate, mortality, and cardiovascular disease. N Engl J Med 1986 Dec 11; 315 (24): 1519–24.

Beal M.F., et al. Neuroprotective effects of creatine in a transgenic animal model of amylotrophic lateral sclerosis. Nat Med 1999 Mar; 5:347.

Beckman J.S., Carson M., Smith C.D., Koppenol W.H. ALS, SOD and peroxynitrite (letter). Nature 1993 Aug 12; 364 (6438): 584.

Bensimon G., Lacomblez L., Meininger, and the ALS/Riluzole Study Group. A controlled trial of riluzole in amyotrophic lateral sclerosis. N Engl J Med 1994 Mar 3; 330 (9): 585–91.

Bergeron C., Muntasser S., Somerville M.J., Weyer L., Percy M.E. Copper/zinc superoxide dismutase mRNA levels are increased in sporadic amyotrophic lateral sclerosis motor neurons. Brain Res 1994 Oct 3; 659 (1–2): 272–6.

Bologa L., Sharma J., Roberts E. Dehydroepiandrosterone and its sulfated derivative reduce neuronal death and enhance astrocytic differentiation in brain cultures. J of Neuroscience Res 1987; 17: 225–34.

Borras-Blasco J., et al. Riluzole as a treatment for amyotrophic lateral sclerosis. (In Italian). Rev Neurol 1998 Dec; 27:1021.

Bowling A.C., Schulz J.B., Brown R.H., Beal M.F. Superoxide dismutase activity, oxidative damage, and mitochondrial energy metabolism in familial and sporadic amyotrophic lateral sclerosis. J Neurochem 1993 Dec; 61 (6): 2322–5.

Bristol L.A., Rothstein J.D. Glutamate transporter gene expression in amyotrophic lateral sclerosis motor cortex. Ann Neurol 1996 May; 39: 676–9.

Brooks N. In vitro evidence for a role of glutamate in CNS toxicity of mercury. Toxicology 1992; 76: 245–6.

Chaudhry V., Corse A.M., Cornblath D.R., et al. Multifocal motor neuropathy: response to human immune globulin. Ann Neurol 1993 Mar; 33 (3): 237–42.

Choi D.W. Methods for antagonizing glutamate neurotoxicity. Cerebrovascular and Brain Metabolism Rev 1990; 2: 105–47.

Colasanti M., Persichini T., Menegazzi M., et al. Introduction of nitric oxide synthase mRNA expression. Suppression by exogenous nitric oxide. J Biol Chem 1995 Nov 10; 270 (45): 26731–3.

Darley-Usmar V., Wiseman H., Halliwell B. Nitric oxide and oxygen radicals: a question of balance. FEBS Lett 1995 Aug 7; 369 (2–3): 131–5.

Dawsen T.M., et al. The immunosuppressant FK506 enhances phosphaphoralation of nitric oxide synthase and protects against glutamate neurotoxicity. Proc Nat Acad Sci 1993; 90: 9808–12.

Dawsen T.M., et al. Mechanisms of nitric oxide mediated neurotoxicity in primary brain cultures. J Neurosci 1993; 13: 2651–61.

DiSilvestro, R.T., et al. Effects of copper supplementation on ceruloplasmin and copper-zinc superoxide dismutase in free-living rheumatoid arthritis patients. J Am Coll Nutr 1992; 11: 177.

Eisen A., Pearmain J., Stewart H. Dehydroepiandrosterone sulphate (DHEAS) concentrations and amyotrophic lateral sclerosis. Muscle & Nerv 1995 Dec; 18: 1481–1483.

Fagni L., Lafon-Cazal M., Lerner-Natoli M., et al. J Pharm Belg 1995 Mar-Jun; 50 (2–3): 204–12.

Fisman, M. Hepatic ultrastructural change and liver dysfunction in amyotrophic lateral sclerosis. Arch Neurol 1987 Oct; 44 (10): 103–6.

Garafolo O., et al. Superoxide dismutase activity in lymphoblastoid cells from motor neuron disease/amyotrophic lateral sclerosis (MND/ALS) patients. J Neurol Sci 1995 May; 129 (Suppl): 90–2.

Gredal O. and Moller S.E. Effect of branched-chain amino acids on glutamate metabolism in amyotrophic lateral sclerosis. J Neurol Sci 1995 Mar; 129 (1): 40–3.

Greenhaff P.L., Bodin K., Soderlund K., Hultman E. The effect of oral creatine supplementation on skeletal muscle phosphocreatine resynthesis. Am J Physiol 1994; 266: E725–E730.

Greenhaff P.L., Casey A., Short A.H., et al. Influence of oral creatine supplementation of muscle torque during repeated bouts of maximal voluntary exercise in man. Clin Sci 1993; 84: 565–71.

Gurney M.E., Cutting F.B., Zhai P., Doble A., et al. Benefit of vitamin E, riluzole, and gabapentin in a transgenic model of familial amyotrophic lateral sclerosis. Ann Neurol 1996 Fed; 39 (2): 147–57.

Harris R.C., Soderlund K., Hultman E. Elevation of creatine in resting and exercised muscle of normal subjects by creatine supplementation. Clin Sci 1992; 83: 367–74.

Ihara Y., Mori A., Hayabara T., Kawai M., et al. Superoxide dismutase and free radicals in sporadic amyotrophic lateral sclerosis: relationship to clinical data. J Neurol Sci 1995 Dec; 134 (1–2): 51–6.

Ikeda K., Linkosz B., Greene T., et al. Effects of brain-derived neurotropic factor on motor dysfunction in wobbler mouse motor neuron disease. Ann Neurol 1995 Apr; 37 (4): 505–11.

The Italian Study Group. Branched-chain amino acids and amyotrophic lateral sclerosis: a treatment failure? Neurology 1993 Dec; 43 (12): 2466–70. Comment in: Neurology 1993 Dec; 43 (12): 2437–8.

Kasarskis E.J., Tandon I.., Lovell M.A., Ehmann W.D. Aluminum, calcium and iron in the spinal cords of patients with sporadic amyotrophic lateral sclerosis using laser microprobe mass spectroscopy: a preliminary study. J Neurol Sci 1995 Jun; 130 (2): 203–8.

Kellcr G. and Snodgrass HR. Human embryonic stem cells: the future is now. Nat Med 1999 Feb; 5:151.

Lang D.J. Recombinant human insulin-like growth factors in ALS. Neurol 1996; 47: S93–5.

Lincoln R. Successful transplantation of human neural stem/progenitor cells in preclinical model. BW Healthwire July 15, 1999.

Lindsay R.M. Trophic protection of motor neurons: clinical potential in motor neuron diseases. J Neurol 1994 Dec; 242 (Suppl 1): S8–S11.

Lipton S.A. and Rosenberg P.A. Excitatory amino acids as a final common pathway for neurologic disorders. N Engl J Med 1994 Mar 3; 330 (9): 613–22.

Louwerse E.S., Buchet J.P., Van Diijik M.A., et al. Urinary excretion of lead and mercury after oral administration of meso-2, 3-dimercaptosuccinic acid in patients with motor neuron disease. Int Arch Occup Environ Health 1995; 67 (2): 135–8.

Louwerse E.S., Weverling G.J., Bossuyt P.M., Meyjes F.E., de Jong

J.M. Randomized, double-blind, controlled trial of acetylcysteine in amyotrophic lateral sclerosis. Arch Neurol 1995 Jun; 52 (6): 559–64.

Lyons T.J., Liu H., Goto J.J., Nersissian A. et al. Mutations in copper-zinc superoxide dismutase that cause amyotrophic lateral sclerosis alter the zinc binding site and the redox behavior of the protein. Proc Natl Acad Sci 1996 Oct 29; 93 (22): 12240–4.

Malessa S., Leigh P.N., Bertel O., Sluga E., Hornykiewicz O. Amyotrophic lateral sclerosis: glutamate dehydrogenase and transmitter amino acids in the spinal cord. J Neurol Neurosurg Psychiatry 1991 Nov; 54 (11): 984–8.

Marx J. Gene linked to Lou Gehrig's disease. Science 1993 Mar 5; 259 (5100): 1393.

McNamara J.O. and Fridovich, I. Did radicals strike Lou Gehrig? Nature 1993 Mar 4; 362: 20–1.

Mennini T., et al. Biochemical and pharmacological evidence of a functional role of AMPA receptors in motor neuron dysfunction in mnd mice. Eur J Neurosci 1999 May; 11:1705.

Mitani K. Relationship between neurological diseases due to aluminum load, especially amyotrophic lateral sclerosis, and magnesium status. Magnes Res 1992 Sept.; 5 (3): 203–13.

Morales A.J., Nolan J.J., Nelson J.C., Yen S.S. Effects of replacement dose of dehydroepiandrosterone in men and women of advancing age. J Clin Endocrinol Metab 1994 Jun; 78 (6): 1360–7.

Moriwaka F., Satoh H., Ejima A., Watanabe E. et al. Mercury and selenium contents in amyotrophic lateral sclerosis in Hokkaido, the northernmost island of Japan. J Neurol Sci 1993 Aug; 118 (1): 38–42.

Nagano S., et al. Benefit of a combined treatment with trientine and ascorbate in familial amyotrophic lateral sclerosis model mice. Neurosci Lett 1999 Apr 23; 265:159.

Nakano Y., Hirayama K., Terao K. Hepatic ultrastructural changes and liver dysfunction in amyotrophic lateral sclerosis. Arch Neurol 1987 Jan; 44 (1): 103–6.

Nishida C.R., Gralla E.B., Valengine J.S. Characterization of three yeast copper-zinc superoxide dismutase mutants analogous to those coded for in familial amyotrophic lateral sclerosis. Proc Natl Acad Sci 1994 Oct 11; 91 (21): 9906–10.

Paakkari I. and Lindsberg P. Nitric oxide in the central nervous system. Ann Med 1995 Jun; 27 (3): 369–77.

Park S.T., Lim K.T., Chung, Y.T., Kim S.U. Methylmercury-induced neurotoxicity in cerebral neuron culture is blocked by antioxidants and NMDA receptor antagonists. NeuroToxicology 1996; 17 (1): 37–46.

Pestronk A., Adams R.N., Clawson L., et al. Serum antibodies to GM1 ganglioside in amyotrophic lateral sclerosis. Neurology 1988; 38: 1457–61.

Piccardo P., Yanagiahara R., Garruto R.M., Gibbs C.J., Gajdusek D.C. Histochemical and x-ray microanalytical localization of aluminum in amyotrophic lateral sclerosis and parkinsonism-dementia of Guam. Acta Neuropathol 1988; 77 (1): 1–4.

Plaitikis A. and Carascio J.T. Abnormal glutamate metabolism in ALS. Ann Neurol 1987; 22: 5755–9.

Plaitakis A. and Constantakakis E. Altered metabolism of excitatory amino acids, n-acetyl-aspartate and n-acetyl-aspartyl-glutamate in amyotrophic lateral sclerosis. Brain Res Bull 1993; 30 (3–4): 381–6.

Plaitakis A., Constantakakis E., Smith J. The neuroexcitoxic amino acids glutamate and aspartate are altered in the spinal cord and brain in amyotrophic lateral sclerosis. Ann Neurol 1988 Sept.; 24 (3): 446–9.

Postam C.T., Hoefnagels W.H.L., Thien Th., DeBoo Th. Zinc, glutamate receptors, and motorneuron disease. Lancet 1987 Nov 7: 1082–84.

Przedborski, S., et al. Brain superoxide dismutase, catalase, and glutathione peroxidase activities in amyotrophic lateral sclerosis. Ann Neurol 1996; 39 (2): 158–65.

Ratan R.R., Murphy T.H., Baraban J.M. Macromolecular synthesis inhibitors prevent oxidative stress-induced apoptosis in embryonic cortical neurons by shunting cysteine from protein synthesis to glutathione. J Neuroscience 1994 Jul; 14 (7): 4385–92.

Reiner A., Medina L., Figueredo-Cardenas G., Anfinson S. Brainstem motorneuron pools that are selectively resistant in amyotrophic lateral sclerosis are preferentially enriched in parvalbumin: evidence from monkey brainstem for a calcium-mediated mechanism in sporadic ALS. Exp Neurol 1995 Feb; 131 (2): 239–50.

Reinholz M.M., et al. Therapeutic benefits of putrescine modified catalase in a transgenic mouse model of familial amyotrophic lateral sclerosis. Exp Neurol 1999 Sep; 159:204.

Rosen D.R., Siddique T., Patterson D., et al. Mutations in Cu/Zn superoxide dismutase gene are associated with familial amyotrophic lateral sclerosis. Nature 1993 Mar 4; 362: 59–62.

Rothstein J.D., Bristol L.A., Hosler B., Brown R.H., Kunci R.W. Chronic inhibition of superoxide dismutase produces apoptotic death of spinal neurons. Proc Natl Acad Sci 1994 May; 91: 4155–59.

Rothstein J.D. and Kunch R.W. Neuroprotective strategies in a model of chronic glutamate-mediated motor neuron toxicity, J Neurochem 1995 Aug; 65 (2): 643–51.

Rothstein J.D., Martin L.J., Kunch R.W. Decreased glutamate transport by the brain and spinal cord in amyotrophic lateral sclerosis. N Engl J Med 1992 May 28; 326 (22): 1464–95.

Rowland L.P. Amyotrophic lateral sclerosis. Cur Opin Neurol 1994 Aug; 7 (4): 310–15.

Sarafian T.A., Bredesen D.E., Verity M.A. Cellular resistance to methylmercury. NeuroToxicology 1996; 17 (1): 27–36.

Seeburger J.L. and Springer J.E. Experimental rationale for the therapeutic use of neurotrophins in amyotrophic lateral sclerosis. Exp Neurol 1993 Nov; 124 (1): 64–72.

Smith R.G. and Appel S.H. Molecular approaches to amyotrophic lateral sclerosis. Ann Rev Med 1995; 46: 133–45.

Szerb J.C. and O'Regan P.A. Glutamine enhances glutamate release in preference to gamma-aminobutyrate release in hippocampal slices. Can J Physiol Pharmcol 1984 Aug; 62 (8): 919–23.

Testa D., Carceni T., Fetoni V. Branched-chain amino acids in the treatment of amyotrophic lateral sclerosis. J Neurol 1989 Dec; 236 (8): 445–7.

Trieu V.N. and Uckun F.M. Genistein is neuroprotective in murine models of familial amyotrophic lateral sclerosis and stroke. Biochem Biophys Red Commun 1999 May 19; 258:685.

Uchino M., Ando Y., Tanaka Y., Nakamura T., et al. Decrease in Cu/Zn- and Mn-superoxide dismutase activities in brain and spinal cord of patients with amyotrophic lateral sclerosis. J Neurol Sci 1994 Dec 1; 127 (1): 61–7.

Wakai M.,Mokuno K., Hashizume Y., Kato K. An immunohistochemical study of the neuronal expression of manganese superoxide dismutase in sporadic amyotrophic lateral sclerosis. Acta Neuropathol 1994; 88 (2): 151–8.

Wei H., et al. Scavenging of hydrogen peroxide and inhibition of ultraviolet light-induced oxidative DNA damage by aqueous extracts from green and black teas. Free Radic Biol Med 1999 Jun; 26:1427.

Weiss R. Brain cell that multiplies is isolated. Washington Post, October 31, 1998.

Wiedau-Pazos M., Goto J.J., Rabizadeh S., Gralla E.B., et al. Altered reactivity of superoxide dismutase in familial amyotrophic lateral sclerosis. Science 1996 Jan 26; 271 (5248): 515–8.

Woznicki F.T. and Walker J.B. Utilization of the synthetic phosphagen cyclocreatine phosphate by a simple brain model during stimulation by neuroexcitatory amino acids. J Neurochem 1988 May; 50:1640.

Yasui M., Ota K., Garruto R.M. Concentrations of zinc and iron in the brains of Guamanian patients with amyotrophic lateral sclerosis and parkinsonism-dementia. NeuroToxicology 1993 Winter; 14 (4): 445–50.

Yasui M., Yase Y., Kihira T., Adachi K., Suzuki Y. Magnesium and calcium contents in CNS tissues of amyotrophic lateral sclerosis patients from the Kii Peninsula, Japan. Eur Neurol 1992; 32: 95–8.

Yasui M., Yase Y., Ota K., Garruto R.M. Aluminum deposition in the central nervous system of patients with amyotrophic lateral sclerosis from the Kii Peninsula of Japan. NeuroToxicology 1991 Fall; 12 (3): 615–20.

Yasui M., Yase Y., Ota K., Mukoyama M., Adachi K. High aluminum deposition in the central nervous system of patients with amyotrophic lateral sclerosis from the Kii Peninsula, Japan: two case reports. NeuroToxicology 1991 Summer; 12 (2): 277–83.

Yee S. and Choi B.H. Oxidative stress in neurotoxic effects of methylmercury poisoning. NeuroToxicology 1996; 17 (1): 17–26.

Yim M.B., Kang J.H., Yim H.S., Kwak H.S., et al. A gain-of-function of an amyotrophic lateral sclerosis–associated Cu, Zn-superoxide dismutase mutant: an enhancement of free radical formation due to a decrease in Km for hydrogen peroxide. Proc Natl Acad Sci 1996 Jun 11; 93 (12): 5709–14.

Yoshida S., Mitani K., Wakayma I., Kihira T., Yase Y. Bunina body formation in amyotrophic lateral sclerosis: a morphometric-statistical and trace element study featuring aluminum. J Neurol Sci 1995 May; 130 (1): 88–94.

• Chapter 9: Attention Deficit Hyperactivity Disorder

American Psychiatric Association Diagnostic and Statistic Manual of Mental Disorders, 3rd Ed., Revised (DSM3R). American Psychiatric Association, Washington, D.C., 1987.

Agostini C., Trojan S., Bellu R., Riva E., Giovannini M. The Neurodevelopmental quotient of healthy term infants at 4 months and feeding practice: the role of long-chain polyunsaturated fatty acids. Ped Res 1995 Aug; 38: 262–6.

Amaducci L., Angst J., Bech P., Benkert O., et al. Consensus conference on the methodology of clinical traits of "Nootropics," Pharmacopsychiatry 1990; 23: 171–5.

Arnsten A,F., Steer J.C., Hunt R.D. The contribution of alpha 2-noradrenergic mechanisms of prefrontal corticol cognitive function. Potential significance for attention-deficit hyperactivity disorder. Arch Gen Psychiatry 1996 May; 53 (5): 448–55.

Banfi S. and Dorigotti L. Experimental behavioral studies with oxiracetam on different types of chronic cerebral impairment. Clin Neuropharmacol 1986; 9 Suppl: 19–26.

Bekaroglu M., Aslan Y., Gedik Y., Deger O., et al. Relationships between serum free fatty acids and zinc, and attention deficit hyperactivity disorder: a research note. J. Child Psychol. Psychiatry 1996 Fed; 37 (2): 225–7.

Benson D.F. The role of frontal dysfunction in attention deficit hyperactivity disorders. J of Child Neurol 1991; 6: 9–12.

Berry C., et al. Girls with attention deficit disorder, a silent minority? A report on behavioral and cognitive characteristics. Pediatrics 1985; 76: 801–9.

Boris M. and Mandel F.S. Foods and additives are common causes of the attention deficit hyperactive disorder in children. Ann Allergy 1994 May; 72 (5): 462–8.

Carter C.M., Urbanowicz M., Hemsley R., Mantilla L., et al. Effects of a new food diet in attention deficit disorder. Arch Dis Child 1993 Nov; 69 (5): 564–8.

Chopin P. and Briley M. Effects of four non-cholinergic cognitive enhancers in comparison with tacrine and galantamine on scopolamine-induced amnesia in rats. Psychopharmacology 1992; 106: 26–30.

Colburn T., Dumanosky D., and Myers J.P. Our Stolen Future. Penguin 1991; 185–9.

Egger J., Carter C.M., Graham P.J., Gumley D., Soothill J.F. Controlled trial of oligoantigenic treatment in the hyperkinetic syndrome. Lancet 1985 Mar 9: 540–5.

Egger J., Stolla A., McEwen L.M. Controlled trial of hyposensitization in children with food-induced hyperkinetic syndrome. Lancet 1992 May 9; 339: 1150–3.

Eisenberg J., Asnis G.M., van Praag H.M., Vela R.M. Effects of tyrosine on attention deficit order with hyperactivity. J Clin Psychiatry 1988 May; 49 (5): 193–5.

Eppright T.D., Sanfacon J.A., Horwitz E.A. Attention deficit hyperactivity disorder, infantile autism, and elevated blood-lead: a possible relationship. Mo Med 1996 Mar; 93 (3): 136–8.

Ernst M. and Zametkin A. The interface of genetics, neuroimaging and neurochemistry in attention deficit disorder. In Psychopharmacology, Fourth Generation of Progress. Blum F.E. and Kupfer D.J., eds. Raven Press, 1995.

Feingold, B. Why Your Child is Hyperactive. Random House, 1975.

Feingold, B. Hyperkinesis and learning disabilities linked to the ingestion of artificial food colors and flavors. J Learn Disabil 1976 (9): 551–59.

Findling R.L., Schwartz M.A., Flannery D.J., Manos M.J. Venlafaxine in adults with attention-deficit/hyperactivity disorder: an open clinical trial. J Clin Psychiatry 1996 May; 57 (5): 184–9.

Funk K.F. and Schmidt J. Effect of nootropics on choline uptake. Biomed Biochim Acta 1988; 47: 417–21.

Gibson R.A., Neumann M.A., Makrides M. Effect of dietary docosa-hexaenoic acid on brain composition and neural function in term infants. Lipids 1996; 31: S177–S93.

Girardi N.L., Shaywitz S.E., Shaywitz B.A., Marchione K., et al. Blunted catecholamine responses after glucose ingestion in children with attention deficit disorder. Ped Res 1995 Oct; 38 (4): 539–42.

Golub M.S., Keen C.L., Gershwin M.E., Hendrickx A.G. Developmental zinc deficiency and behavior. J Nutr 1995; 125: 2263S–2271S.

Gouliaev A.H. and Senning A. Piracetam and other structurally related nootropics. Brain Res Rev 1994; 19: 180–22.

Grau M., Montero J.L., Balasch J. Effect of piracetam on electrocorti-gram and local cerebral glucose utilization in the rat. Gen Pharmacol 1987; 18: 207–11.

Guilarte T.R., Miceli R.C., Jett D.A. Biochemical evidence of an interaction of lead at the zinc allosteric sites of the NMDA receptor complex: effects of neuronal development. NeuroToxicology 1995; 16 (1): 63–72.

Hauser P. Attention deficit hyperactivity disorder in people with generalized resistance to thyroid hormone. N Engl J Med 1993; 328: 997–1001.

Hjorther A., Browne E., Jakobsen K., et al. Organic brain syndrome treated with oxiracetam. A double-blind randomized controlled trial. Acta Neurol Scand 1987; 75: 271–6.

Joffe R.T. and Sokolov S.T.H. Thyroid hormones, the brain, and affective disorders. Critical Rev in Neurobiol 1994; 8(½): 46–53.

Kahn C.A., Kelly P.C., Walker W.O. Lead screening in children with attention deficit hyperactivity disorder and developmental delay. Clin Pediatr 1995 Sept; 34 (9): 498–501.

Kaneko M., et al. Hypothalamic-pituitary-adrenal axis function in children with attention deficit hyperactivity disorder. J Autism Dev Disord 1993 Mar; 23 (1): 59–65.

Lecaillon J.B., Dubois J.P., Coppens H., et al. Pharmacokinetics of oxiracetam in elderly patients after 800 mg oral doses, comparison with non-geriatric healthy subjects. Eur J Drug Metab Pharmacokinet, 1990; 15: 223–30.

Lenegre A., Chermat R., Avril I., et al. Specificity of piracetam's anti-amnesic activity in three models of amnesia in the mouse. Pharmacol Biochem Behav 1988; 29: 626–9.

Marret S., Gressens P., Gadisseux J.F., Evrard P. Prevention by magnesium of excitotoxic neuronal death in the developing brain: an animal model for clinical intervention studies. Dev Med Child Neurol 1995 Jun; 37 (6): 473–84.

McConnell H. Catecholamine metabolism in the attention deficit disorder: implications for the use of amino acid precursor therapy. Med Hypotheses 1985 Aug; 17 (4): 305–11.

Mefforid I.N. et al. A neuroanatomical and biochemical basis for attention deficit disorder with hyperactivity in children. A defect in tonic adrenal mediated inhibition of locus ceruleus stimulation. Med Hypotheses 1989; 29: 33–42.

Michals K. and Matalon R. Phenylalanine metabolites, attention span and hyperactivity. Am J Clin Nutr 1985 Aug; 42 (2): 361–5.

Mitchell E.A., Aman M.G., Turbott S.H. Clinical characteristics and serum essential fatty acid levels in hyperactive children. Clin Pediatr 1987 Aug; 26 (8): 406–11.

Needleman H.L., Riess JA., Tobin M.J., et al. Bone lead levels and delinquent behavior. JAMA 1996 Feb 7; 275 (5): 363–9.

Oades R.D. Attention deficit disorder with hyperactivity. The contribution of catecholinergic activity. Prog in Neurobiol 1987; 29: 365–91.

Piercey M.F., Vogelsang G.D., Franklin S.R., Tang A. H. Reversal of scopolamine-induced amnesia and alterations in energy metabolism by the nootropic piracetam: implications regarding identification of brain structures involved in consolidation of memory traces. Brain Res 1987; 424: 1–9.

Pliszka S.R., Hatch J.P., Borcherding S.H., Rogeness G.A. Classical conditioning in children with attention deficit hyperactivity disorder (ADHD) and anxiety disorders: a test of Quay's model. J Abnorm Child Psychol 1993 Aug; 21 (4): 411–23.

Refetoff S., Weiss R.E., Usala S.J. The syndromes of resistance to thyroid hormone. Endocrine Rev 1993; 14 (3): 348–90.

Reimherr F.W., Wender P.H., Wood D.R., Ward M. An open trial of L-tyrosine in the treatment of attention deficit disorder, residual type. Am J Psychiatry 1987 Aug; 144 (8): 1071–3.

Rowe K.S. Synthetic food colourings and "hyperactivity": a double-blind crossover study. Aust Ped J 1988 Apr; 24 (2): 143–7.

Shanaz M.T. and Yang J. A time course of altered thyroid states on the noradrenergic system in rat brain by quantitative autoradiography. Neuroendocrinology 1994; 59: 235–44.

Shekim W.O., Antun F., Hanna G.L., McCracken J.T., Hess E.B. S-adenosyl-l-methionine (SAMe) in adults with ADHD. Psychopharmacol Bull 1990; 26 (2): 249–53.

Stevens L.J., Zentall S.S., Deck J.L., Abate M.L., et al. Essential fatty acid metabolism in boys with attention deficit hyperactivity disorder. Am J Clin Nutr 1995 Oct; 62 (4): 761–8.

Tuthill, R.W. Hair lead levels related to children's classroom attention-deficit behavior. Arch Environ Health 1996 May-Jun; 51 (3): 214–20.

Tritschler H.J., Packer L., Medori R. Oxidative stress and mitochondrial dysfunction in neurodegeneration. Biochem Mol Biol Int 1994 Aug; 34 (1): 169–81.

Uauy R., Peirano P., Hoffman D., Mena P., Birch D., Birch E. Role of essential fatty acids in the function of the developing nervous system. Lipids 1996; 31: Supplement.

Ward N.I., et al. The influence of the chemical additive tartrazine on the zinc status of hyperactive children—a double-blind placebo-controlled study. J of Nutr Med 1990; 1: 51–57.

Weiss R.E., Stein M.A., Trommer B., Refetoff, S. Attention-deficit hyperactivity disorder and thyroid function. J Ped 1993 Oct; 123 (4): 539–45.

Wender E.H. and Solanto M.V. Effects of sugar on aggressive and inattentive behavior in children with attention deficit disorder with hyperactivity and normal children. Pediatrics 1991 Nov; 88 (5): 960–6.

Wilens T.E., Biederman J., Spencer T.J., Prince J. Pharmacotherapy of adult attention deficit/hyperactivity disorder: a review. J Clin Psychopharmacol 1995; 15 (4): 270–8.

Williams L.R. Oxidative stress, age-related neurodegeneration, and the potential for neurotrophic treatment. Cerebrovas Brain Metab Rev 1995 Spring; 7 (1): 55–73.

Wood D.R., Reimherr F.W., Wender P.H. Treatment of attention deficit disorder with DL-phenylalanine. Psychiatry Res 1985 Sept; 16 (1): 21–6.

Zametkin, Alan J. Cerebral glucose metabolism in adults with hyperactivity of childhood onset. N Engl J Med 1990 Nov 15; 323 (20): 1361–6.

• Chapter 10: Chronic Fatigue Syndrome

Amarakoon A.M., Tappia P.S., Grimble R.F. Endotoxin induced production of interleukin-6 is enhanced by vitamin E deficiency and reduced by black tea extract. Inflamm Res 1995 Jul; 44 (7): 301–5.

Araki R., Inoue S., Osborne M.P., Telang W. T. Chemoprevention of mammary preneoplasia. In vitro effects of a green tea polyphenol. Ann NY Acad Sci 1995; 768: 215–22.

Arora D. and Ross A.C. Antibody response against tetanus toxoid is enhanced by lipopolysaccharide or tumor necrosis factor-alpha in vitamin A-sufficient and deficient rats. Am J Clin Nutr 1994; 59 (4): 922–8.

Barnes P.R., Taylor D.J., Kemp G.J., Radda G.K. Skeletal muscle bioenergetics in the chronic fatigue syndrome. J Neurol Neurosurg Psychiatry 1993 Jun; 56 (6): 679–83.

Baum C.G., Szabo P., Siskind G.W., et al. Cellular control of IGE induction by a polyphenol-rich compound. Preferential activation of TH2 cells. J Immunol 1990; 145 (3): 779–84.

Behan P.O., Haniffah A.G., Doogan D.P., Loudon M. A pilot study of sertraline for the treatment of chronic fatigue syndrome. Ann Int Med 1992 Nov; 117 (10): 854–63.

Behan W.M. and Behan P.O. The role of viral infection in polymyositis dermatomyositis and chronic fatgue syndrome. Clin Neurol 1993 Nov; 2 (3): 637–57.

Bell S.J., Chavali S., Bistrian B.R., et al. Dietary fish oil and cytokine and eicosanoid production during human immunodeficiency virus infection. J Parenter Enteral Nutr 1996 Jan-Feb; 20 (1): 43–9.

Benfield T.L., van Steenwijk R., Nielsen T.L., et al. Interleukin-8 and eicosanoid production in the lung during moderate to severe Pneumocystis carinii pneumonia in AIDS: a role of interleukin-8 in the pathogenesis of P. carinii pneumonia. Respir Med 1995 Apr; 89 (4): 285–90.

Blomhoff H.K., et al. Vitamin A is a key regulator for cell growth, cytokine production, and differentiation in normal B cells. J Biol Chem 1992; 267 (33): 23988–92.

Bou-Holaigah I., Rowe P.C., Kan J., Calkins H. The relationship between neurally mediated hypotension and the chronic fatigue syndrome. JAMA 1995 Sept 27; 274 (12): 961–7.

Bowles N.E., Bayston T.A., Zhang H.Y., Dowyl D., et al. Persistance of enterovirus RNA in muscle biopsy samples suggest that some cases of chronic fatigue syndrome result from a previous, inflammatory viral myopathy. J Med 1993; 24 (2–3): 145–60.

Brechel M.M., Lozano Y., Wright M.A., et al. Immune modulation by interleukin-12 in tumor-bearing mice receiving vitamin D_3 treatments to block induction of immunosuppressive granulocyte/macrophage progenitor cells. Cancer Immunol Immunother 1996 May; 42 (4): 213–20.

Brohee D. and Neve P. Effect of dietary high doses of vitamin E on the cell size of T and B lymphocyte subsets in young and old CBA mice. Mech Aging Dev 1995 Nov 24; 85 (2–3): 147–55.

Buchwald D., Cheney P.R., Peterson D.L., Henry B., et al. A chronic illness characterized by fatigue, neurologic and immunologic disorders, and active human herpesvirus type 6 infection. Ann Int Med 1992 Jan; 116 (2): 103–13.

Buffi O., Ciaroni S., Guidi L., Cecchini T., Bombardelli E. Morphological analysis on the adrenal zona fasciculata of Ginseng, Ginsenoside Rb1 and Geinsenoside Rg1 treated mice. Boll Soc Ital Biol Sper 1993 Dec; 69 (12): 791–7.

Bukovsky M., et al. Immunomodulating activity of echinacea gloriosa L., echinacea angustifolia DC. and rudbeckia speciosa Wenderoth ethanol-water extracts. J Pharmacol 1995 Mar-Apr; 47 (2): 175–7.

Bukovsky M., Vaverkova S., Kostalova D., Magnusova R. Immunomodulating activity of ethanol-water extracts of the roots of echinacea gloriosa L., echinacea angustifolia D.C. and rudbeckia speciosa Wenderoth tested on the immune system in C57BL6 inbred mice. Cesk Farm 1993 Aug; 42 (4): 184–7.

Calabrese L.H., Danao T., Camara E.G., Wilde W.S. Chronic fatigue and immune dysfunction. Cleve Clin J Med 1992 Mar-Apr; 59 (2): 123–4.

Carrick J.B., Schnellmann R.G., Moore J.N. Dietary source of omega-3 fatty acids affects endotoxin-induced peritoneal macrophage tumor necrosis factor and eicosanoid synthesis. Shock 1994; 2 (6): 421–6.

Carver J.D. Dietary nucleotides: cellular immune, intestinal and hepatic system effects. J Nutr 1994; 124: 144S–146S.

Chung F.L., XU Y., Ho C.T., Han C. Possible mechanism of inhibition of tobacco-specific nitrosamine-induced lung tumorigenesis in A/J mice by green tea and its polyphenol. Proc Ann Meet Am Assoc Cancer Res 1992; 33: A962.

Clague J.E., et al. Intravenous magnesium loading and chronic fatigue syndrome. Lancet 1992 Jul 11; 340: 124–5.

Cox I.M., et al. Red blood cell magnesium and chronic fatigue syndrome. Lancet 1991 Mar 30; 337 (8744): 757–60.

Coyle P.K., Krupp L.B., Doscher C., Amin K. Borrelia burgdorferi reactivity in patients with severe persistent fatigue who are from a region in which Lyme disease is endemic. Clin Infectious Disease 1994; 18 (Suppl 1): 24–7.

De Caterina R., Cybulsky M.I., Clinton S.K., et al. The omega-3 fatty acid docosahexaenoate reduces cytokine-induced expression of proatherogenic and proinflammatory proteins in human endothelial cells. Arterioscler Thromb 1994; 14 (11): 1829–36.

Demitrack, M.A. Chronic fatigue syndrome: a disease of the hypothalamic-pituitary-adrenal axis? Ann Med 1994 Feb; 26 (1): 1–5.

Demitrack M.A., et al. Evidence for impaired activation of the hypothalamic pituitary-adrenal axis in patients with chronic fatigue syndrome. J Clin Endocrinology and Metabolis 1991; 73: 1224–34.

de Vries H.E., Hoogendoorn K.H., van Dijk J., et al. Eicosanoid production by rat cerebral endothelial cells: stimulation by lipopolysaccharide, interleukin-1 and interleukin-6. J Neuroimmunol 1995 Jun; 59 (1–2): 1–8.

Dorsch W. Clinical application of extracts of echinacea purpurea or echinacea pallida. Z Arztl Fortbild 1996 Apr; 90 (2): 117–22.

Forsyth, L.M., et al. Therapeutic effects of oral NADH on the symptoms of patients with chronic fatigue syndrome. Ann Allergy Asthma Immunol 1999 Feb; 82:185.

Fujibayashi S., Suzuki S., Okano K., Naitoh T., et al. The weak calcemic vitamin D_3 analogue 22-oxacalcitriol suppresses the production of tumor necrosis factor-alpha by peripheral mononuclear cells. Immunol Lett 1991; 30 (3): 307–11.

Fukui H., Goto K., Tabata M. Two antimicrobial flavanones from the leaves of glycyrrhiza glabra. Chem Pharm Bull 1988 Oct; 36 (10): 4174.

Goldenberg D.L. Fibromyalgia and its relation to chronic fatigue syndrome, viral illness and immune abnormalities. J Rheumatol 1989 Nov; 19: (Suppl) 91–3.

Gray J.B. and Martinovic A.M. Eicosanoids and essential fatty acid modulation in chronic disease and the chronic fatigue syndrome. Med Hypotheses 1994 Jul; 43 (1): 31–42.

Guo Q., Peng T.Q., Yang Y.Z. Effect of Astragalus membranaceous on Ca2+ influx and coxsackie virus B3 RNA replication in cultured neonatal rat heart cells. Chung Kuo Chung Hsi I Chieh Ho Tsa Chih 1995 Aug; 15 (8): 483–5.

Haverty T., Haddad J.G., Neilson E.G. 1,25-dihydroxyvitamin D_3 stimulates interleukin-2 production by a T cell lymphoma line (MLA-144) cultured in vitamin D-deficient rat serum. J Leukoc Biol 1987 Feb; 41 (2): 177–82.

Hiai S., Sasayama Y., Oguro C. Chronic effects of ginseng saponin, glycyrrhizin and flavin adenine dinucleotide on adrenal and thymus weight in normal and dexamethasone-treated rats. Chem Pharm Bull 1987 Jan; 35 (1): 241–8.

Hibino Y., Konishi Y., Koike J., Tabata T., et al. Productions of interferon-gamma and nitrite are induced in mouse splenic cells by a heteroglycan-protein fraction from culture medium of Lentinus edodes mycelia. Immunopharmacol 1994 Jul-Aug; 28 (1): 77–85.

Hilgers A. and Frank J. Chronic fatigue syndrome: immune dysfunction, role of pathogens and toxic agents and neurological and cardial changes. Wien Med Wochenschr 1994; 144 (16): 399–406.

Hirata A., Adachi Y., Itoh W., et al. Monoclonal antibody to proteoglycan derived from grifola frondosa (maitake). Biol Pharm Bull 1994 Apr; 17 (4): 539–42.

Hishida I., Nanba H., Kuroda H. Antitumor activity exhibited by orally administered extract from fruit body of grifola frondosa (maitake). Chem Pharm Bull 1988; 36 (5): 1819–27.

Holt S. Colostrum as a dietary supplement. Alternative and Complementary Therapies 1998 Aug:276.

Howard J.M., et al. Magnesium and chronic fatigue syndrome. Lancet 1992 Aug 15; 340: 426.

Huang Z., Quin N.P., Ye W. Effect of astragalus membranaceous on T-lymphocyte subsets in patients with viral myocarditis. Chung Kuo Chung Hsi I Chieh Ho Tsa Chih 1995 Jun; 15 (6): 328–30.

Jones J.F., Streib J., Baker S., Herberger M. Chronic fatigue syndrome: I. Epstein-Barr virus immune response and molecular epidemiology. J Med Virol 1991 Mar; 33 (3): 151–8.

Ju H.S., Li X.J., Zaho B.L., et al. Effects of glycyrrhiza flavonoid on lipid peroxidation and active oxygen radicals. Yao Hsueh Pao 1989; 24 (11): 807–12.

Jyonouchi H. Nucleotide actions on humoral immune responses. J Nutr 1994; 124: 138S–140S.

Katiyar S.K., Agarwal R., Mukhtar H. Inhibition of both stage I and stage II skin tumor promotion in SENCAR mice by a polyphenolic fraction isolated from green tea: inhibition depends on the duration of polyphenol treatment. Carcinogenesis 1993; 14 (12): 2641–3.

Keller R.H., Lane J.L., Klimas N., Reiter W.M., et al. Association between HLA class II antigens and the chronic fatigue immune dysfunction syndrome. Clin Infect Dis 1994 Jan; 18 (Suppl 1): S154–6.

Kent-Braun J.A., Sharma K.R., Weiner M.W., Massie B., Miller R.G. Central basis of muscle fatigue in chronic fatigue syndrome. Neurol 1993 Sept; 43 (9): 1866–7.

Komaroff A.L. Chronic fatigue syndromes: relationship to chronic viral infections. J Virol Methods 1988 Sept; 21 (1–4): 3–10.

Kramer T.R., Udomkesmalee E., Dhanamitta S., et al. Lymphocyte responsiveness of children supplemented with vitamin A and zinc. Am J Clin Nutr 1993 Oct; 58 (4): 566–70.

Kulkarni A.D., Rudolph F.B., Van Buren C.T. The role of dietary sources of nucleotides in immune function: a review. American Institute of Nutrition 1994.

Kuratsune H., Yamaguti K., Takahashi M., et al. Acetylcarnitine deficiency in chronic fatigue syndrome. Clin Infectious Diseases 1994; 18 (Suppl 1): S62–7.

Land J.M., Kemp G.J., Taylor D.J., Standing S.J., et al. Oral phosphate supplements reverse skeletal muscle abnormalities in a case of chronic fatigue with idiopathic renal hypophosphatemia. Neuromuscul Disord 1993 May; 3 (3): 223–5.

Lei L.S. and Lin Z.B. Effects of ganoderma polysaccharides on the activity of DNA polymerase alpha of splenocytes and immune function in aged mice. Yao Hsueh Hsueh Pao 1993; 28 (8): 577–82.

Levine P.H. The use of transfer factors in chronic fatigue syndrome. Biotherapy 1996; 9:77.

Levy J.A. Viral studies of chronic fatigue syndrome. Clin Infect Dis 1994 Jan; 18 (Suppl 1): S1117–20.

Liang H., Wang Z., Tian F., Geng B. Effects of astragalus polysaccharides and ginsenoisides of ginseng stems and leaves on lymphocytes membrane fluidity and lipid peroxidation in traumatized mice. Chung Kuo Chung Yao Tsa Chih 1995 Sept; 20 (9): 558–60.

Lin J.M., et al. Evaluation of the anti-inflammatory and liver-protective effects of anoectochilus formosanus, ganoderma lucidum and gynostemma pentaphyllum in rats. Am J Chin Med 1993; 21 (1): 59–69.

Lloyd A.R. and Klimas N. Summary: immunologic studies of chronic fatigue syndrome. Clin Infectious Diseases 1994; 18 (Suppl 1): S160–1.

Lu Z.W. Psychoneuroimmunological effects of morphine and the immunoprotection of ganoderma polysaccharides peptide in morphinc-dependent mice. Sheng Li Ko Hsueh Chin Chan 1995 Jan; 26 (1): 45–9.

Manu P., Matthews D.A., Lane T.J. Food intolerance in patients with chronic fatigue. Int J Eat Disord 1993 Mar; 13 (2): 203–9.

McCully K.K., Natelson B.H., Iotti S., Sisto S., Leigh J.S. Reduced oxidative muscle metabolism in chronic fatigue syndrome. Muscle Nerve 1996 May; 19 (5): 621–5.

Meydani S.N. Interaction of omega-3 polyunsaturated fatty acids and vitamin E on the immune response. World Rev Nutr Diet 1994; 75: 155–61.

Muller-Jakic B., Brew W., Probstle A., Redl K., et al. In vitro inhibition of cyclooxygenase and 5-lipoxygenase by alkamides from echinacea and achillea species. Planta Med 1994 Feb; 60 (1): 37–40.

Nanba H. Activity of maitake D-fraction to inhibit carcinogenesis and metastasis. Ann NY Acad Sci 1995 Sept 30; 768: 243–5.

Ojo-Amaize F.A., Conley E.J., Peter J.B. Decreased natural killer cell activity is associated with severity of chronic fatigue immune dysfunction syndrome. Clin Infect Dis 1994 Jan; 18 (Suppl 1): S157–9.

Okano M. Viral infection and its causative role for chronic fatigue syndrome. Nippon Rinsho 1992 Nov; 50 (11): 2617–24.

Oxholm A., Oxholm P., Staberg B., Bendtzen K. Expression of interleukin-6-like molecules and tumor necrosis factor after topical treatment of psoriasis with a new vitamin D analogue (MC 903). Acta Derm Venereol 1989; 69 (5): 385–90.

Patarca R., Klimas N.G., Lugtendorf S., Antoni M., Fletcher M.A. Dysregulated expression of tumor necrosis factor in chronic fatigue syndrome: interrelations with cellular sources and patterns of soluble immune mediator expression. Clin Infect Dis 1994 Jan; 18 (Suppl 1): S147–53.

Plioplys A.V. and Plioplys S. Electron-microscopic investigation of muscle mitochondria in chronic fatigue syndrome. Neuropsychobiology 1995; 32 (4): 175–81.

Potaznick W. and Kozol N. Ocular manifestations of chronic fatigue and immune dysfunction syndrome. Optom Vis Sci 1992 Oct; 69 (10): 811–4.

Rosen P. The synergism of gamma-interferon and tumor necrosis factor in whole body hypothermia with vitamin C to control toxicity. Med Hypotheses 1992; 38 (3): 257–8.

Rowe P.C., Bou-Holaigah I., Flynn J., Kan J., Calkins H. Information for physicians. The Johns Hopkins Hospital, 1995 Oct.

Sakamotol K., Reddy D., Hara Y., Milner J.A. Impact of green or black tea polyphenol on canine mammary tumor cells in culture. Proc Annu Meet Am Assoc Cancer Res 1995; 36: A3542.

Sandman C.A., Barron J.L., Nackoul K., et. al. Memory deficits associated with chronic fatigue immune dysfunction syndrome. Biol Psychiatry 1993 Apr 15-May 1; 33 (8–9): 618–23.

Sarkar S., Koga J., Whitley R.J., Chatterjee S. Antiviral effect of the extract of culture medium of Lentinus edodes mycelia on the replication of herpes simplex virus type 1. Antiviral Res 1993 Apr; 20 (4): 293–303.

Shimizu N., Tomoda M., Takada K., Gonda R. The core structure and immunological activities of glycyrrhizin UA, the main polysaccharide from the root of glycyrrhiza uralensis. Chem Pharm Bull 1992 Aug: (40*8): 2125–8.

Stabel J.R. and Goff J.P. Influence of vitamin D3 infusion and dietary calcium on secretion of interleukin 1, interleukin 6, and tumor necrosis factor in mice infected with Mycobacterium paratuberculosis. Am J Vet Res 1996 Jun; 57 (6): 825–9.

Steinmuller C., Roesler J., Grottrup E., et al. Polysaccharides isolated from plant cell cultures of echinacea purpurea enhance the resistance of immunosuppressed mice against systemic infections with candida albicans and Listeria monocytogenes. Int J Immunopharmacol 1993 Jul; 15 (5): 605–14.

Sternberg E., Chrouusos G.P., Wilder R.L., Gold P.W. The stress response and the regulation of inflammatory disease. Ann Internal Med 1992 Nov 15; 117 (10): 854–66.

Sugiura H., Nichida H., Inaba R., Iwata H. Effects of exercise in the growing stage in mice and of astragalus membranaceous on immune functions. Nipon Eiseigaku Zasshi 1993 Feb; 47 (6): 1021–31.

Suzuki I., Hashimoto K., Oikawa S., Sato K., et al. Antitumor and immunomodulating activities of a beta-glucan obtained from liquid-cultured grifola frondosa. Chem Pharm Bull 1989; 37 (2): 410–13.

Tachikawa E., Kudo K., Kashimoto T., Takahashi E. Ginseng saponins reduced acetylcholine-evoked Na+ influx and catecholamine secretion in bovine adrenal chromaffin cells. J Pharmacol Exp Ther 1995 May; 273 (2): 629–36.

Taimi M., Defacque H., Commes T., et al. Effect of retinoic acid and vitamin D on the expression of interleukin-6 in the human monocytic cell line U937. Immunology 1993 Jun; 79 (2): 229–35.

Takahashi H., Imai K., Katanuma A., Sugaya T., et al. A case of chronic fatigue syndrome who showed a beneficial effect by intravenous administration of magnesium sulphate. Arerugi 1992 Nov; 41 (11): 1605–10.

Takeyama T., et al. Host-mediated antitumor effect of grifolan NMF-5N, a polysaccharide obtained from grifola frondosa. J Pharmacobiodyn 1987; 10 (11): 644–51.

Takeyama T., et al. Vitamin E increases interleukin-2 dependent cellular growth and glycoprotein glycosylation in murine cytotoxic T-cell line. Biochem Biophy Res Commun 1993 Jun 30; 193 (3): 872–7.

Telang N.T., Inoue S., Bradlow H.L., Fujiki H., Osborne M.P. Antipromotional effect of a green tea polyphenol on c-myc- transfected mammary epithelial cells. Proc Annu Meet Am Assoc Cancer Res 1994; 35: A3692.

Uchida A. Chronic fatigue immune dysfunction syndrome. Nippon Rinsho 1992 Nov; 50 (11): 2625–9.

Walker W.A. Nucleotides and nutrition: role as dietary supplement. J Nutr 1994; 124: 121S–123S.

Wang Y., Huang D.S., Eskelson C.D., Watson R.R. Long-term dietary vitamin E retards development of retrovirus-induced disregulation in cytokine production. Clin Immunol Immunopathol 1994; 72 (1): 70–5.

Wang Y., Huang D.S., Watson R.R. Dietary vitamin E modulation of cytokine production by splenocytes and thymocytes from alcohol-fed mice. Alcohol Clin Exp Res 1994; 18 (2): 355–62.

Wang Y., Huang D.S., Watson R.R. Vitamin E supplementation modulates cytokine production by thymocytes during murine AIDS. Immunol Res 1993; 12 (4): 358–66.

Wang Y. and Watson R.R. Vitamin E supplementation at various levels alters cytokine production by thymocytes during retrovirus infection causing murine AIDS. Thymus 1994; 22 (3): 153–65.

Weng X.S. Treatment of leucopenia with pure astragalus preparation—an analysis of 115 leukocopenic cases. Chung Kuo Chung Hsi I Chieh Ho Tsa Chih 1995; 15 (8): 462–4.

Wong R., Lopaschuk G., Zhu G., Walker D., et al. Skeletal muscle metabolism in the chronic fatigue syndrome. Chest 1992 Dec; 102 (6): 1716–22.

Xu Y., Ho C.T., Amin S.G., Han C., Chung F.L. Inhibition of tobacco-specific nitrosamine-induced lung tumorigenesis in A/J mice by green tea and its major polyphenol as antioxidants. Cancer Res 1992; 52 (14): 3875–9.

Yamashiki M., Nichimura A., Kosaka Y. Effects of methylcobalamin (vitamin B_{12}) on in vitro cytokine production of peripheral blood mononuclear cells. J Clin Lab Immunol 1992; 37 (4): 173–82.

Yang G. and Yu Y. Immunopotentiating effect of traditional Chinese drugs—ginsenoside and glycyrrhiza polysaccharide. Porc Chin Acad Med Sci Peking Union Med Coll 1990; 5 (4): 188–93.

Yu W., Sanders B.G., Kline K. Modulation of murine EL-4 thymic lymphoma cell proliferation any cytokine production by vitamin E succinate. Nutr Cancer 1996; 25 (2): 137–49.

Zhang L.X., Mong H., Zhou X.B. Effect of Japanese ganoderma lucidum on production of interleukin-2 from murine splenocytes. Chung Kuo Chung Hsi I Chieh Ho Tsa Chih 1993 Oct; 13 (10): 613–15.

Zhao T.H. Positive modulating action of shengmaisan with astragalus membranaceous on anti-tumor activity of LAK cells. Chung Kuo Chung Hsi I Chieh Ho Tsa Chih 1993 Aug; 13 (8): 471–2.

•Chapter 11: Depression

Abou-Saleh M.T. and Coppen A. The biology of folate in depression: implications for nutritional hypotheses of the psychoses. J Psychiatr Res 1986; 20 (2): 91–101.

Abou-Saleh M.T. and Coppen A. Serum and red blood cell folate in depression. Acta Psychiatr Scand 1989 Jul; 80 (1): 78–82.

Altamura C., Maes M., Dai J., Meltzer H.Y. Plasma concentrations of excitatory amino acids, serine, glycine, taurine and histidine in major depression. Eur Neuropsychopharmacol 1995; 5 (Suppl): 71–5.

Amato L., Paolisso G., Cacciatore F., Ferrara N., et al. Non-insulin-dependent diabetes mellitus is associated with a greater prevalence of depression in the elderly. Diabetes Metab 1996 Oct; 22 (5): 314–8.

Anderson I.M., Parry-Billings M., Newsholme E.A., Poortmans J.R., Cowen P.J. Decreased plasma tryptophan concentration in major depression: relationship to melancholia and weight loss. J Affect Disord 1990 Nov; 20 (3): 185–91.

Bartold P.M., et al. Substance P. J Periodontal 1994 Dec; 65:1113.

Bell I.R., Edman J.S., Morrow F.D., Marby D.W., et al. B complex vitamin patterns in geriatric and young adult in patients with major depression. J Am Geriatr Soc 1991 Mar; 39 (3): 252–7.

Bell I.R., Edman J.S., Morrow F.D., Marby D.W., et al. Vitamin B_1, B_2, and B_6 augmentation of tricyclic antidepressant treatment in geriatric depression with cognitive dysfunction. J Am Coll Nutr 1992 Apr; 11 (2): 159–63.

Bell K.M., Plon L., Bunney W.E., Potkin S.G. S-adenosylmethionine treatment of depression: a controlled clinical trial. Am J Psychiatry 1988 Sept; 145 (9): 1110–4.

Bladt S. and Wagner H. Inhibition of MAO by fractions and constituents of hypericum extract. J Geriatr Psychiatry Neurol 1994 Oct; 7 (Suppl 1): S57–9.

Bottiglieri T., Godfrey P., Flynn T., Carney M.W. et al. Cerebrospinal fluid S-adenosylmethionine in depression and dementia: effects of treatment with parenteral and oral S-adenosylmethionine. J Neurol Neurosurg Psychiatry 1990 Dec; 53 (12): 1096–8.

Bottiglieri T. and Hyland K. S-adenosylmethionine levels in psychiatric and neurological disorders: a review. Acta Neurol Scand 1994; Supplement 154: 19–26.

Brambilla F., et al. Effects of phosphatidylserine therapy in geriatric patients with depressive disorders. Acta Psychiatr Scand 1990 Mar; 81:265.

Candito M., Souetre E., Iordache A., Pringuey D., et al. Diurnal variation in total plasma tryptophan in controls and in depression. J Psychiatr Res 1990; 24 (3): 227–30.

Castilla-Cortazar I., et al. Opioid peptides and immunodysfunction in patients with major depression and anxiety disorders. J Physiol Biochem 1998 Dec; 54:203.

Charles H.C., Lazeyras F., Krishnan K.R., Boyko O.B., et al. Brain choline in depression: in vivo detection of potential pharmacodynamic effects of antidepressant therapy using hydrogen localized spectroscopy. Prog Neuropsychopharmacol Biol Psychiatry 1994 Nov; 18 (7): 1121–7.

Chatterjee S.S., et al. Hyperforin as a possible antidepressant component of hypercium extracts. Life Sciences 1998; 63:499.

Chen R.W. and Chuang D.M. Long term lithium treatment suppresses p53 and Bax expression but increases Bcl-2 expression. J Biol Chem 1999 March 5; 174:6039.

Coiro V., et al. Stimulation of ACTH/cortisol by intravenously infused substance P in normal men. Neuroendocrinology 1992 Oct; 56:459.

Coppen A., Swade C., Jones S.A., Armstrong R.A., Blair J.A., Leeming R.J. Depression and tetrahydrobiopterin: the folate connection. J Affect Disord 1989 Mar-Jun; 16 (2–3): 103–7.

Cowen P.J. and Charig E.M. Neuroendocrine responses to intravenous tryptophan in major depression. Arch Gen Psychiatry 1987 Nov; 44 (11): 958–66.

Culman J., et al. Effect of tachykinin receptor inhibition in the brain on cardiovascular and behavioral responses to stress. J Pharmacol Exp Ther 1997 Jan; 280:238.

Delgado P.L., Charney C.S., Price L.H., et al. Neuroendocrine and behavioral effects of dietary tryptophan restriction in healthy subjects. Life Science 1990; 45: 2323–32.

Einat H., et al. Inositol reduces depressive-like behaviors in two different animal models of depression. Psychopharmacology (Berl) 1999 May; 144:158.

Fava M., et al. Neuroendocrine effects of S-adenosyl-L-methionine, a novel putative antidepressent. J Psychiatr Res 1990; 24:177.

Fava M. Rapidity of onset of the antidepressant effect of parenteral S-adenosyl L-methionine. Psych Res 1995; 956: 295–7.

Fuller R.W. The involvement of serotonin in regulation of pituitary adrenal cortical function. Frontiers of Neuroendocrinology 1992; 13: 250–70.

Gelenberg A.J., Wojcik J.D., Falk W.E., Baldessarini R.J., et al. Tyrosine for depression: a double-blind trial. J Affect Disord 1990 Jun; 19 (2): 125–32.

Haleem D.J., Yasmeen A., Haleem M.A., Zafar A. 24h withdrawal following repeated administration of caffeine attenuates brain serotonin but not tryptophan in rat brain: implications for caffeine-induced depression. Life Sci 1995; 57 (19): PL285–92.

Hansgen K.D., Vesper J., Ploch M. Multicenter double-blind study examining the antidepressant effectiveness of the hypericum extract LI 160. J Geriatr Psychiatry Neurol 1994 Oct; 7 (Suppl 1): 215–8.

Harrer G., Hubner W.D., Podzuweit H. Effectiveness and tolerance of the hypericum extract LI 160 compared to maprotiline: a multicenter double-blind study. J Geriatr Psychiatry Neurol 1994 Oct; 7 (Suppl 1): S24–8.

Harrer G. and Schulz V. Clinical investigation of the antidepressant effectiveness of hypericum. J Geriatr Psychiatry Neurol 1994 Oct; 7 (Suppl): S6–8.

Hibbeln J.R. and Salem N. Dietary polyunsaturated fatty acids and depression: when cholesterol does not satisfy. Am J Clin Nutr 1995; 62 (1): 1–9.

Hubner W.D., Lande S., Podzueweit H. Hypericum treatment of mild depressions with somatic symptoms. J Geriatr Psychiatry Neurol 1994 Oct; 7 (Suppl 1): S12–4.

Jeanningros R., Serres F., Dassa D., Azorin J.M., Grignon S. Red blood cell L-tryptophan uptake in depression: kinetic analysis in untreated depressed patients and healthy volunteers. Psychiatry Res 1996 Jul 31; 63 (2–3): 151–9.

Kaehler S.T. et al. Hyperforin enhances the extracellular concentrations of catecholamines, serotonin and glutamate in the rat locus coeruleus. Neurosci Lett 1999 Mar 12; 262:199.

Kagan B.L., Sultzer D.L., Rosenlicht N., Gerner R.H. Oral s-adenosylmethionine in depression: a randomized, double-blind, placebo-controlled trial. Am J Psychiatry 1990 May; 147 (5): 591–595.

Knapp S. and Irwin M. Plasma levels of tetrahydrobiopterin and folate in major depression. Biol Psychiatry 1989 Jun; 26 (2): 156–62.

Kofman O., Bersudsky U., Vinnitsky I., Alpert C., Belmaker R.H. The effect of peripheral inositol injection on rat motor activity models of depression. Isr J Med Sci 1993 Sept; 29 (9): 580–6.

Kramer M.S., et al. Novel strategies for pharmacology of depression. Curr Opin Chem Biol 1999 Aug; 3:481.

Kramer M.S., et al. Distinct mechanism for antidepressant activity by blockade of central substance P receptors. Science 1998 Sep 11; 281:1640.

Kumar A., Newberg A., Alavi A., Berlin J., et al. Regional cerebral glucose metabolism in late-life depression and Alzheimer's disease: a preliminary positron emission tomography study. Proc Natl Acad Sci 1993 Aug 1; 90 (15): 7019–23.

Laakmann G., et al. St. John's wort in mild to moderate depression. Pharmacopsychiat 1998:54.

Levine J., Barak Y., Gonzalves M., Szor H., et al. Double-blind controlled trial of inositol treatment of depression. Am J Psychiatry 1995 May; 152 (5): 792–4.

Levine J., et al. Combination of inostiol and serotonin reuptake inhibitors in the treatment of depression. Biol Psychiatry 1999 Feb 1; 42:270.

Levine J., et al. Double-blind, controlled study of inositol treatment of depression. Am J Psychiatry 1995 May; 152:792.

Lewis R.T., et al. Tryptophan-derived NK1 antagonists. J Med Chem 1995 Mar 17; 38:923.

Lopez J.F., Kathol R.G., Jaeckle R.S., Meller W. The HPA axis response to insulin hypoglycemia in depression. Biol Psychiatry 1987 Feb; 22 (2): 153–66.

Linde K., et al. St. John's wort for depression—an overview and meta-analysis of randomised clinical trials. BMJ 1996 Aug 3; 313 (7052): 253–8.

MacLeod A.M., et al. Identification of L-tryptophan derivatives with potent and selective antagonist activity at the NK1 receptor. J Med Chem 1994 Apr 29; 37:1269.

Maes M. and Meltzer H. The serotonin hypothesis of major depression. In Psychopharmacology, Fourth Generation of Progress, Blum F. and Kupfer B., eds. Raven Press, 1995.

Maes M., et al. The relationship between the viability of L-tryptophan to the brain. The spontaneous HPA axis activity and the HPA axis response to dexamethasone in depressed patients. Amino Acids 1991; 1: 57–65.

Maes M., et al. Suppressant effect of dexamethasone on the availability of plasma L-tryptophan and tyrosine in health control and in depressed patients. Acta Psychiatrica Scand 1990; 81: 19–23.

Maes M., Scharpe S., Meltzer H.Y., Okayli G., et al. Increased neopterin and interferon-gamma secretion and lower availability of L-tryptophan in major depression: further evidence for an immune response. Psychiatry Res 1994 Nov; 54 (2): 143–60.

Maes M., Meltzer H.Y., Scharpe S., Bosmans E., et al. Relationships between lower plasma L-tryptophan levels and immune-inflammatory variables in depression. Psychiatry Res 1993 Nov; 49 (2): 151–65.

Maes M., Smith R., Cristophe A., Cosyns P., et al. Fatty acid composition in major depression: decreased omega 3 fractions in cholesteryl esters and increased C20: 4 omega 6/C20:5 omega 3 ratio in cholesteryl esters and phospholipids. J Affect Disord 1996 Apr 26; 38 (1): 35–46.

Maes M., Wauters A., Verkerk R., Demedts P., et al. Lower serum L-tryptophan availability in depression as a marker of a more generalized disorder in protein metabolism. Neuropsychopharmacology 1996 Sept; 15 (3): 243–51.

Martinez B., Kasper S., Ruhrmann S., Moller H.J. Hypericum in the treatment of seasonal affective disorders. J Geriatr Psychiatry Neurol 1994 Oct; 7 (Suppl 1): S29–33.

Maurizi C.P. The therapeutic potential for tryptophan and melatonin: possible roles in depression, sleep, Alzheimer's disease and abnormal aging. Med Hypotheses 1990 Mar; 31 (3): 233–42.

McCarty, M.F. Enhancing central and peripheral insulin activity as strategy for the treatment of endogenous depression—an adjuvant role for chromium picolinate? Med Hypotheses 1994 Oct; 43 (4): 247–52.

Moller S.E., et al. Plasma ratio tryptophan to neutral amino acids in relation to clinical response to paroxetine and clomipramine in patients with major depression. J Psychiatric Disord 1990; 18: 59–66.

Moore T.C., et al. Substance P increases and prolongs increased output of T4 (DC4) lymphocytes from lymph nodes of sheep in vivo. Immunopharmacology 1990 Nov-Dec; 20:207.

Moore T.C., et al. Substance P increased lymphocyte traffic and lymph flow through peripheral lymph nodes of sheep. Immunology 1989 May 67:109.

Muller W.E. and Rossol R. Effects of hypericum extract on the expression of serotonin receptors. J Geriatr Psychiatry Neurol 1994 Oct; 7 (Suppl 1): S63–4.

Quintana J., et al. Platelet serotonin and plasma tryptophan decreases in endogenous depression. Clinical, therapeutic, and biological correlations. J Affect Disord 1992 Feb; 24 (2): 55–62.

Rasmussen H.H., Mortensen P.B., Jensen I.W. Depression and magnesium deficiency. Int J Psychiatry Med 1989; 19 (1): 57–63.

Rauch T.M. and Lieberman H.R. Tyrosine pretreatment reverses hypothermia-induced behavioral depression. Brain Res Bull 1990 Jan; 24 (1): 147–50.

Raucoules D., Azorin J.M., Barre A., Tissot R. Plasma levels and membrane transports in red blood cell of tyrosine and tryptophane in depression. Evaluation at baseline and recovery. Encephale 1991 May-Jun; 17 (3): 197–201.

Rosenbaum J.F., et al. The antidepressant potential of oral S-adenosyl-L-methionine. Acta Psychiatr Scand 1990 May; 81:432.

Schiffer, R.B. Depressive syndromes associated with diseases of the central nervous system. Seminars in Neurology 1990 Sept; 10 (3): 239–44.

Schmidt U. and Sommer H. St. John's wort extract in the ambulatory therapy of depression. Attention and reaction ability are preserved. Fortschr Med 1993 Jul 10; 111 (19): 339–42.

Simpson P.B. and Russell J.T. Mitochondria support inositol 1,4,5-

triphosphate-medicated CA2+ waves in cultured oligodendrocytes. J Biol Chem 1996 Dec 27; 271:33493.

Sommer H. and Harrer G. Placebo-controlled double-blind study examining the effectiveness of an hypericum preparation in 105 mildly depressed patients. J Geriatr Psychiatry Neurol 1994 Oct; 7 (Suppl 1): S9–11.

Stoll A.L., et al. Omega-3 fatty acids in bipolar disorder. Arch Gen Psychiatry 1998 (in press).

Van Praag H.M. In search of the mode of action of antidepressants: 5-HTP/tyrosine mixtures in depression. Adv Biochem Psychopharmacol 1984; 39: 301–14.

Vorbach E.U., Hubner W.D., Arnoldt K.H. Effectiveness and tolerance of the hypericum extract LI 160 in comparison with imipramine: randomized double-blind study with 135 outpatients, J Geriatr Psychiatry Neurol 1994 Oct; 7 (Suppl 1): S19–23.

Winokur A., Maislin G., Phillips J.L. Insulin resistance after oral glucose tolerance testing in patients with major depression. Am J Psychiatry 1988 Mar; 145 (3): 325–30.

Winokur A., Maislin G., Phillips J.L., Amsterdam J.D. Insulin resistance after oral glucose tolerance testing in patients with major depression. Am J Psychiatry 1988 Mar; 145 (3): 325–30.

Wolkowitz O.M., et al. Double-blind treatment of major depression with dehydroepiandrosterone. Am J Psychiatry 1999 Apr; 156:646.

Yamauchi A., Takei I., Kasuga A., Kitamura Y., et al. Depression of dehydroepiandrosterone in Japanese diabetic men—comparison between non-insulin-dependent diabetes mellitus and impaired glucose tolerance. Eur J Endocrinol 1996 Jul; 135 (1): 101–4.

Young S.N. Tryptophan depletion causes a rapid lowering of mood in normal males. Psychopharmacol 1985; 87: 173–7.

Zuker R.S. Calcium- and activity-dependent synaptic plasticity. Curr Opin Neurobiol 1999 Jun; 9:305.

• Chapter 12: Autism

Bolman W.M. and Richmond J.A. A double-blind, placebo-controlled, crossover pilot trial of low dose dimethylglycine in patients with autistic disorder. J Autism Dev Discord 1999 Jun; 29:191.

Centers for Disease Control. Literature review on autism. December 1998.

Carlsson M.L. Hypothesis: is infantile autism a hypoglutamatergic disorder? J Neural Transm 1998; 105:525.

Cazzulo A.G., et al. Beta-endorphin levels in peripheral blood mononuclear cells and long-term naltrexone treatment in autistic children. Eur Neuropsychopharmacol 1999 Jun; 9:361.

Connors, J. Secretin and Autism. J Am Acad Child Adolesc Psychiatry 1999 Jul; 38:7.

Edelson S.B. and Cantor D.S. Autism: xenobiotic influences. Toxicol Ind Health 1998 Jul-Aug; 14:553.

Feldman H.M., et al. Naltrexone and communication skills in young children with autism. J Am Acad Child Adolesc Psychiatry 1999 May; 38:587.

Horvath K., et al. Improved social and language skills after secretin administration in patients with autism spectrum disorders. J Assoc Acad Minor Phys 1998; 9:9.

Kolmen B.K., et al. Naltrexone in young autistic children. J Am Acad Child Adolesc Psychiatry 1997 Nov; 36:1570.

Launay J.M., et al. Serotonin metabolism and other biochemical parameters in infantile autism. Neuropsychobiology 1988; 20;1.

Lombard J. Autism: A mitochondrial disorder? Med Hypotheses 1998 Jun; 50:497.

Nicholson R., et al. An open trial of risperidone in young autistic children. J Am Acad Child Adolesc Psychiatry 1998 Apr; 37:372.

McDougle C.J., et al. A double-blind, placebo-controlled study of risperidone in adults with autistic disorder and other pervasive developmental disorders. Arch Gen Psych 1998 Jul; 55:633.

Nanson J.L. Autism in fetal alcohol syndrome. Alcohol Clin Exp Res 1992 Jun; 16:558.

Rapin I. and Katzman R. Neurobiology of Autism. Ann Neurol 1998;43:7.

Rapin I. Autism. New Engl J Med 1997 Jul 10; 337:97.

Schreir H.A. Risperidone for young children with mood disorders and aggressive behavior. J Child Adolesc Psychopharmacol 1998; 8:49.

Steingard R.J., et al. Sertraline treatment of transition-associated anxiety and agitation in children with autistic disorder. J Child Adolesc Psyhopharmacol 1997 spring; 7:9.

Van Gent T., et al. Autism and the immune system. J Child Psychol Psychiatry 1997 Mar; 38:337.

INDEX

350   Index

352   Index

ABOUT THE AUTHORS

DR. JAY LOMBARD is chief of neurology at Westchester Square Medical Center, assistant clinical professor of neurology at Cornell University Medical College, and voluntary attending physician at Albert Einstein College Hospital. He is certified in neurology by the American Board of Psychiatry and Neurology. As a private practitioner in Bronx, New York and Rockland County, New York, he specializes in neurodegenerative disease, multiple sclerosis, and autism.

CARL GERMANO, R.D., C.N.S., L.D.N., is a registered and certified clinical nutritionist and practitioner of Chinese herbology. With a master's degree in clinical nutrition from New York University and over 22 years experience developing and using innovative, complementary nutritional therapies, he has been instrumental in bringing cutting-edge nutritional substances and formulations to the dietary supplement market. Today, he continues his efforts in product development and research and is responsible for providing the dietary supplement industry with the next generation of clinically important nutritional substances. In addition, he is adjunct professor of nutrition at New York Chiropractic College, author of the bestselling books *Nature's Pain Killers* and *The Osteoporosis Solution,* and has served as Vice President of Product Development and Research at Solgar Vitamin and Herb Company for many years. Presently, he is Senior Vice President of Research and Product Development for Nutratech, Inc.